PROTEINS IN HUMAN NUTRITION

Based on
The Proceedings of a
NATO ADVANCED STUDY INSTITUTE
on
The Chemistry, Biology and Physics of Protein Evaluation
held in Reading, England, March 20–24, 1972

Organized on behalf of the International Union
of Food Science and Technology and the
International Union of Nutritional Sciences

PROTEINS IN HUMAN NUTRITION

Edited by

J. W. G. PORTER

and

B. A. ROLLS
National Institute for Research in Dairying, Shinfield, Reading, England

1973

ACADEMIC PRESS – LONDON AND NEW YORK

ACADEMIC PRESS INC. (LONDON) LTD.
24/28 Oval Road,
London NW1

United States Edition published by
ACADEMIC PRESS INC.
111 Fifth Avenue
New York, New York 10003

Second printing 1974

Library of Congress Catalog Card Number: 72-12277
ISBN: 0 12 562950 8

PRINTED IN GREAT BRITAIN BY
T. & A. CONSTABLE LTD
EDINBURGH

List of Contributors

Numbers in parentheses indicate the pages on which the authors' contributions begin.

J. C. ABBOTT Rural Institutions Division, FAO, Via delle Terme di Caracalla, 00100-Rome, Italy (75).

F. X. AYLWARD Department of Food Science, University of Reading, England (122).

A. E. BENDER Nutrition Department, Queen Elizabeth College (University of London), Campden Hill Road, London W8, England (167).

RICARDO BRESSANI Division of Agricultural and Food Sciences, Instituto de Nutricion de Centro America Y Panama, Oficina Sanitaria Panamericana, Carretera Roosevelt, Zona 11, Guatemala, Central America (293).

J. A. CAMPBELL Department of National Health and Welfare, Tunney's Pasture, Ottawa K1A OL2, Canada (353).

K. J. CARPENTER Department of Applied Biology, University of Cambridge, Downing Street, Cambridge, England (343, 531).

J. J. DREYER Biological Evaluation Division, National Food Research Institute, P O Box 395, Pretoria, RSA (245).

BJØRN O. EGGUM Landøkonomisk Forsøgslaboratorium, Afdelingen for Dyrefysiologi, Biokemi OG Analytisk Kemi, Rolighedsvej 24, 1958 København V, Denmark (317).

L. G. ELÍAS Division of Agricultural and Food Sciences, Instituto de Nutricion de Centro America Y Panama, Oficina Sanitaria Panamericana, Carretera Roosevelt, Zona 11, Guatemala, Central America (293).

H. ERBERSDOBLER Institut für Tierphysiologie der Universität München, Veterinarstrasse 13, 8 München 22, GFR (453).

P. A. FINOT Nestlé Products Technical Assistance Co. Ltd, CH–1814, La Tour de Peilz, Switzerland (501).

HANS FISHER Department of Nutrition, Rutgers University, College of Agriculture and Environmental Science, Thompson Hall, New Brunswick (P O Box 231), New Jersey 08903, USA (263).

J. E. FORD National Institute for Research in Dairying, Shinfield, Reading, England (207, 515).

H. HAENEL Deutsche Akademie der Wissenschaften zu Berlin, Zentralinstitut für Ernährung, Potsdam-Rehbrücke, 1505 Bergholz-Rehbrucke Arthur-Scheunert-Allee 114–116, GDR (195).

BO HALLGREN Astra Nutrition AB, Fack, 431 20 Mölndal 1, Sweden (369).

A. E. HARPER Nutritional Sciences Department, The University of Wisconsin, College of Agricultural and Life Sciences, Madison, Wisconsin 53706 608, USA (349).

D. M. HEGSTED Harvard University, School of Public Health, Department of Nutrition 665 Huntington Avenue, Boston 15, Massachusetts, USA (275, 356).

ANNE-MARIE HERMANSSON Chemical Center, The Lund Institute of Technology, (P O Box 740), S–220 07, Lund 7, Sweden (407).

M. E. JALIL Crop and Grassland Production Service (Field Food Crops), Plant Production and Protection Division, FAO, Via delle Terme di Caracalla, 00100-Rome, Italy (35).

S. G. KHARATYAN Institute of Organo-Element Compounds, Soviet Academy of Sciences, Vavilova 28, Moscow, USSR (195).

A. L. LAKIN Department of Food Science, University of Reading, England (179).

IRVIN E. LIENER Department of Biochemistry, College of Biological Sciences, 140 Gortner Laboratory, St Paul, Minnesota 55101, USA (481).

JOHN B. LONGENECKER Graduate Nutrition Division, The University of Texas at Austin, Austin, Texas 78712, USA (155).

J. MAURON Nestlé Products Technical Assistance Co. Ltd, CH–1814, La Tour de Peilz, Switzerland (1, 139).

D. S. MILLER Nutrition Department, Queen Elizabeth College (University of London), Campden Hill Road, London W8, England (93).

P. R. PAYNE Department of Nutrition, London School of Hygiene and Tropical Medicine, Keppel Street (Gower Street), London WC1E 7HT, England (119).

D. PEARSON National College of Food Technology (University of Reading), St George's Avenue, Weybridge, Surrey, England (397).

P. L. PELLETT Department of Nutrition and Food, The Commonwealth of Massachusetts, University of Massachusetts, Amherst 01002 USA (225).

T. PERSSON Swedish Institute for Food Preservation Research, Kallebäck, Göteborg 16, Sweden (421).

R. PION Institute National de la Recherche Agronomique, Station d'Études des Métabolismes, CRZV Métabolismes à Theix par Saint-Genes-Champanelle 63, France (329).

N. W. PIRIE Biochemistry Department, Rothamsted Experimental Station, Harpenden, Herts, England (537).

I. QVIST Swedish Institute for Food Preservation Research, Kallebäck Göteborg 16, Sweden (421).

E. J. ROLFE National College of Food Technology (University of Reading), St George's Avenue, Weybridge, Surrey, England (439).

G. D. ROSEN Birchwood Lodge, The Birches, Farnborough, Kent, England (383).

P. SHERMAN Department of Food Science, Queen Elizabeth College (University of London), Campden Hill Road, London W8, England (425).

C. SHORROCK* National Institute for Research in Dairying, Shinfield, Reading, England (207).

LARS-BÖRJE SJÖBERG Astra Nutrition AB, Fack, 431 20 Mölndal 1, Sweden (369).

JAN STELLEMAN Astra Nutrition AB, Fack, 431 20 Mölndal 1, Sweden (369).

BRUCE R. STILLINGS US Department of Commerce, National Oceanic and Atmospheric Administration, National Marine Fisheries Service, College Park Fishery Products Technology Laboratory, Regents Drive, University of Maryland Campus, College Park, Maryland 20740, USA (11).

W. M. TAHIR Crop and Grassland Production Service (Field Food Crops), Plant Production and Protection Division, FAO, Via delle Terme di Caracalla, 00100-Rome, Italy (35).

F. VITERI Division of Agricultural and Food Sciences, Instituto de Nutricion de Centro America Y Panama, Oficina Sanitaria Panamericana, Carretera Roosevelt, Zona 11, Guatemala, Central America (293).

E. VON SYDOW Swedish Institute for Food Preservation Research, Kallebäck, Göteborg 16, Sweden (421).

R. G. WHITEHEAD Medical Research Council Child Nutrition Research Unit, Mulago Hospital (P O Box 6717), Kampala, Uganda (103).

J. T. WORGAN National College of Food Technology (University of Reading), St George's Avenue, Weybridge, Surrey, England (47).

H. ZUCKER Sandoz Forschungsinstitut, Gesellschaft MBH, Brunnerstrasse 59, A 1235 Vienna, Austria (469).

* Present address: Colborn Group Limited, Barton Mills, Canterbury, Kent, England.

Preface

World food production lags behind the needs of the ever-increasing population, and whilst it can be argued whether the greater demand is for additional supplies of dietary energy or dietary protein, there is no doubt that in many parts of the world substantial numbers of individuals are short of both.

The particular problems associated with the effective use of proteins in human nutrition formed the subject of the NATO Advanced Study Institute held in Reading in March, 1972 and organized on behalf of the International Union of Food Science and Technology and the International Union of Nutritional Sciences. The groups of papers presented during that meeting and the discussions arising from them are collected in this book.

The principal objectives of the meeting were to review existing knowledge of world protein resources in relation to human requirements, to discuss factors affecting protein utilization in the body, to assess critically the usefulness in human nutrition of methods currently used for the evaluation of protein quality, and to consider the role of the food scientist and technologist in the development and use of new protein foods.

To ensure consistency in preparing the manuscripts for publication we have adopted the metric units, conversion factors and nomenclature recommended in the Report of the Sub-committee on Metrication of the British National Committee for Nutritional Sciences (Royal Society, London, 1972). Among the consequent alterations are that values for the energy content of diets are given in joules (4·184 J = 1 calorie) and the common ratios such as digestibility (d.), biological value (b.v.) and net protein utilization (n.p.u.) are expressed as decimals rather than as percentages.

We are most grateful to all those who contributed material for this book. We also wish to thank Mr B. F. Bone for preparing the index.

November, 1972

J. W. G. P.
B. A. R.

Contents

The Role of Food Science and Technology

Some Factors Affecting the Utilization of Proteins

Concluding Remarks

CHAPTER 1

Some Current Problems in Protein Nutrition

J. MAURON

Nestlé Products Technical Assistance Co. Ltd, La Tour de Peilz, Switzerland

I. INTRODUCTION

When the prevalence of protein malnutrition in many parts of the world became known after World War II, a great boom in protein research began that has lasted more or less ever since. The result has been a great increase in basic knowledge of protein metabolism, requirements and evaluation, the preparation of numerous "high protein foods" for "developing" countries and even the manufacture of new kinds of protein material. The basic assumption was that protein malnutrition was essentially a matter of ignorance and could therefore be overcome by science and technology. Two decades of very limited success, if not overt failure, in the fight against protein malnutrition have taught us that this approach was over-optimistic. We are now aware that protein malnutrition is more an economic problem than a medical one, more a matter of food distribution than of production, more linked to the slowness of land reform than to the introduction of sophisticated technology. Present scientific knowledge is already capable of eliminating protein deficiency in most underdeveloped countries. The crucial problem is to overcome the formidable obstacles that impede the proper use of this knowledge in the underdeveloped countries, not to elaborate still more refined techniques. The euphemistic replacement of "developing" countries for "underdeveloped" countries does not change their status: quite the contrary, the gap between rich and poor nations is increasing, not diminishing. The formulation of new vegetable protein mixtures, the production of fish protein concentrate, the development of single cell protein, the amino acid fortification of staple foods, the refinements of methodology in protein evaluation and amino acid determination, and so on, do not *per se* improve the protein supply among the poorer classes. We must realize that in few fields is there such a distressing gap between knowledge and its implementation, between a worthy intent and practical achievement.

Why then does research in protein nutrition still attract support? Although we are aware that the ultimate cause of malnutrition is poverty, we cannot afford to wait for full economic development before we begin to attack the problem, since reducing the ravages of severe malnutrition should itself accelerate economic development and thus contribute to the elimination of poverty. The green revolution is an example of this approach. Moreover, as time goes on and present knowledge is not implemented, the situation may deteriorate to the point where only radically new technology will be able to reverse the trend. Lastly, the drive for new knowledge is a part of human nature and nutrition research often reveals more problems than it solves. The present situation in protein nutrition is one in which we have lost most of our illusions, but not the hope that a more realistic approach will be of some benefit to mankind.

These critical remarks are not meant to discourage but to put the problem into perspective. However brilliant our scientific achievements, we have every reason to remain modest indeed.

II. PROTEIN REQUIREMENTS

What are the logical steps to achieve a proper evaluation of the protein situation? First we need a standard of reference, which can be found in the protein requirements of man. To establish these requirements we need methods to evaluate protein quality. Then, we have to relate these protein requirements with the actual supply in different populations. This should enable us to identify the vulnerable groups, in which food supply and/or protein is deficient. Means must then be sought to make more food and protein available. The specialized methodology of protein evaluation is again needed for screening the new protein foods.

There is considerable controversy about the protein needs of man, and even about the criteria by which they are judged. The man in the field who has to evaluate diets and food supply is faced with a difficult situation. He must apply recommendations for human protein requirements that are based on assumptions for which experimental proof is not yet forthcoming.

III. PROTEIN SUPPLIES

Theoretically there is no protein shortage in the world. In fact, maldistribution is such that wide disparities occur between developed and underdeveloped countries, particularly with animal protein. Moreover, national food consumption data are not very meaningful since the distribution of the available supplies among different social classes is extremely uneven. Even in the USA there are indications that 10% of the population does not properly cover its nutritional needs.

To improve protein nutrition we should have to improve on production and distribution. Some consider that there is no lack of protein, merely a lack of food that happens to contain a normal amount of protein. Although this might be so where cereals are the staple food, it is not the case where cassava is the staple. Moreover, the green revolution may increase cereal production at the expense of pulses, leading to a relative secondary protein deficiency.

The most logical way to increase the world protein supply would be to make more plant proteins available for human consumption and to develop production of unconventional proteins for animal feed. However, great difficulties—generally economic—are encountered when such simple schemes are attempted. Thus, great efforts have been made to divert some oilseeds from animal to human consumption, but with limited success. The textured protein foods, on the other hand, do not contribute to the protein supply in underdeveloped countries, but are introduced into Western markets. Fish protein concentrate and leaf protein have not even reached this stage.

The development of totally new, unconventional proteins, such as single cell proteins (SCP), has been comparatively rapid. Even so, SCP cannot compete with oilseed meals in animal feed without governmental support, and it will probably be another decade or so before SCP products appear on the market, because of the need for long term safety evaluations.

However, even if they are successful, these unconventional foods will be relatively expensive and will not immediately benefit the underdeveloped countries.

The enhancement of protein quality by amino acid supplementation of staples has been envisaged as a way of improving protein supply. There is no doubt about the efficiency of amino acid fortification of cereals for animals or for human subjects in a metabolic unit. It is much more difficult to prove its effectiveness in field trials, because of the complex variables in any ecological system.

Others have proposed that the major sources of energy of a population should be converted as far as possible into complete foods. Those millions reduced by circumstances to eating cheap diets consisting largely of the staple would then be adequately nourished, provided that they consumed sufficient of the food to obtain their requirements of energy.

None of these proposals provides a solution of the protein problem on its own. Each must be studied to find whether it provides a worthwhile contribution that is the most feasible way of achieving adequate nutrition in a given ecological context.

IV. PROTEIN EVALUATION

Protein evaluation in the strict sense comprises the determination of the nutritive value by direct biological methods or by indirect methods such as amino acid analysis. In the broader sense it includes the appraisal of organoleptic qualities, as well as the detection of possible toxic factors that accompany certain protein foods. Essentially, there are only two parameters used to evaluate nutritive value, growth and nitrogen balance. However, there is considerable variation in methodology and much controversy about the adequacy of the different procedures.

It has been suggested that the measurement of protein quality under standardized conditions is of little practical importance because they are unrelated to normal dietary conditions. Clearly, measurement of nutritive value gives a protein's full nutritional potential, not its actual utilization in a concrete situation. However, to conclude that protein quality is meaningless because it is not universally applicable is an unjustified oversimplification. More serious is the objection that nutritive value gives no information on the complementary value of a protein. For this we need its amino acid composition, which will disclose any excess or deficit of individual essential amino acids as well as the ratio of essential to non-essential amino acids (important because non-specific N can spare essential N). Some measure of amino acid availability should also be made, especially in heat-processed protein foods.

The interrelationships between the efficiency of protein utilization and the dietary energy are of great importance. The protein-sparing effect of energy is sometimes considered greater than that of a balanced amino acid supply, although probably both are important.

Protein quality is a factor even for an adult in N equilibrium, in whom protein is apparently used as a source of energy, since it is involved in metabolic processes for which the amino acid composition is relevant. It may be true that in the past too much emphasis was put on nutritive value and not enough on the organoleptic properties which are decisive for practical application. Texture and flavour are crucial factors in the success of new protein foods.

V. BIOCHEMICAL ASSESSMENTS OF PROTEIN QUALITY

Nitrogen balance studies do not yield information relevant to protein requirements unless the N intake is limiting. Derivation of the requirements for optimal nutrition from such data is an uncertain process, involving considerable extrapolation. It would, therefore, be a great advance to have parameters to define nutritional status accurately. Those investigated include the chemical composition of biological fluids, muscles or liver, and the activity of selected enzymes. Although it has been shown that the level of xanthine oxidase is related to the intake of utilizable protein (Muramatsu and Ashida, 1962), it remains uncertain what the optimal enzyme activity should be.

The enzymic *adaptation* of the organism to changes in protein quantity and quality may be a more profitable field of study. Mauron *et al.* (1972) have investigated the adaptation of the rat to dietary protein concentration by measuring the level of two model enzymes in liver, serinedehydratase (involved in the serine–pyruvate pathway in the conversion of protein to carbohydrate) and 3-phosphoglyceratedehydrogenase (involved in the opposite pyruvate–serine pathway in the conversion of carbohydrate to protein). Rats became adapted to increasing dietary concentrations of casein by induction of serinedehydratase and repression of phosphoglyceratedehydrogenase; a logical regulatory mechanism, since with a high-protein diet the excess amino acids are converted to carbohydrate to produce energy, and with a low-protein diet carbohydrate must be converted to amino acids as far as possible. Thus, serinedehydratase level indicates the catabolic state and phosphoglyceratedehydrogenase the anabolic state. Both enzymes react in an opposite but perfectly symmetrical way and can be used as "markers" of the state of protein metabolism. Both enzyme activities were in equilibrium at a relatively low level when maximal growth was achieved at the 22% casein concentration. At lower casein concentrations anabolism prevailed, at high concentrations catabolism (Fig. 1A). With gluten, a protein of low nutritive value, growth could still be attained at a gluten level of about 4% but, since enzyme activities remained unchanged, the animal was now in a permanent state of protein catabolism (Fig. 1B). This is the price the body has to pay for using a low-quality protein. With SCP, a protein of intermediate nutritive value, we found that the animal had adapted its protein metabolism to the lower protein quality (as compared to casein) by displacing the equilibrium point towards higher dietary protein concentrations, so that near maximum growth again coincided with metabolic equilibrium (Fig. 1C), as with casein. Thus, with SCP the lower nutritive value paralleled a lower inducing power for serinedehydratase and a lower repressing power for phosphoglyceratedehydrogenase, whereas with gluten the lower nutritive value was not accompanied by a change in enzyme regulatory power.

Since the first limiting amino acid in gluten is lysine, whereas in SCP it is methionine, we tested the hypothesis that not all ten amino acids essential for growth of the rat were active in regulating the level of these two enzymes. This proved to be the case. Methionine, tryptophan, threonine and valine induced serinedehydratase and repressed phosphoglyceratedehydrogenase; all the other amino acids were inactive. This explains why gluten has the same enzyme regulating activity as casein: lysine is not an "active" amino acid. We therefore make a tentative distinction between essential and regulatory amino acids: the latter are responsible for the enzymic adaptation of the animal to variations in the protein supply. Thus, the concentration of regulatory amino acids in a given diet would monitor the adaptive response of the body, whereas the concentration of the essential amino acids would control N retention. This distinction might one day provide an additional parameter for protein

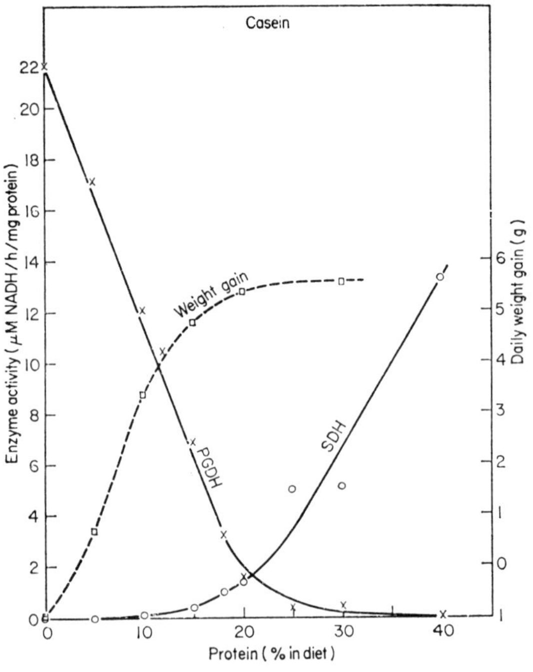

(A)

FIG. 1. The weight gains of rats given (A) casein, (B) gluten or (C) SCP at various dietary levels and the levels of serinedehydratase (SDH) and 3-phosphoglyceratedehydrogenase (PGDH) in their livers

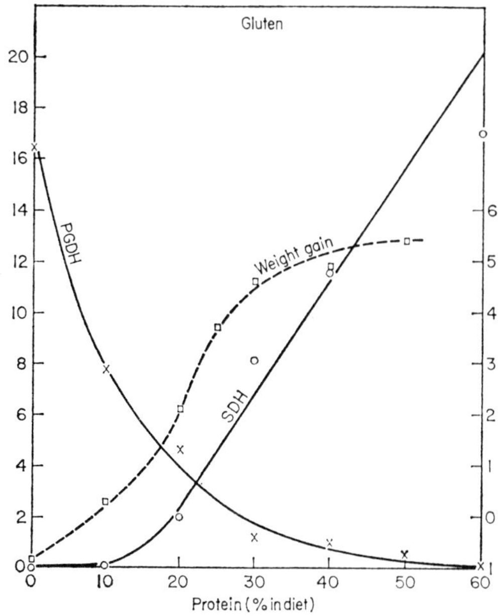
Gluten
PGDH
Weight gain
SDH
20
18
16
14
12
10
8
6
4
2
0
6
5
4
3
2
1
0
1
0
10
20
30
40
50
60
Protein (% in diet)

(B)

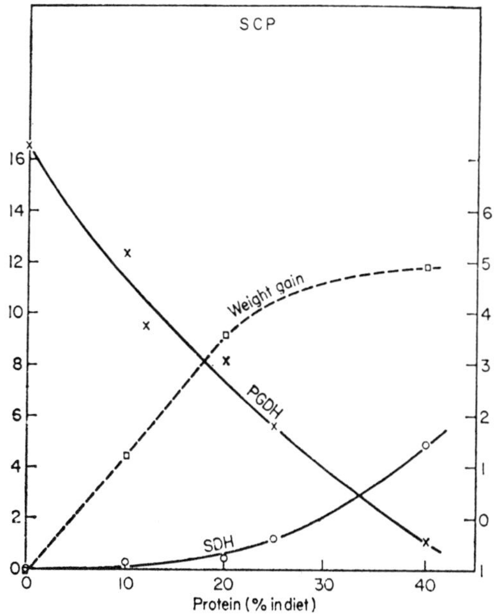
SCP
Weight gain
PGDH
SDH
16
14
12
10
8
6
4
2
0
6
5
4
3
2
1
0
1
0
10
20
30
40
Protein (% in diet)

(C)

evaluation, but the concept of regulatory amino acids first needs confirmation.

It is not justifiable to apply the classic criteria of maximum growth or N retention uncritically to man, pertinent though they are to the raising of farm animals. The purpose of human nutrition is quite different: to ensure a long life with minimum disease and maximum intellectual capacity, objectives that have little to do with mere size and rate of growth. Indeed, a negative correlation between maximum growth rate and longevity might even be expected from the results of McCay *et al.* (1939) who showed that restriction of food serious enough to interfere markedly with growth allowed animals not only to live longer but also to remain physiologically younger at the same chronological age as the controls. Moreover, the incidence of practically all the common causes of death of rats was greatly diminished. The results of Ross (1961) suggested that some protein restriction may contribute to a longer life in rats. Ross and Batt (1957) have put forward the hypothesis that biological ageing may be the manifestation of naturally occurring enzymatic changes and that, by retarding these changes through diet, it may be possible to retard biological ageing. Rats given a low-casein (8%) diet grew suboptimally, maintained an enzyme pattern characteristic of that of the young animal and had a longer life span.

In our own assays (Mauron, 1967) we found that the response of some enzymes to age is similar to their response to increased dietary protein quantity or quality (Fig. 2). In practical terms this means that a diet

Correlation between age and diet enzyme patterns

Enzyme	*Age* ↗	*Protein Content* ↗	*Protein Quality* ↗
Succinoxidase	↗	↗	↗
D-Amino acid oxidase	↗	↗	↗
Xanthine oxidase	↗	↗	↗
Transamidinase (kidney)	↗	↗	↗
Alkaline phosphatase	↘	↘	↘

↗ increase ↘ decrease

FIG. 2. Effect on certain enzymes of age, dietary protein level and dietary protein quality

adequate in utilizable protein will provoke more rapid ageing, including enzyme pattern modifications, than a protein-restricted diet, and will eventually reduce life span.

Of course, it would be unjustified to extend such limited results with experimental animals to man. This example is intended only to emphasize that the classic criteria of protein evaluation do not give the final answer to the problem of protein nutrition in man. Our ignorance is such that many more meetings on the subject can easily be justified.

REFERENCES

Mauron, J. (1967). *Int. Congr. Nutr. F, Hamburg* **7**, 367–481. (J. Kühnau, ed.) Viehweg & Sohn, Braunschweig; Pergamon Press, Oxford.

Mauron, J., Mottu, F. and Spohr, G. (1972). *Eur. J. Biochem.* (submitted for publication).

McCay, C. M., Maynard, L. A., Sperling, G. and Barnes, L. L. (1939). *J. Nutr.* **18**, 1–13.

Muramatsu, K. and Ashida, K. (1962). *J. Nutr.* **76**, 143–150.

Ross, M. H. (1961). *J. Nutr.* **75**, 197–210.

Ross, M. H. and Batt, W. G. (1957). *J. Nutr.* **61**, 39–49.

CHAPTER 2

World Supplies of Animal Protein

BRUCE R. STILLINGS

National Marine Fisheries Service, US Department of Commerce, University of Maryland, USA

I. INTRODUCTION

Animal protein in the form of meat and fish was of major importance in man's hunting days, before the origin of agriculture and aquaculture. Domestication of animals appears to have started at about the same time as the growing of crops, and was complete before the dawn of history. The British ecologist, Charles Elton (1936), has called animals that live directly off plants "key industry animals" because all of the rest of the animal's system depends on them. They can also be called "first order consumers", which, in turn, are eaten by "second order consumers" and so on (Bates, 1969). A similar analogy can be made for fish that feed at different trophic levels. As a meat eater, man becomes a "second order consumer", whereas in largely vegetarian societies he is a "key industry animal".

Proteins of animal origin have traditionally been used by man to balance his diet. Foods of animal origin such as meat, milk, eggs and fish provide the essential amino acids as well as minerals, fats and vitamins. Moreover, at least in western societies and some eastern societies, animal products are desired because of their flavour and texture.

Currently, proteins from animal sources play a major role in meeting the protein requirements of man. There are, however, gross imbalances in the supplies of animal proteins between various regions of the world.

Correction of these imbalances is a key to improving the nutritional status of populations in the less developed regions. The purpose of this discussion is to review the dietary requirements for animal protein, to assess the production and supplies of animal protein in various regions of the world during the past two decades, and to assess the potential for increasing supplies in the future.

II. REQUIREMENTS FOR ANIMAL PROTEIN

Although there is no requirement for animal protein in the diet *per se*, the quantity of dietary protein from animal sources is usually accepted as being indicative of the overall protein quality of the diet. Moreover, supply of adequate quantities of animal products is generally recognized as being an ideal way to improve world protein nutrition.

Human beings and other monogastric animals do not distinguish between amino acids of plant, animal, or other origin as long as adequate quantities of each essential amino acid are present. As shown in Table I,

TABLE I. Protein quality of selected foods

Food	*Chemical Score*[a, b]	*Limiting amino acid*[a, b]	*Net protein utilization*[a]	*Biological value*[c]	*Protein efficiency ratio*[c]
Egg	1·00	—	1·00	0·99	4·2
Beef muscle	0·80	Sulphur AA	0·80	0·74	2·4
Milk (cow's)	0·60	Sulphur AA	0·75	0·85	3·2
Fish	0·75	Tryptophan	0·83	0·85	3·1
Rice	0·75	Lysine	0·57	0·70	2·1
Maize meal	0·45	Tryptophan	0·55	0·54	0·9
Wheat flour	0·50	Lysine	0·52	0·64	1·6

[a] FAO (1965)
[b] Based on essential amino acid pattern of whole egg
[c] FAO (1964)

meat, milk, eggs, and fish protein are higher in quality than proteins of plant origin, in that they contain the balance of the amino acids essential to man, whereas plant proteins are usually deficient in one or more essential amino acids. To the extent that plant proteins are deficient in essential amino acids, the latter can be supplied adequately in the human diet by combining vegetable proteins having a complementary pattern of essential amino acids or by supplementing with animal protein. As is well known, however, the proportion of essential amino acids in the proteins of animal origin comes closer to meeting the human needs than does that in most plant sources.

Protein needs include the essential amino acids that must be supplied from the diet because they cannot be synthesized by the body, and the N in non-essential amino acids that is also necessary for the synthesis of body protein. Although most emphasis has been placed on the need for essential amino acids, under certain conditions the amount of non-essential N in the diet may be limiting. In the case of both cow's milk and eggs, the minimum quantity that will maintain N balance in the adult human being provides more than double the estimated requirement of each essential amino acid (FAO, 1965). Thus, to meet protein needs, animal proteins can be used most efficiently as dietary supplements to proteins of vegetable origin, which often are not only deficient in one or more essential amino acids but which also contain a higher proportion of non-essential amino acids.

III. SUPPLIES OF ANIMAL PRODUCTS AND PROTEINS

There is no shortage of animal protein in the world, and the potential for expansion is great. Because of poor distribution, however, there is a large discrepancy in the supplies of total and animal protein in developing regions as compared with developed regions of the world. Table II shows the populations and the daily energy and protein supplies *per caput* in various regions of the world and in the developed and developing areas. Based on 1969 figures, the population in the developing regions accounted for nearly 75% of the total world population. Energy and protein supplies are derived from food balance sheets and are based on 1963–5 data. These figures overestimate actual dietary intakes, but can be considered indicative of relative differences and changes in dietary intakes. For the developing regions, the average daily supply of animal protein was about 11 g compared with 48 g in the developed regions. Total protein supply was 58 g in the developing regions and 89 g in the developed areas.

It should be pointed out that the deficiency of animal protein in the developing regions is not as great as would be implied from the difference in animal protein supplies between developed and developing regions. The reason for this is that in the developed regions the supplies of animal protein are clearly in excess of the minimum requirements. As pointed out earlier, there is no fixed requirement for animal protein, since protein requirements are, in effect, based on the need for adequate quantities of essential amino acids, whether from plant or animal sources. Altschul (1965) has suggested, however, that diets that contain an average of

30 g per day of protein from animal sources will be adequate in quality regardless of the source of the remainder of the protein. An average of less than 30 g per day will result in a diet of questionable quality, and an average of less than 15 g of animal protein per day poses the near certainty of protein malnutrition for part of the population. Based on these assumptions, the gap in quality of dietary protein between developed and developing regions, although large, is considerably less than would be indicated from the data in Table II.

The contribution of all animal protein and of the protein from individual animal products to the total protein supply on a world and regional basis is shown in Table III. Total animal protein accounts for 32% of the world's protein supplies. Protein from meat, milk, eggs and fish contribute 15, 11, 2 and 4% of the world's protein supplies, respectively. There are considerable variations between regions, however. In the developing regions, total animal protein and protein from meat, milk, eggs and fish contribute 19, 8, 5, 1 and 4%, respectively, of the total protein supplies. In the developed regions, comparable figures are 54, 25, 20, 4 and 4%, respectively.

TABLE II. Energy and protein supplies (1963–5) *per caput* per day

Region	*Population* (1969)[a] (million)	*Energy* (kJ)[b]	*Animal protein*[b] (g)	*Total protein*[b] (g)
Far East[c]	1966	8580	8·6	54·8
Near and Middle East	166	10 080	14·0	71·6
Africa	297	9080	10·9	58·5
Latin America	276	10 840	24·1	67·6
DEVELOPING REGIONS	2705	8950	10·7	57·6
Europe[d]	698	12 760	42·8	87·6
North America	224	13 140	65·3	93·1
Oceania	19	13 510	63·9	95·4
DEVELOPED REGIONS	941	12 850	48·3	89·1
WORLD	3646	9960	21·0	66·1

[a] FAO (1971a)
[b] Autret (1970)
[c] Includes Mainland China
[d] Includes USSR

Figures on total and animal protein supplies in the developed and developing regions are based on the 1963–5 period. Recent information, however, indicates that the situation has not improved. In fact, on a *per caput* basis, it appears that the gap in supplies of total and animal protein between the developed and the developing regions has widened. Figure 1 shows the total and animal protein in the food supplies and the

TABLE III. Percentage contribution of animal products to the total protein supply (1963–5)[a]

Region	*Animal proteins*	*Protein contributed by*			
		Meat	*Eggs*	*Fish*	*Milk*
Far East[b]	15·7	6·6	0·7	4·6	3·8
Near and Middle East	19·6	8·0	0·7	1·4	9·5
Africa	18·6	9·2	0·5	4·1	4·8
Latin America	35·7	18·3	1·9	2·7	12·7
DEVELOPING REGIONS	18·6	8·3	0·9	4·0	5·4
Europe[c]	48·5	21·5	3·8	4·2	18·8
North America	69·9	36·3	5·8	2·9	24·9
Oceania	66·9	36·8	4·2	3·1	22·5
DEVELOPED REGIONS	54·2	25·4	4·3	3·9	20·4
WORLD	31·8	14·7	2·1	3·9	10·9

[a] Autret (1970)
[b] Includes Mainland China
[c] Includes USSR

populations during the last 20 years in selected countries in developed and developing regions of the world. The developed countries included in the graph are the USA, UK, France, West Germany and Italy. The selected countries in the developing region include the UAR, India, Pakistan, Ceylon, Venezuela and Mexico. In the developed regions, there has been a steady increase in the daily *per caput* supplies of animal protein for the past 20 years. In the early 1950s the supplies of animal protein were about 46 g *per caput* per day; and in the late 1960s the value had risen to about 60 g. In contrast, very little change occurred in the developing countries. There was a slight increase from 6·8 to 7·7 g *per caput* per day from the early 1950s to the early 1960s. However, a slight decrease to 7·4 g occurred from the early 1960s to the late 1960s.

In terms of total protein, the pattern is similar. Again, supplies *per caput* per day increased in the developed countries. In the developing region, although the supply increased from the early 1950s to the early

1960s, during the last few years the supplies of total protein available *per caput* per day have decreased slightly. Also shown in Fig. 1 are the population figures for these selected countries. In contrast to the available supplies of total and animal protein, the developing countries excelled in terms of increases in population. In the selected developed countries,

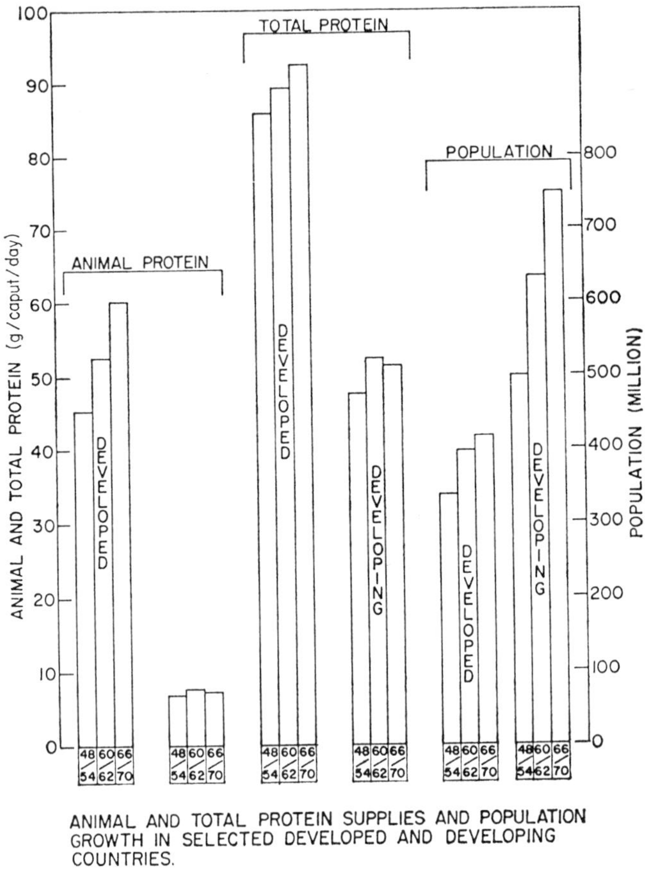

FIG. 1. Animal and total protein supplies and population growth in selected developed and developing countries (FAO, 1971a)

total population increased by about 23% from the early 1950s to the late 1960s. The population increase in the selected developing countries for the same time period was about 50%. As is well known, one of the major hindrances to increasing the supplies and intakes of total protein and animal protein in the developing countries is the rapid increase in population.

Based on the data discussed above, it would appear that the intakes of total and animal protein have increased in the developed regions of the world and remained rather static in the developing regions during the last two decades. This assumes, of course, that the countries selected are representative of the two regions, and that the estimated protein content of the food supply is indicative of changes in consumption patterns.

Obviously, average values for protein supplies in a country or region are inadequate to describe the specific conditions within the area. Part of the population in all areas has a level of nutrition far in excess of the average. This means that, especially in areas where the average nutrition level is less than adequate, many people have grossly inadequate diets.

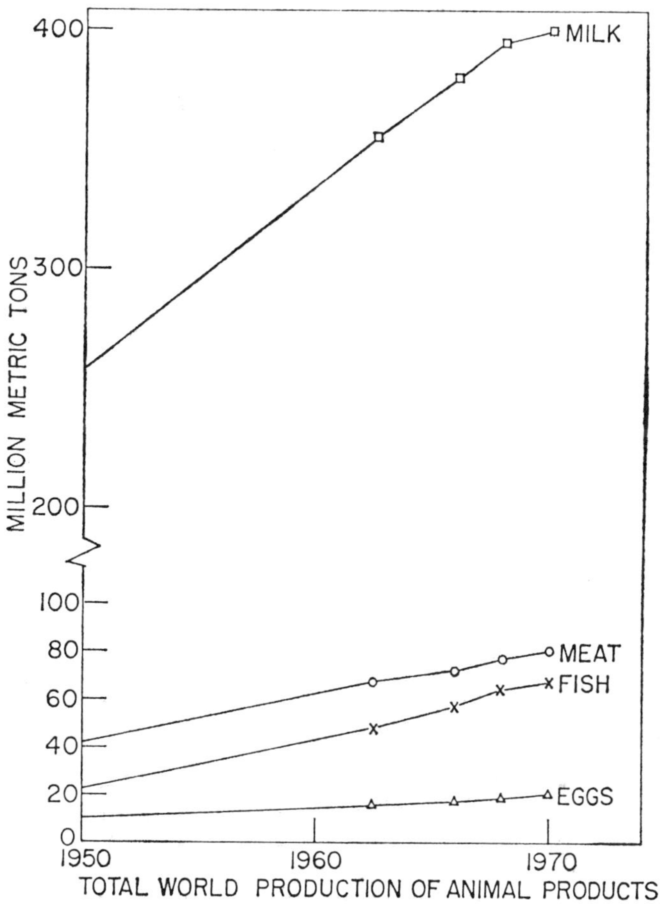

FIG. 2. Total world production of animal products (FAO, 1970b, 1971a, b)

IV. PRODUCTION OF ANIMAL PRODUCTS AND PROTEIN

A. World Production

Figure 2 shows the world production of the major animal products during the last 20 years. Total production of all commodities has increased substantially during this period. The greatest increase in total production has been with milk, which increased from 258 million metric tons in 1950 to 399 million metric tons in 1970. During this period, meat increased from 41 to 80 million metric tons, fish from 22 to 68 million metric tons, and eggs from 10 to 20 million metric tons. The production figures for meat are based on dressed carcass weight and include beef, veal, mutton, lamb and pork but do not include poultry. If the production for poultry

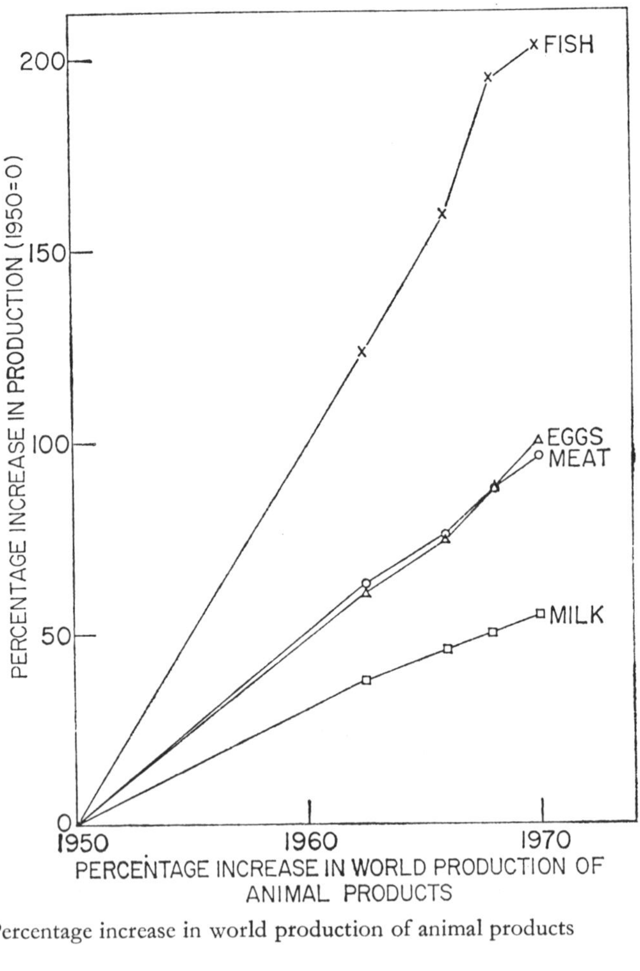

FIG. 3. Percentage increase in world production of animal products

meat were included in the total meat figures, they would be increased by about 12–15%.

As shown in Fig. 3, fish has shown the greatest improvement in terms of percentage increase in production of the four major animal products. From 1950 to 1970, fish catch has increased over 200%. A large portion of this increased catch, however, has been used for animal feed, as will be discussed later. Meat and egg production have increased about 100% during this period, whereas milk has increased only about 55%.

Based on the total world production of animal products, the available protein from these major animal products has been calculated on a daily *per caput* basis. The protein values used were as follows: dressed carcass meat, 14%; milk, 3·5%; egg, 11%; and fish, 18% (FAO, 1967). Figure 4 shows the total protein supplies from each of the major animal products during the last 20 years, expressed as g *per caput* per day. *Per caput* supplies of protein from meat increased from 6·3 g in 1950 to 8·3 g by the late 1960s. Nearly all of this supply was available for human consumption. *Per caput* supplies of protein from milk have shown little change during

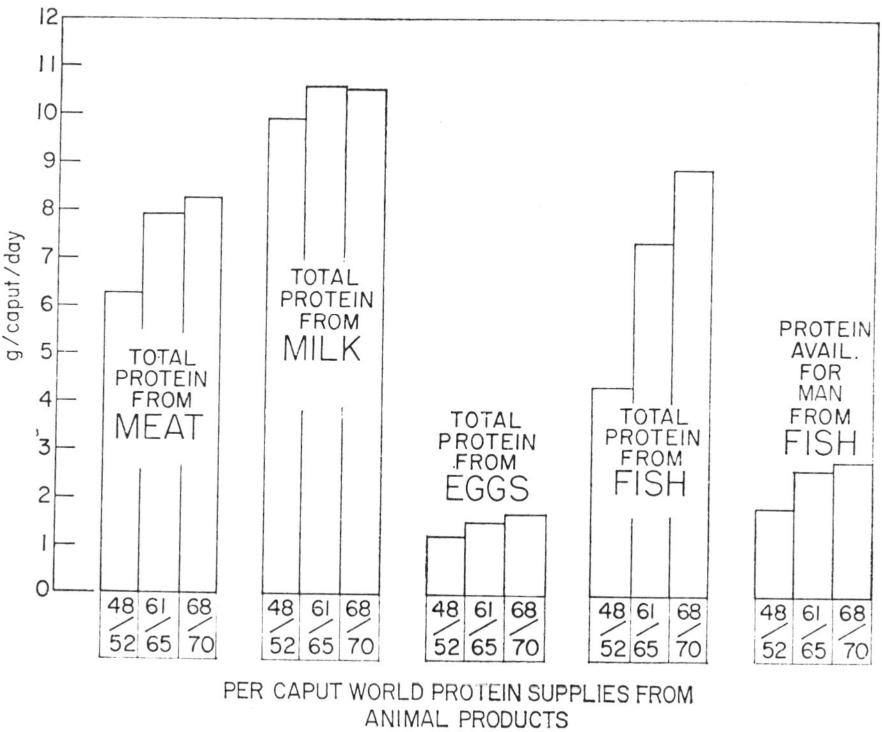

FIG. 4. *Per caput* world protein supplies from animal products

the past two decades. From 1950 to the early 1960s, the supply increased from 9·9 g to 10·5 g and then decreased to 10·4 g in the late 1960s. About 90% of the milk protein was available for human consumption, since about 8–10% was used for animals. Protein from eggs increased slightly during the past two decades, and ranged from 1·2 g to 1·6 g *per caput* per day. Essentially all protein from eggs was available for human consumption.

The largest increase in *per caput* protein supplies occurred with fish. The supplies of protein increased from about 4·3 g in 1950 to 7·4 g in the early 1960s and up to 8·9 g *per caput* per day in the late 1960s. A large portion of this increase was not, however, directly available for human consumption. In large part, the increase was due to the tremendous stocks of fish converted to fish meal, primarily for animal feeds. The last column shown in Fig. 4 is a more accurate estimate of the amount of protein from fish available for human consumption. These values have been obtained by subtracting the amount of fish used for producing fish meal from the total catch. Moreover, according to Finch (1970), about 50% of the protein is lost between the ocean and the consumer during processing of fish for human consumption. Thus, of the fish remaining after the subtraction of that processed into fish meal, an additional 50% has been subtracted to arrive at the values shown for protein available for human beings from fish. Examining these values, it is clear that only a slight increase has occurred during the last 20 years in the *per caput* supply of protein from fish for direct human consumption. It should be pointed out that in addition to the protein available for direct human consumption, approximately one-third of the protein from fish meal is converted to meat protein for human consumption. If this protein were added to that derived directly from fish, the *per caput* world supply of fish protein for human consumption in 1968–70 would be increased from 2·8 g to 3·5 g per day.

B. Regional Production

The total production of meat and the *per caput* protein supplies from meat on a regional basis are shown in Figs 5 and 6. Total production of meat has increased in all regions during the last 20 years. Total production and increases in production have been greatest in Europe and the USSR, North America and the Far East. On a *per caput* basis, protein supplies from meat have also increased during the last 20 years in Europe and the USSR, North America and Oceania. In Latin America, although the total production has increased during the last 20 years, the *per caput* supplies of protein from meat have actually decreased. Moreover, the supplies of meat in Latin America are not totally available for indigenous

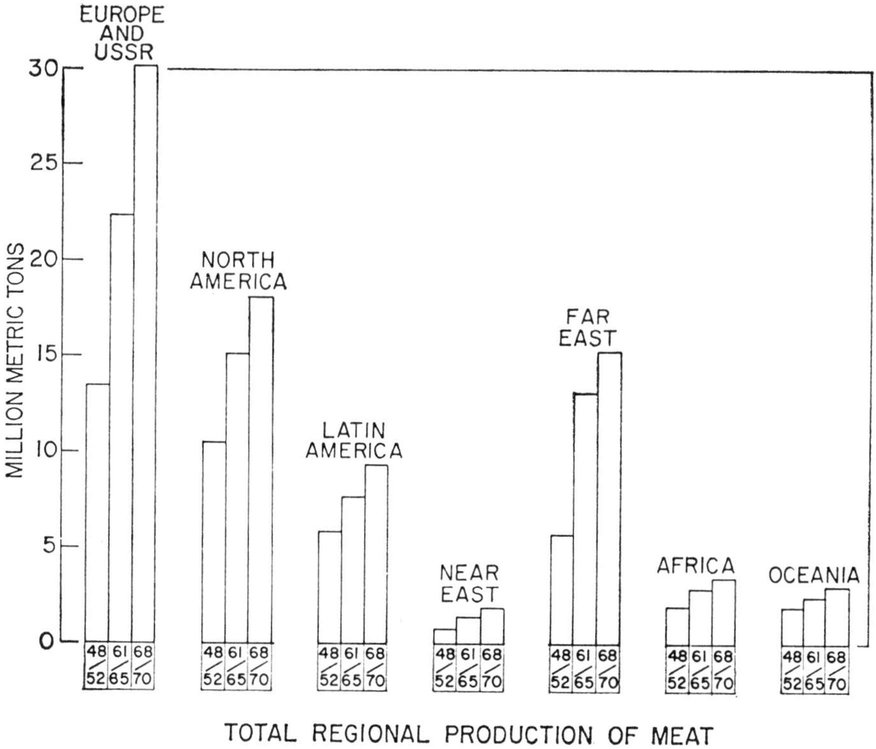

FIG. 5. Total regional production of meat (FAO, 1971a)

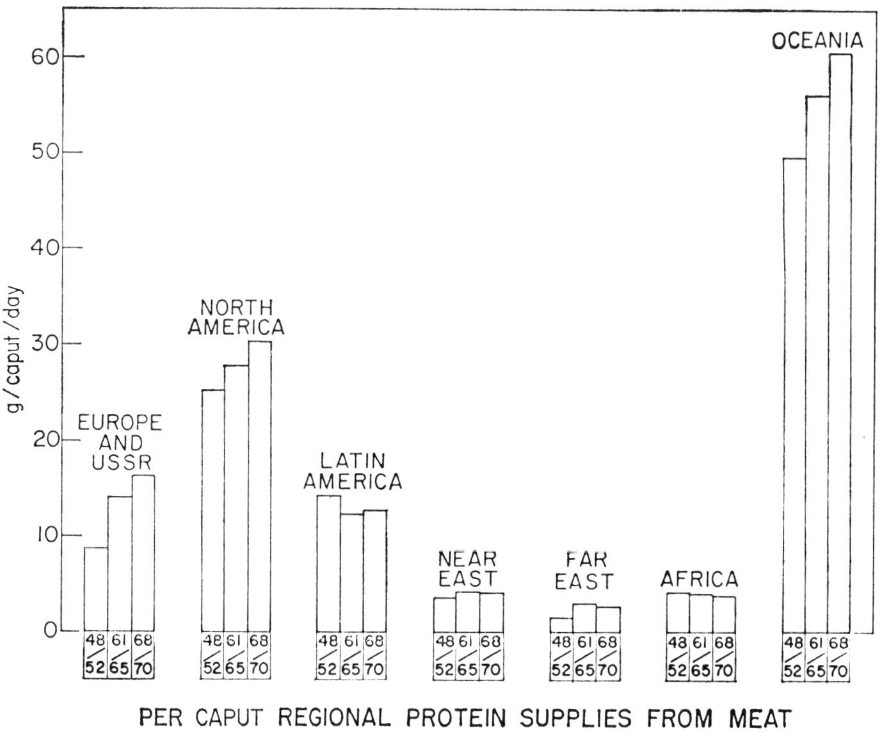

FIG. 6. *Per caput* regional protein supplies from meat

consumption, since during the last decade about 7% of the supplies have been exported. On a *per caput* basis, meat furnishes only small amounts of protein in the Near East, Far East and in Africa. During the last two decades, only slight changes have occurred in the *per caput* protein supplies from meat in these regions. In Oceania, approximately one-third of the total meat produced has been exported in recent years. Thus, the *per*

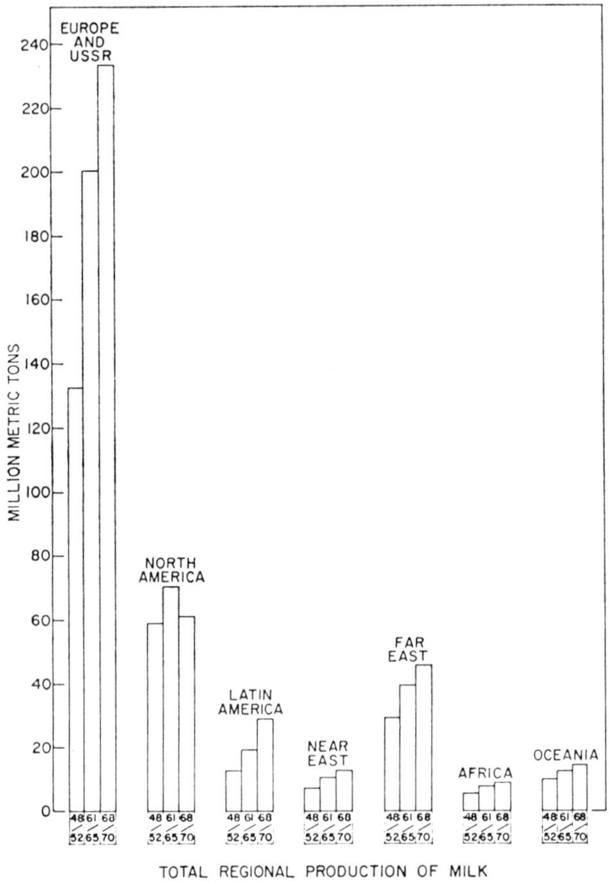

Fig. 7. Total regional production of milk (FAO, 1971a)

caput protein supplies from meat available for consumption in Oceania are considerably less than those shown in Fig. 6. These figures illustrate the large resources for the production of protein from meat on a *per caput* basis in Oceania compared with the apparently more limited potential for the production of protein from meat in the Near East, Far East and Africa.

Figures 7 and 8 show the total production of milk and the *per caput* regional supplies of protein from milk. As is evident, Europe and the USSR exceeds any other region in its total production of milk, and production has increased substantially during the past few decades. North America is second in the production of milk, but total production has decreased during the past decade. Latin America and the Far East produced somewhat smaller quantities, but production has increased in both of these areas during the past two decades. Total production in the

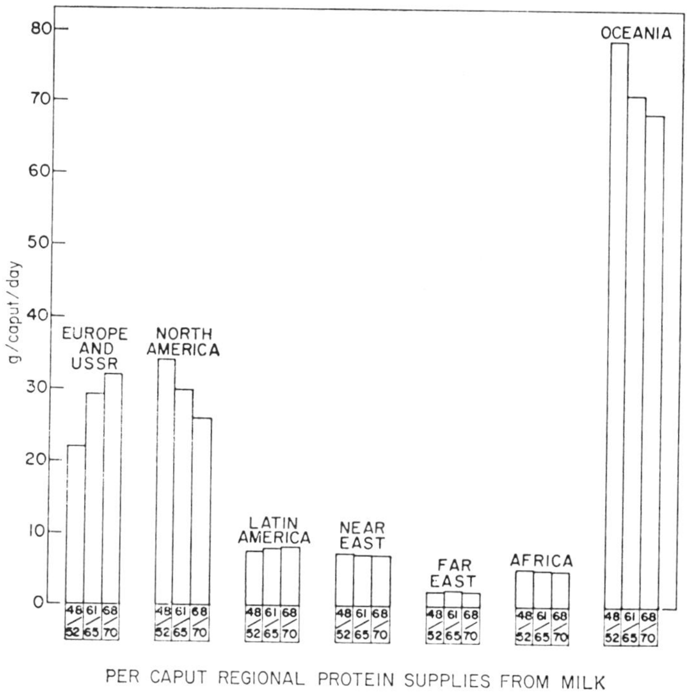

FIG. 8. *Per caput* regional protein supplies from Milk

Near East, Africa and Oceania is relatively small compared with the other regions. In terms of *per caput* protein supplies from milk, however, Oceania far exceeds any other region in the world. *Per caput* protein supplies from milk have decreased during the last two decades in Oceania and North America. Protein supplies have increased in Europe and the USSR and have remained relatively stable in Latin America, the Near East, the Far East and Africa.

With both meat and milk, these figures illustrate the marked discrepancy in *per caput* protein supplies between the developed regions of

Europe and the USSR, North America and Oceania, and the developing regions of Latin America, the Near East, the Far East and Africa. In terms of total production, countries in Latin America, the Near East, the Far East and Africa account for 74% of the total world population, but they account for only 36% and 22% of the world production of meat and milk, respectively.

As shown in Fig. 9, production of eggs is greatest in Europe and the USSR, North America and the Far East. Production has increased in all regions during the last two decades, particularly in Europe and the

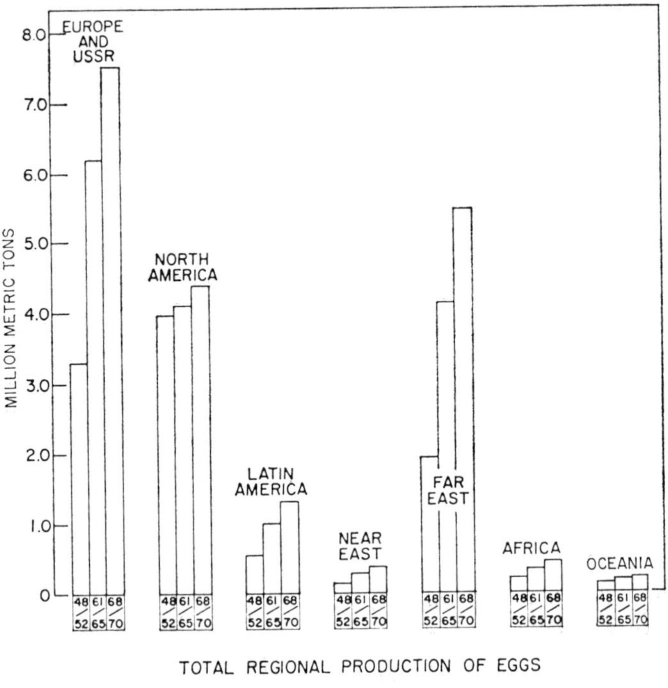

FIG. 9. Total regional production of eggs (FAO, 1971a)

USSR and the Far East. In 1969, 38% of the world production of eggs was in countries with 74% of the world population, i.e., Latin America, the Near East, the Far East and Africa. On a *per caput* basis supplies of protein from eggs were highest in North Africa and Oceania (Fig. 10). In both of these areas, however, supplies have either decreased or have remained relatively static during the last two decades. Increases in supplies of protein from eggs have occurred in Europe and the USSR, Latin America, and to a lesser extent in the Near East, Far East and Africa.

Figure 11 shows the total regional fish catch during the last two decades. Particularly significant developments have occurred in total production in Europe and the USSR, South America and Asia. In these three regions, the fish catch has increased over 200% during the last two decades. A large proportion of this increased catch, however, has been used for reduction to fish meal for animal feed rather than for use directly as human food. As shown in Table IV, 32% of the catch in Europe and the USSR in 1968–70 was used for reduction to fish meal for animal feed rather than for use directly as human food. The situations in South America and Asia offer contrasting pictures. In South America the fish

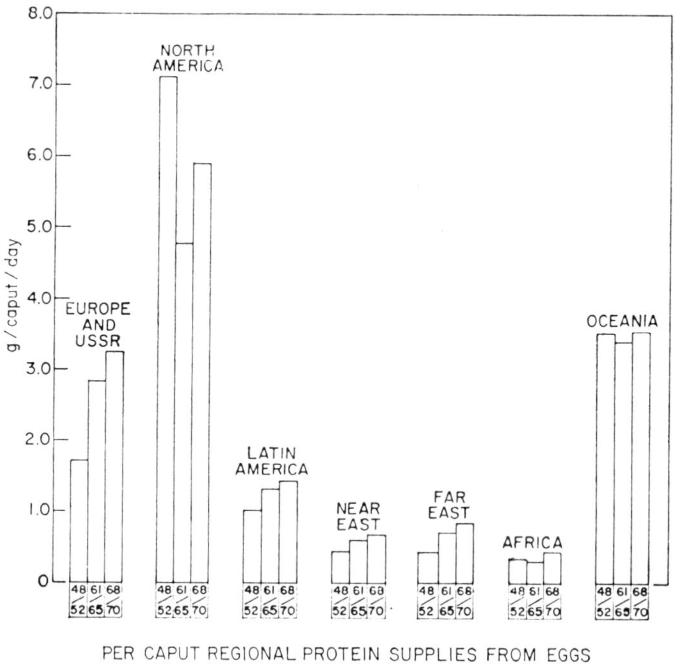

FIG. 10. *Per caput* Regional protein supplies from eggs

catch increased from about 0·5 million metric tons in 1950 to 12·9 million metric tons in 1968–70. During this latter period, however, 76% of the catch was used for reduction to fish meal. In Asia, the catch increased from 8·2 million metric tons in 1950 to 24·7 million metric tons in 1968–70. During 1968–70, only about 11% was used for the preparation of fish meal.

The *per caput* regional protein supplies from fish, shown in Fig. 12, are based on the total fish catch in each of the regions rather than on the amount of protein available for direct human consumption. The figures indicate the great potential in South America for increasing dietary intake of animal protein from fish if a large portion of the catch presently reduced to fish meal and exported were used for direct human consumption within the region. This point is emphasized by figures in Table IV which show that about 34 g of fish protein were available *per caput* per day based on the total catch, but only 4 g were available after subtraction of the catch used for fish meal and subtraction of an additional 50% of the

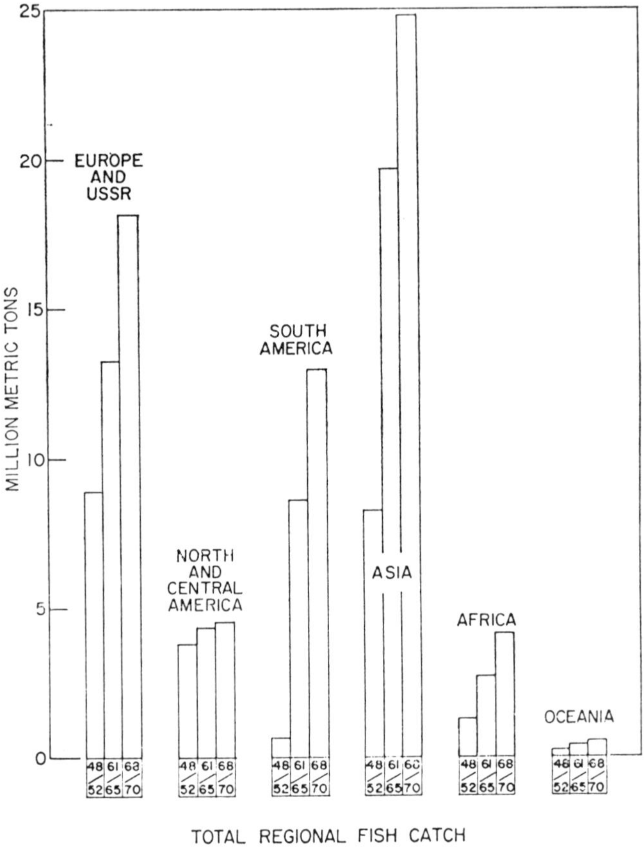

FIG. 11. Total regional fish catch (FAO, 1970b, 1971b)

protein to allow for processing losses. In Asia, on the other hand, even though the total catch of fish exceeded that in any other region, only about 6 g of fish protein *per caput* per day were available based on the total fish catch in 1968–70. Since only 11% was used for the preparation of fish meal, the potential for increasing the amount of fish protein for direct human consumption is not nearly as great as in South America. In

TABLE IV. Total fish catch and protein available from fish (1968–70)

Region	*Total fish catch* (million metric tons)	*Amount used for reduction purposes*[a] (% of total)	*Protein available based on total catch* (g/caput/day)	*Protein available from fish for direct human consumption*[b] (g/caput/day)
Europe and USSR	18·22	32·3	12·9	4·4
North and Central America	4·50	41·3	7·1	2·1
South America	12·91	76·1	34·2	4·1
Asia	24·74	10·8	5·9	2·6
Africa	4·52	53·1	6·4	1·5
Oceania	0·19	10·5	4·9	2·2

[a] FAO (1970, 1971b)

[b] Calculated by subtracting the amount of fish used for reduction purposes from the total catch and by subtracting an additional 50% of the protein due to processing losses

other regions, the protein available from fish, based on the total catch in 1968–70, ranged from 5 g in Oceania to 13 g in Europe and the USSR. However, after subtraction of the fish catch used for fish meal and the protein lost during processing, the protein available for direct human consumption ranged from 1·5 g in Africa to 5·5 g in Europe and the USSR.

In summary, world milk production increased only slightly in recent years. In some European countries and in North America, policy action has been taken to reduce production. Production and market demand for milk are expected to increase slightly in Europe but decrease in North America in the 1970s. Although output is expected to increase in the developing regions, it will lag far behind demand. Thus, in the main dairying countries—developed countries—policies have been instituted to prevent production from exceeding demand. At the same time, developing countries are struggling to increase production to meet demands.

World meat production has increased in recent years (about 4% per year) and is expected to continue to increase because of strong consumer demand. Increases can be expected from meat in the developing countries, especially poultry and pork. Beef and veal production has increased only slightly (1%) in developing countries and it is not expected to rise substantially in the 1970s.

Fisheries production during the past two decades has increased at a greater rate (about 7% per year) than the increase in world population. The growth rates tend to be higher in the developing countries than in

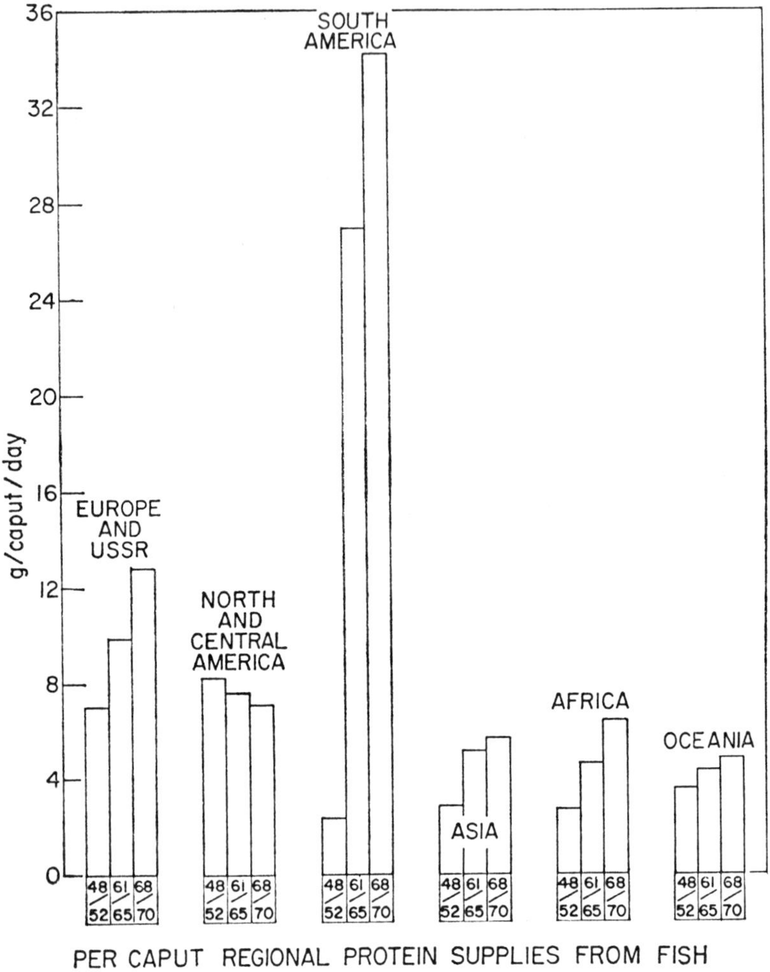

FIG. 12. *Per caput* regional protein supplies from fish

the developed high-income countries. As pointed out earlier, however, most of this increase has had little impact on dietary deficiencies in the developing world. Fishery production is expected to increase in the 1970s but at a lower rate of growth than during the past two decades.

V. PROSPECTS FOR INCREASING SUPPLIES OF ANIMAL PROTEIN

Increased supplies of animal protein can be obtained by increasing production of animal products through the use of more land, by increasing the productivity of land and water resources now used and by increasing the efficiency of use of animal protein now produced.

A. Increased Supplies from Land Animals

Any attempt to assess future land availabilities to increase the production of animal products is hampered by many imponderables. About one-fourth of the world's 32×10^9 acres is potentially arable, that is, suitable for cultivated crops (Table V). Another one-fourth of the world's land area can best be used for grazing, since it would yield little additional food in crops. Somewhat less than half ($3{\cdot}5 \times 10^9$ acres) of the world's potentially arable land is now cultivated, and much of the rest is used for grazing and the production of livestock. Of the land suitable only for grazing, more than half is currently used (Hendricks, 1969). The projected increase in world population is such that land available per person for food production must shrink substantially below present levels regardless of efforts to bring new land into cultivation and grazing. Even

TABLE V. Total arable and grazing land available

Region	*Total*[a]	*Arable land*			*Additional grazing land*[b] (10^9 acres)
		Potentially arable[a] (10^9 acres)	*At present cultivated*[b]	*Percentage cultivated of potentially arable*	
Europe and USSR	6·70	1·31	0·94	72	1·16
North and Central America	5·21	1·15	0·63	55	0·92
South America	4·33	1·68	0·22	13	1·11
Asia	6·76	1·55	1·11	72	1·11
Africa	7·46	1·81	0·50	28	2·08
Oceania	2·03	0·38	0·12	32	1·14
TOTAL	32·49	7·88	3·52	—	7·52

[a] President's Science Advisory Committee Report (1967)
[b] FAO (1971a)

if all the additional arable land, amounting to just over 3×10^9 acres, could be brought into cultivation by the year 2000, the amount of arable land per person would be somewhat less than in 1960, while the amounts of pasture and forest lands projected for 2000 would be substantially lower than in 1960 because of conversion of some of these lands to crop production. In Africa and South America, considerable potential exists for increasing the land for crop and animal production. In Europe and the USSR and in Asia, however, little additional land is available for food production.

In considering an increase in production of food from a finite quantity of land, scepticism is often met regarding the role of animals. Animals are notoriously inefficient in the conversion of feed protein into protein for human consumption. As shown in Table VI, the efficiency of conversion ranges from 5 to 24%. The premise is often stated that land can be used more efficiently for production of crops than for animals. Blaxter (1968) has pointed out several reasons why animals, especially ruminants, will play a major role in the future. Ruminants, as herbivores, use plant material, simple nitrogenous compounds and agricultural wastes that man cannot use for his own food. Herbivores can use land suitable for

TABLE VI. Percentage feed converted to edible food protein from various animal sources[a]

Eggs	23·5
Beef and Veal	4·6
Pork	12·5
Poultry	17·7
Cow's milk	22·9

[a] President's Science Advisory Committee Report (1967)

grazing but not suited to cultivation. As noted in Table V, about one-fourth of the world's land area is best suited for grazing. Although some grazing land could be used for crops, the advantage in terms of protein may not be as great as sometimes thought. On a comparable area of land, about 15–20% more protein can be produced from wheat than from milk production. The greater nutritive quality of protein from milk more than compensates for the small difference in production.

There is a large potential for increasing the efficiency of production of animal products in the developing countries. For example, in 1969, the average milk production per cow in the USA and Japan was 4154 kg and 4320 kg, respectively. In developing countries, average production generally was less than 1000 kg, i.e., India 450 kg and Brazil 460 kg. Most of the developing countries, and others as well, are not producing food at anywhere near their potential. The developing countries have about 60% of the world's livestock and domestic fowl, yet they produce only about 22% of the world's supply of meat, milk and eggs. The United States produced about 15% of the world's meat, milk and egg products in 1969. This was almost as much as all of the 70 developing countries throughout the world. Further, the USA produced this amount of animal products on about 6% of the world's land area and with about 6% of the world's population.

B. Increased Supplies from Fisheries

There is considerable controversy over the extent to which the sustainable yield of the oceans can be increased. Based on 17 estimates, Schaefer and Alverson (1968) concluded that a sustainable world potential existed of 180 million metric tons annually with foreseeable extensions of present harvesting techniques. FAO (1970a) has estimated a somewhat lower potential: 118 million metric tons. It may be reasonable to assume that the total potential for world fisheries is between these two estimates, or about 140 million metric tons. Approximately seven-eights of the world's supply of fish and shellfish comes from the oceans; the remainder from fresh or brackish waters (Finch, 1970). The rapidly growing application of aquacultural techniques may increase the future supply of fish from fresh water sources.

The potential for increasing available protein from fish in the future rests either in increasing the fish catch or in more efficient utilization of the protein harvested. As pointed out earlier, the potential fish catch is approximately double the 1970 figure. More efficient utilization of harvested fish protein would also significantly increase the protein from fish available for man. A loss of 50% of the fish protein between the ocean and the consumer represents a high level of waste, which is a feature unique to the fish processing industry and one which would not be tolerated by other food industries, such as the meat industry (Finch, 1970). New methods of processing are becoming available to convert some of this currently wasted protein into useful and attractive foods for human consumption. Firstly, methods have been developed for converting fish flesh into fish protein concentrates or isolates that can be used as protein supplements in the manufacture of new or traditional foods. In recent years, a considerable amount of effort has been made in the processing and utilization of fish protein concentrate (Library of Congress, 1970) and these efforts are discussed in more detail in Chapter 27. Secondly, more efficient separation and recovery of flesh from fish processing operations can result in 50% more fish protein recovered for human consumption. Flesh separating machines are available to recover flesh from fish frames, which are the bony skeleton left after filleting (King and Carver, 1970).

In addition to the 50% loss of protein that occurs during the processing of fish for human consumption, approximately one-third of the total catch is converted to fish meal. When consumed by chickens, approximately one-third of the protein in the diet is converted to tissue protein. In terms of edible protein, approximately 6 units of feed protein are required to produce 1 unit of cooked, boned meat protein.

The utilization of fish protein could be significantly increased by increasing the amount of fish used for direct human consumption and by decreasing the wastage in the fish processing industry. The world supply of fish protein is currently about 3·5 g *per caput* per day, which includes fish protein converted to animal protein and consumed by man. This value could be increased to about 6·2 g of protein *per caput* per day if fish used for direct human consumption were increased from 62% (current proportion) to 80% of the total catch and if wastage in the fish processing industry were reduced from 50% to 20%. Taking this one step further, the amount of protein available for human consumption could be increased by an additional 100% or up to about 12 g *per caput* per day, based on present world population figures, if the total world potential catch of about 140 million metric tons were realized. Unless the problem of pollution of the oceans receives immediate and serious attention, however, the supplies of fish protein for human consumption may fall considerably below the predicted potential.

VI. CONCLUSIONS

There is a large potential for increasing supplies of animal protein. To a limited extent, additional land can be used to increase production. The greatest potential, however, is in increasing the efficiency of production of the resources now in use and in increasing the efficiency of use of animal protein now produced. The probability of this potential being realized in the developing countries is not encouraging.

It is generally conceded that increased supplies of animal protein in developing regions must be produced indigenously, rather than produced and imported from developed countries. Thus, the problem of increasing animal protein supplies in developing areas is one of stimulating agricultural development.

Animal products in general have a high-income elasticity and there is considerable evidence to show a direct relationship between income and quantity and quality of food consumed among the poor classes of developing countries (President's Science Advisory Committee, 1967). In one study of this relationship in Madras, India, the average intakes of total protein and animal protein were 41 g and 2 g, respectively, when *per caput* income was $17 per year; and 56 g and 8 g, respectively, when the average *per caput* income was $242 per year. From this and other studies, it seems clear that dietary adequacy is directly tied to income. Thus, one can argue that the problem of providing adequate nutrition is an economic problem. To a large extent this is true, and economic development is a prerequisite for a long-term solution to the problem of providing food of adequate quantity and quality.

REFERENCES

ALTSCHUL, A. M. (1965). "Proteins: Their Chemistry and Politics." Basic Books, New York.

AUTRET, M. (1970). *In* "Proteins as Human Food" (R. A. Lawrie, ed.) pp. 3–19. (*Easter Sch. agric. Sci. Univ. Nott.* **16**, 1969). Butterworths, London.

BATES, M. (1969). *In* "Resources and Man" (NAS-NRC) pp. 21–30. Freeman, San Francisco.

BLAXTER, K. L. (1968). *Sci. J.* **1**, 53–59.

ELTON, C. (1936). "Animal Ecology." Macmillan, New York.

FINCH, R. (1970). *CRC Critical Rev. Fd Technol.* **1**, 519–580.

FAO (1964). "Protein. At the Heart of the World Food Problem." *World Food Problems* no. 5.

FAO (1967). Agricultural Commodities—Projections for 1975 and 1985, Vol. 2.

FAO (1970a). Provisional Indicative World Plan for Agricultural Development, Vol. 1.

FAO (1970b). *Yb. Fish. Statist.* **28** (1969).

FAO (1971a). *Prod. Yb. F.A.O.* **24** (1970).

FAO (1971b). *Commodity Review and Outlook*, 1970–1971.

FAO/WHO (1965). "Protein Requirements." *F.A.O. Nutr. Mtg Rep. Ser.* no. 37.

HENDRICKS, S. B. (1969). *In* "Resources and Man" (NAS-NRC) pp. 65–85. Freeman, San Francisco.

KING, F. J., and CARVER, J. H. (1970). *Comml Fish. Rev.* **32** (12), 12–21.

LIBRARY OF CONGRESS (1970). Fish Protein Concentrate: A Comprehensive Bibliography, Washington, D.C.

PRESIDENT'S SCIENCE ADVISORY COMMITTEE (1967). "The World Food Problem", Vol. 2 U.S. Government Printing Office, Washington, D.C., p. 364.

SCHAEFER, M. E., and ALVERSON, D. L. (1968). *In* "The Future of the Fishing Industry of the United States". University of Washington, Seattle.

CHAPTER 3

World Supplies of Plant Proteins*

M. E. JALIL AND W. M. TAHIR

FAO, Rome, Italy

I. INTRODUCTION

World food production between 1952–6 and 1969 increased by 50% (3·0% per annum), but due to rising population the *per caput* increase was only 18% (1·2% per annum). Table I shows that developed and developing regions achieved practically the same increases in total food crop production, but due to disparities in the population growth the *per caput* increase in food crop production was 24% (1·6% per annum) in the developed region and only 14% (0·8% per annum) in the developing countries. Incidentally, in Africa practically no increase was achieved. The situation is further aggravated by the fact that the marginal increase in food production in developing countries is absorbed by the considerable losses of products in storage, transportation, and so on, as well as by deterioration in the nutritional quality of food products.

There is at present a general awareness of the world food situation, of the population explosion, and of the critical task of closing the protein gap. Protein production is below the world average in the developing countries. This phenomenon is related to the quantity and quality of protein in the staple food and shows a well-defined pattern when the countries are classified into dietary groups according to the foods which constitute their primary source of protein. Classifying the countries according to diets based on animal products; wheat; millet and sorghum; maize; rice; roots, tubers and plantain, shows that from the first to the last group the quality of dietary protein declines, the protein/energy ratio becomes

* Presented at the meeting by Dr B. M. Nicol, FAO, Rome.

TABLE I. Index numbers of total and *per caput* food production, 1957–1969[a]

	(1952–6 = 100)												
	1957	1958	1959	1960	1961	1962	1963	1964	1965	1966	1967	1968	1969
A. DEVELOPED REGIONS[b]													
Total production	107	115	117	120	121	125	127	131	133	142	146	151	148
Per caput production	103	109	109	111	110	113	113	115	116	122	125	128	124
B. DEVELOPING REGIONS[c]													
Total production	109	114	117	121	124	128	132	135	136	138	145	150	151
Per caput production	102	106	106	107	106	106	108	109	108	111	113	114	114

[a] Cereals, starchy roots and tubers, grain legumes, edible oil crops, sugar, fruits and vegetables, livestock and livestock products

[b] Europe, USSR, North America, Oceania

[c] Latin America, Near East, Africa, Far East excluding Mainland China

Source: FAO Production Year Book, 1970

unfavourable, and the gap between protein requirements and intake widens. It is of interest to note that the countries where diets are based on millet and sorghum, maize, rice, roots and tubers and plantains (Africa, Far East and Central America) are mainly the developing countries.

II. DISTRIBUTION OF PROTEIN PRODUCTION

Using the crop production estimates for 1968, Jalil and Tahir (1970) calculated total and *per caput* production of protein from various crop groups in different regions. These are given in Table II, and Table III indicates the relative importance of the main crop groups at regional and world level.

The total world protein production from plant sources for direct human consumption in 1968 was 153·85 million metric tons *per caput* production was 43·04 kg/year (Table IIB). Developed regions (North America—156·36 kg, Oceania—117·23 kg, USSR—87·78 kg, Europe—44·0 kg) produced above average and developing countries below average *per caput* protein. The situation was serious in the Far East (24·09 kg); Africa (26·02 kg), Mainland China (31·1 kg) and the Near East (32·94 kg). Severe population pressure in the Far East resulted in very low *per caput* protein supply from almost all plant protein sources.

The highest total contribution (22·6%) to world plant protein production was from North America (Table IIIA), followed by the Far East (17·3%) and Mainland China (16·5%). Cereals produced over two-thirds (68·5%) and grain legumes just under one-fifth (18·0%) of world plant protein supply. The remaining crop sector (root and tuber crops, fruits, vegetables, treenuts) contributed only 13·5%. North America and the Far East (including Mainland China) were respectively responsible for 14·0 and 22·9% cereal protein and for 7·6 and 6·7% grain legume protein production. The distribution of crop groups within the regions indicates that Oceania, Europe, the Near East, USSR and the Far East were more dependent on cereal protein production than other regions (Table IIIB). Grain legumes played a significant part in North America, Mainland China and Africa, whereas roots and tubers were important in Europe, Africa, China and the USSR. Other crops such as oilseeds were important in the USSR, North America, Latin America and the Near East. Fruits have also made an appreciable contribution to protein production in Latin America. It must be pointed out that whereas in the developing regions most of cereals and grain legumes are for human consumption, in Europe, North America and the USSR a major part of cereals, except wheat and rice, and almost all the proteins from groundnuts and soya-bean are used as animal feed.

TABLE II. Food crop protein production, 1968

Crops	*Europe*	*North America*	*Latin America*	*Near East*	*Far East*	*Africa*	*Oceania*	*USSR*	*China Mainland*	*World total*
A. TOTAL PRODUCTION (million metric tons)										
Cereals	15·59	21·55	6·78	4·09	19·35	4·82	2·06	15·47	15·78	105·49
Grain legumes	0·63	11·72	1·56	0·35	4·13	1·45	0·02	1·84	6·15	27·85
Roots and tubers	2·40	0·28	0·53	0·05	0·67	0·74	0·02	1·74	2·23	8·66
Oilseeds	0·28	0·74	0·72	0·51	0·69	0·19	0·01	1·58	0·58	5·30
Fruits	0·34	0·08	1·50	0·09	0·76	0·15	0·02	0·02	0·02	2·98
Vegetables	0·68	0·30	0·12	0·19	0·65	0·05	0·01	0·23	0·59	2·82
Treenuts	0·08	0·02	0·08	0·03	0·39	0·12	0·03	—	—	0·75
TOTAL	20·00	34·69	11·29	5·31	26·64	7·52	2·17	20·88	25·35	153·85
Population (millions)	454·26	222·03	267·80	161·021	105·82	289·31	18·51	237·81	814·60	3571·16
B. PER CAPUT PRODUCTION (kg/year)										*Mean*
Cereals	34·31	97·08	25·31	25·41	17·50	16·67	111·29	65·04	19·37	29·50
Grain legumes	1·38	52·76	5·83	2·15	3·74	5·02	1·08	7·74	7·54	7·79
Roots and tubers	5·29	1·26	1·97	0·32	0·61	2·55	1·08	7·30	2·74	2·42
Oilseeds	0·62	3·33	2·69	2·17	0·62	0·66	0·54	6·64	0·71	1·49
Fruits	0·75	0·35	5·60	0·56	0·69	0·53	1·08	0·07	0·02	0·84
Vegetables	0·49	1·33	0·46	1·17	0·59	0·16	0·54	0·96	0·72	0·79
Treenuts	0·02	0·07	0·29	0·16	0·35	0·43	1·62	—	—	0·21
TOTAL	44·00	156·36	42·16	32·94	24·09	26·02	117·23	87·78	31·10	43·04

Source: FAO Production Year Book, 1969

Cereals: Wheat, Barley, Rice, Maize, Sorghum, Millets

Grain Legumes: Beans, Cowpeas, Groundnuts, Lentils, Peas, Chick-peas, Pigeon peas, Soya-bean, Lupins, Vetch

Roots and Tubers: Cassava, White Potatoes, Sweet Potatoes, Yams

Oilseeds: Cottonseed, Sesame, Sunflower

Fruits: Bananas, Citrus, Grapes, Olives, Pineapples, Dates

Treenuts: Coconuts, Palm Kernels, other nuts

TABLE III. Percent contribution of crop groups to total protein production, 1968

Crops	*Europe*	*North America*	*Latin America*	*Near East*	*Far East*	*Africa*	*Oceania*	USSR	*China Mainland*	*World total*
TOTAL PROTEIN PRODUCTION										
A. *Percent of Total World Protein Production*										
Cereals	10·1	14·0	4·4	2·7	12·6	3·1	1·3	10·1	10·3	68·5
Grain Legumes	0·4	7·6	1·0	0·2	2·7	0·9	—	1·2	4·0	18·0
Roots and Tubers	1·6	0·2	0·3	—	0·4	0·5	—	1·1	1·4	5·6
Others	0·9	0·8	1·6	0·5	1·6	0·3	0·2	1·2	0·8	7·9
TOTAL	13·0	22·6	7·3	3·4	17·3	4·8	1·5	13·6	16·5	100·0
B. *Percent of Total Regional Protein Production*										
Cereals	78·0	62·1	60·1	77·2	72·7	64·0	86·2	74·1	62·3	—
Grain Legumes	3·2	33·8	13·8	6·6	15·5	19·3	0·8	8·8	24·3	—
Roots and Tubers	11·9	0·8	4·7	0·1	2·5	9·8	0·1	8·3	8·8	—
Others	6·9	3·3	21·4	16·1	9·3	6·9	12·9	8·8	4·6	—

Source: FAO Production Year Book, 1969

It has been shown that cereals play a predominant role in the production of plant protein. Therefore it will be worthwhile to consider past trends in this group of crops. Table IV shows world population, total and *per caput* cereal protein production between 1959 and 1968. It will be seen that except for 1960 and 1961 there was a general upward trend in the total cereal protein production. By 1968 the production had increased by 25% (2·5% per annum) over 1959, but this was almost all absorbed by an increase in population so that 1968 *per caput* protein production registered an increase of only 2% (0·2% per annum) over 1959 and during 1960 and 1965 population increase outstripped the supply.

It will be seen in Table V that wheat was the major supplier of protein (38·4%) in 1968 followed by maize (22·5%) and rice (20·9%). This was not only due to its higher world production (about 332 million tons) as compared with maize (250 million tons) and rice (285 million tons) but also because of the higher protein content of wheat (12·2%) relative to maize (9·5%) and rice (7·5%). Developed regions produced 72·7% (29·5 million tons) of wheat protein with a *per caput* production of 31·6 kg/year as against 4·2 kg/year produced by the developing countries. The Far East and China (Mainland) produced 87·4% (19·3 million tons) of rice protein with *per caput* production of 10 kg/year. Developed regions produced 64·8% (about 7 million tons) of protein from barley and 61·9% (14·7 million tons) from maize and used it mostly as animal feed. Sorghum and millet protein in Africa (1·75 million tons) accounted for 21·1% of world plant protein from this source and gave the highest (6 kg/year) *per caput* return of all the cereals in that region.

During the 1959–1968 period the highest increase in the world protein production was from wheat (33·1%) and the lowest from barley (3·7%) while the increases for rice and maize were 29·5 and 27·8% respectively. Regional trends in the contributions made by different cereals between 1959–1968 are given in Table VI. In all regions except Latin America and the USSR there was a shift away from barley and towards wheat. This was particularly noticeable in North America, the Near East and Oceania. Latin America and the USSR increased the share of barley at the cost of wheat. Among the summer cereals Africa and the Far East increased the share of maize relative to sorghum and millet whereas the reverse was the case in Latin America and, to some extent, in North America. Rice had become more important in the USSR in 1968 than in 1959.

III. CONCLUSIONS

It has been shown that although the overall increase in food production during 1957–1969 in the developed and developing regions was practically

TABLE IV. World population: Total and *per caput* cereal protein production, 1959–1968

Year	*Population* (1000 millions)	*Total cereal protein production* (million metric tons)	Per Caput *cereal protein production* (kg)	Index Numbers (1959 = 100) *Total cereal protein production*	Per Caput *cereal protein production*
1959	2·94	84·69	28·81	100	100
1960	3·00	84·38	28·13	100	98
1961	3·08	81·62	26·50	96	92
1962	3·11	87·47	28·13	103	98
1963	3·22	88·07	27·35	104	95
1964	3·29	91·79	27·90	108	97
1965	3·36	90·18	26·84	106	93
1966	3·43	98·36	28·68	116	100
1967	3·50	101·91	29·12	120	101
1968	3·58	105·48	29·46	125	102

Source: FAO Production Year Books

TABLE V. Protein production from different cereals, 1959 and 1968 (million metric tons)

Region	*Wheat* 1959	*Wheat* 1968	*Barley* 1959	*Barley* 1968	*Rice* 1959	*Rice* 1968	*Maize* 1959	*Maize* 1968	*Sorghum/Millet* 1959	*Sorghum/Millet* 1968
Europe	6·91	8·90	2·86	3·44	0·13	0·11	2·45	3·10	0·01	0·04
North America	5·10	7·37	1·55	1·21	0·18	0·36	9·30	10·75	1·40	1·86
Latin America	1·15	1·30	0·21	1·03	0·56	0·79	2·11	3·22	0·15	0·44
Near East	1·99	2·56	0·66	0·52	0·20	0·34	0·32	0·39	0·25	0·28
Far East	1·90	3·06	0·68	0·53	9·72	12·48	0·92	1·47	1·69	1·81
Africa	0·45	0·83	0·29	0·40	0·21	0·34	0·89	1·50	1·26	1·75
Oceania	0·69	1·84	0·09	0·13	0·01	0·02	0·02	0·02	0·03	0·04
USSR	8·43	11·39	1·12	2·17	0·02	0·80	1·14	0·84	0·31	0·27
China (Mainland)	3·82	3·29	—	1·28	6·00	6·83	2·04[a]	2·47	—	1·91
TOTAL	30·44	40·54	7·46[b]	10·71	17·03	22·07	19·19	23·76	5·10[b]	8·40
Percentage of Total Cereal Protein Production[c]	35·90	38·40	8·80	10·20	20·10	20·90	22·60	22·50	6·00	ε·00

[a] 1957
[b] Excluding Mainland China
[c] Total world cereal protein production in 1959 was 84·69 million metric tons (without Mainland China = 78·89) and percentages are based on this figure

TABLE VI. Comparative protein contribution of different cereal crops, 1959 and 1968

Region	*Percentage of total cereal protein contribution within each region*									
	Wheat		*Barley*		*Rice*		*Maize*		*Sorghum/Millet*	
	1959	1968	1959	1968	1959	1968	1959	1968	1959	1968
Europe	55·9	57·1	23·2	22·0	1·0	0·7	19·8	19·9	0·1	0·3
North America	29·0	34·2	9·9	5·6	1·0	1·7	53·1	49·9	8·0	8·6
Latin America	27·5	19·2	5·0	15·2	13·5	11·7	50·5	47·5	3·5	6·4
Near East	53·3	62·6	19·3	12·7	5·8	8·2	9·2	9·6	7·4	6·9
Far East	12·8	15·8	4·5	2·7	65·2	64·5	6·2	7·6	11·3	9·4
Africa	14·5	17·2	9·2	8·4	6·9	7·0	28·8	31·2	40·6	36·3
Oceania	82·2	89·5	11·2	6·4	1·4	0·9	2·2	1·1	3·0	2·0
USSR	78·7	73·7	10·4	14·0	0·2	5·2	10·7	5·4	—	1·7
China (Mainland)	38·9	20·9	—	8·1	61·1	43·3	—	15·7	—	12·1

Source: FAO. Production Year Book, 1969

the same, a high population growth during this period appreciably reduced the *per caput* production in the developing countries. A similar situation existed as far as plant protein is concerned. The developed and developing regions produced 78·0 and 76·1 million tons of plant protein, respectively, in 1968 to be divided among 932·6 and 2638·6 million people, respectively. This vast disparity in population gave 83·6 and 28·8 kg *per caput* protein respectively to developed and developing countries. The Far East and Mainland China produced 33·7% of the total world protein from plant sources to be shared by almost 54% of the world population. The Far East with the highest population (1106 millions) produced the lowest *per caput* plant protein (24 kg) in 1968. Unfortunately, regions with low protein production have the higher rates of growth of population further to accentuate the problem.

This analysis of plant protein production has indicated that the problem of low *per caput* production of plant protein exists only in developing regions. Of course, there are disparities also between different countries within the same region as there are between different socio-economic classes in any country but, by and large, the lack of protein is without question the most serious qualitative deficiency in the nutrition of developing countries. The great mass of the population of these countries subsists mainly on foods derived from plants frequently deficient in protein, which results in poor health and low productivity per man. It may be that protein deficiencies will be completely overcome only when the countries have reached a certain level of income. There is a tendency to equate high-protein foods with livestock products, and certainly the high income elasticity of demand for animal products shows that this form of protein food enjoys strong consumer preference. In fact, however, about 70% of the world supply of edible protein comes from plant sources, notably cereals and grain legumes, and in developing countries the percentage is usually higher. Although in principle a more equitable distribution of existing supplies of protein food would often greatly reduce the incidence of kwashiorkor and other less acute manifestations of protein deficiency, the most practical short-term solution lies in the increased production of plant protein food.

The question arises whether agriculture is capable of achieving the needed dimensions of increased production. Positive and quick results can be achieved by a balanced combination of investment, education, research and organization. Without investment, neither can existing resources be developed nor can the hitherto unexplored resources be rendered productive. Without interdisciplinary research the factors limiting crop productivity cannot be eliminated and, without education, including technical education and training, the farming communities in the developing countries cannot be made aware of the possibilities of increasing productivity nor can they derive full benefit from science and technology. And without organization, which includes the creation of those institutions for agricultural research and development, extension services, credit and marketing, there would neither be adequate infrastructure for increasing productivity, nor an assurance of the return that the farmer would expect from his extra effort.

The role of science and technology in agricultural development should be viewed against this background. There are two main aspects of the application of scientific techniques to inefficient and subsistence agriculture, one which involves the transfer of knowledge and skill from the advanced countries to the less developed parts of the world, and the other concerned with the discovery and utilization of new sources of food. Meanwhile, the most immediate need is to find ways and means of applying known scientific facts to improve the production and utilization of existing food sources.

It has been recognized that, skilfully handled, the breakthrough in plant breeding (the so-called "green revolution") would help achieve better balance between growing populations and their food needs, at least for the time being. It is important, therefore, to assist Governments in: (a) furthering the spread of successful new technology in order to help ensure that the momentum already gained by the "green revolution" is not lost; (b) finding ways and means to promote development of improved agricultural technology for areas and crops that cannot benefit from the particular techniques which have thus far been evolved.

A two-pronged approach seems necessary here. The first and most immediately attainable goal would be to spread the extent and benefits of the already developed high-yielding varieties of wheat, maize and rice, by improving their nutritive quality and consumer acceptability, increasing their resistance to pests and diseases, and making them more readily available together with an appropriate input "package" to all classes of farmers. This implies both continued multi-disciplinary research and expanded "outreach" programmes and pioneer projects to sort out and overcome the technical problems encountered in the field and the socio-economic obstacles to the wider adoption of successful new techniques.

Highest priority needs to be given to increasing yields of sorghum and the various species of millet, which for instance occupy 40 million hectares in India and Pakistan (double that under wheat), and over 30 million hectares in Africa, and are largely grown in relatively unfavourable environmental conditions where they cannot easily be substituted by other crops. They provide the staple diet to an estimated 400 million people, and also make an important contribution to feed-grain supplies.

In respect of grain legumes, research is still far from adequate and, as a result, yields of these crops have hardly increased since the mid-fifties. High priority needs to be accorded to chick-peas and pigeon peas (mainly in drier areas of the Near East and South Asia), to cowpeas (mainly in tropical latitudes) and to haricot beans (genus *Phaseolus*) especially in Latin America.

At present these protein-rich crops are often grown in the areas of lower ecological potential, to which they are increasingly being pushed by competition from more profitable high-yielding cereal varieties in the better areas. This is likely to continue unless their yields can be appreciably improved by developing improved varieties and husbandry practices and by proper plant protection measures.

This makes it all the more important to seek additional approaches and probably the most promising of these is through multiple cropping. Experiments on multiple cropping in India, the Philippines and Taiwan show the practical possibilities of obtaining at least two cereal crops and a crop of grain legumes from the same piece of land and thus obtaining very high outputs of protein per unit of time. Given the short-maturing varieties of cereals and grain legumes, there is every reason that the concept of multiple cropping would be adopted on a large scale in countries with favourable climatic conditions and irrigation facilities. Large-scale adoption of multiple cropping, which includes protein-rich food legumes, would also permit diversification of the diet. Thus although the progress in the past to raise the level of protein production has been slow and disappointing in the developing regions of the world, there is a solid basis for optimism that rapid progress can now be made in closing the protein gap.

REFERENCE

Jalil, M. E. and Tahir, W. M. (1970). Paper presented at the "Symposium on Plant Protein Resources: Their Improvement through the Application of Nuclear Techniques", International Atomic Energy Agency, Vienna. pp. 21–32.

CHAPTER 4

World Supplies of Proteins from Unconventional Sources

J. T. WORGAN

National College of Food Technology (University of Reading), Weybridge, Surrey, England

I. INTRODUCTION

Between the years 1960 and 1970, world population continued to increase at a more rapid rate than the most pessimistic estimates made by the UN in 1960 (Benjamin, 1963; Thoday, 1969; FAO, 1971). If this trend continues then in less than thirty years the world population will be double that of today. Since it is improbable that, in the foreseeable future, effective measures can be taken to stabilize the population, it must be assumed that food output will have to be doubled to meet the increasing demand.

Ultimately the population will be limited by food supplies unless some other form of control becomes effective or can be adopted throughout the world as a matter of deliberate policy. To resort to food supplies as a control measure is both unwieldy and inhuman, since man has become adapted to survive and reproduce when living in an almost permanent state of malnutrition. The possibility of future food shortages is unlikely to act as an initial deterrent to population growth, since the food intake of the newly born child is negligible when compared with the amount it will require when it is sixteen to eighteen years old. There is therefore an inevitable time lag between population increase and maximum food requirements. Seasonal variations in the yields of crops will also disguise a situation where the limits of the food supply in a given area have been reached and a crisis may become apparent only in a year of poor harvests. Food shortages are therefore more likely to control the number of people by starvation than by limiting the birth rate.

The bulk of the additional food required will continue to be produced by conventional agricultural methods. Quantities can be increased by cultivating additional land and by improving the yields of food per unit area. It is important that the magnitude of the problem of doubling the world's supply of food should not be underestimated. Willcox (1959) has drawn attention to the fallacy of assuming that the high yields obtained by sophisticated methods of agriculture can be maintained in many areas of the developing countries, since these yields are made possible only by mechanization and by the excessive use of pesticides, weed killers and fertilizers. Tropical soils are less stable than those in temperate climates and it is doubtful whether they will withstand the intensive methods of cultivation which are used in Europe and North America. The failure of the groundnut scheme in East Africa and the attempt to mechanize rice cultivation in Gambia are examples which should serve as warnings. The total area of land which could be cultivated has been estimated to be about 3000 million hectares (Stamp, 1960) and the area cultivated in 1967 was estimated to be 1400 million hectares (Ewell, 1969). Thus if there are no improvements in the yield of food per unit area then in 30 years' time there will be just sufficient arable land to feed the population. Although improvements in the yields of conventional crops will undoubtedly be made, land could become a limiting factor in the production of sufficient food unless measures are taken both to conserve and to utilize to the full the arable land available.

Supplies of protein must be considered in relation to total food output, since without a sufficient supply of energy in the diet protein cannot be effectively utilized. In view of the need to make the maximum use of arable land for food production, supplies of animal protein may need to be curtailed since they require nearly four times as much arable land as plant protein sources. It is doubtful, therefore, whether animal protein supplies can be increased on the scale that will be required to maintain the present proportion of animal protein in the diet. The use of additional grazing land for the rearing of ruminants and the adoption of more efficient systems for the rearing of livestock may partially offset this possible deficit. To meet any deficiency of protein which may occur from the output of conventional agriculture, methods of production which do not require the use of arable land should therefore be given priority.

In addition to land, water and energy are the other basic resources which are required for food production. By systems of recovery and recycling, the water used in the methods for producing unconventional sources of protein could be kept to a minimum and should not be a limiting factor in production. The energy required to operate the recovery systems may be a more critical requirement. Although sunlight is the source of energy for plant growth in conventional agricultural systems the input of other forms of energy is by no means negligible and greater quantities will be needed if food output per unit area is to be increased. The production of 1 ton of fertilizer nitrogen, for example, requires 1·5 tons of oil or 4 tons of coal (Fleck, 1961).

Energy is also needed for the manufacture of pesticides and weed killers, for mechanization and for the transport and processing operations associated with agricultural production. To maintain the industrialized societies which are continuing to grow and extend to other areas of the world inputs of large quantities of energy are also essential. In the more advanced industrial societies the energy consumption per head of population is increasing because of the rising standard of living. The consumption of energy resources is therefore increasing at a much faster rate than the growth of the population. Coal and oil are the two main sources of energy in present-day use and world supplies of both these sources are not unlimited. King-Hubbert (1971) has estimated that the maximum annual production of oil will be reached about the year 1990 and the maximum output of coal in the year 2150. If a population of 7000 million people is to be sustained for any period of time in the future, then both these resources will have to be available to maintain sufficient food output, unless alternative sources of energy are developed on a large scale. Atomic energy and hydro-electric power are the only feasible alternative sources which have been developed at the present time.

II. SOURCES OF UNCONVENTIONAL PROTEINS

Almost by definition the term "unconventional sources" implies that supplies of these proteins are not currently available. In the past a number of projects for their production have been abandoned on the grounds of their unfavourable cost at the time the studies were made. To assess their potential contribution to supplies of protein for human consumption in the future, the requirements for the resources of energy and arable land involved in their production should be used to select the most appropriate sources on which to concentrate production. These criteria are not incompatible with economic assessments since costs in the future must reflect the increasing demands upon limited resources. Possible sources of unconventional proteins are listed in Table I.

TABLE I. Unconventional sources of protein

Source	*Estimated potential annual yield of protein* (×10^{-3}, tons)
SCP (Hydrocarbon substrates)	23 000
Oilseed Protein Residues	22 000
Fish Protein Products (Fish Protein Concentrate, FPC)	4800
Plankton (Krill)	2200
Game Meat	500
	(kg/hectare)
Algae	24 800
SCP (Carbohydrate substrates)	11 230
Leaf Protein	5000
Fish Culture	800
Other sources:	
Synthetic Amino Acids	
Recovery from Wastes	
Plant and Animal Cell Tissue Culture	
Plant Growth in Controlled Environments	

A. Oilseed Protein Residues

In the past, as their name implies, the oilseeds have been used primarily as a source of oils. The processes used for oil extraction have reflected this emphasis and, after removal of the oil, most of the residues are unfit for human consumption. In addition to protein many of these residues contain fibre and some also contain toxins. Excessive heat developed during several of the oil extraction processes reduces the nutritional value of the proteins in the residues. In all cases improved standards of hygiene in the methods of operation of the processes and in the design of the equipment are necessary to produce material suitable for human consumption.

By the development of new technologies for oil extraction, protein concentrates of improved quality could be produced. Processes for most of the oilseeds are being developed. In comparatively small amounts, relative to the total available, soya-bean, groundnut and cottonseed protein concentrates are being used for human food. The total quantity of protein which could be made available from all sources has been estimated to be 22 million tons/year (Altschul, 1970). The salvaging of this protein for use in human food would not require additional arable land or the use of significant amounts of energy.

B. Leaf Protein Concentrates

The leaves of plants contain appreciable quantities of protein which are at a maximum during the period of rapid growth. Although the leaves of some plants are digestible by human beings most contain sufficient fibre to prevent effective utilization. By crushing or by disintegrating the leaves, protein can be separated from the fibre and is extracted in the leaf juice. Heat or the addition of acid precipitates a concentrate from the juice containing about 60% protein. The possibilities of producing leaf protein as human food are referred to in a series of articles by Pirie (1966, 1969a, b, 1971). Investigations on the production of leaf protein on a large scale are described by Kohler and Bickoff (1971) and by Hollo and Koch (1971).

In experimental trials the yields of protein per unit area of land have been improved since the process was first developed. The selection of plant species and the assessment of the optimum frequency of harvesting are two important factors involved in these improvements. Yields of 2000 kg protein/hectare are possible in the UK and 5000 kg protein/hectare in the wet tropics (Arkcoll, 1971). The poor nutritional value in feeding trials of some of the earlier protein concentrates was due to the presence of traces of toxic compounds from the leaves of some species, and to the unsatisfactory conditions which were used during the drying of the product. More recent assessments show considerable improvements and biological values of approximately 0·80 are reported for wheat and barley leaf proteins. Leaf protein concentrates are good supplements to the seed proteins of wheat, rice and maize (Woodham, 1971). Both the biological value and the true digestibility of leaf protein may improve with increasing maturity of the leaf (Henry and Ford, 1965).

The growth of a leafy crop specifically for the purpose of producing leaf protein will be in direct competition with conventional crops for the use of arable land. However, by comparison with a conventional cropping system, more efficient use of the energy received on the land surface will be made by a system of frequent harvesting of the leaves. Throughout the year the land surface will be covered with foliage and photosynthesis will be continually taking place. If leaf protein, associated with a high-yielding crop such as cassava, is considered as a food production unit then a greater output of nutritionally balanced food per unit area of land can be obtained than that from a conventional cropping system. This possibility is illustrated in Table II. The carbohydrate is based on a yield of 10 tons of cassava per acre (8650 kg/hectare) containing 35% carbohydrate (Nicholls *et al.*, 1961), and the leaf protein on the yield of 5000 kg protein/hectare referred to above (Arkcoll, 1971). The maize yield is an average one for that of hybrid maize in North America (Stamp, 1960). The total output of food per hectare, while still maintaining approximately the same protein/energy ratio, is 3·3 times greater from the leaf protein/cassava

TABLE II. Comparison of yields from a maize crop, a cassava/SCP system and a cassava/leaf protein system

	Yield (kg/hectare)			*Approximate protein/ carbohydrate ratio*
	Carbohydrate	*Protein*	*Total food output*	
MAIZE	2000	300	2300	1 : 7
CASSAVA	8650			
Less 3150 kg carbohydrate	5500		6287	1 : 7
Conversion of 3150 kg carbohydrate to SCP		787		
	From 0·8 hectare	From 0·2 hectare		
CASSAVA	6920		7920	1 : 7
Leaf protein (separate crop)		1000		

system than that from the conventional maize crop. No account in these calculations has been taken of the potential yields of leaf protein from the cassava or maize plants or of the cassava protein.

When most conventional crops are harvested only a proportion of the plant is used for human food. Extraction of protein from the leaves of the plant would increase the food output per unit area of land (see p. 67).

Hollo and Koch (1971) estimate that 45 kWh of electricity and 40 kg of fuel oil are required to process one ton of green matter which should yield 100 kg of leaf protein concentrate. Assuming that the protein content of the concentrate is 60% and that one ton of oil is equivalent to 11 332 kWh of electricity (Fleck, 1961) then 733 kg of oil are required to supply the power to extract 1000 kg of leaf protein.

C. Synthetic Amino Acids

Most of the amino acids can be synthesized from the basic raw materials carbon, oxygen, water and nitrogen; in addition, sulphur is needed for the synthesis of cystine and methionine. To overcome the problem of the utilization of free amino acids from the diet, Fox (1963) has investigated the synthesis of amino acid polymers. In contrast to most other methods for the production of food these processes do not make any use of the energy provided by sunlight. Several of the large-scale processes that have been developed by-pass the earlier stages of the synthesis by starting from coal or oil as raw materials. Stored energy originating from photosynthesis is therefore being utilized. Synthesis by either of these procedures will be less efficient in terms of energy conservation than methods which utilize directly or indirectly the energy derived from the sun. Ottenheym (1971) has listed the starting materials which could be used for amino acid syntheses. Many of these could be derived from biologically replenishable sources. Synthetic processes have the disadvantage that racemic mixtures of optical isomers are produced only one of which may be biologically active.

Microbiological syntheses of amino acids are in reality a process of conversion, since the micro-organism must be supplied with an organic compound as a carbon skeleton and as a source of energy. Metabolic products other than amino acids are produced in the process, in addition to the cell biomass which is not utilized. These processes will therefore be less efficient than the production of Single Cell Proteins (SCP) from the same substrates. Where the amino acids synthesized are used as supplements their contribution to the nutritional value of a deficient diet can be considerable and this aspect is discussed in Chapter 32. The synthesis of amino acids for the supplementation of proteins will be an effective use of the energy required for their synthesis. Lysine and methionine are the amino acids most frequently required for this purpose. Methionine is synthesized chemically on a large scale and the production of a racemic mixture is of no significance since both optical isomers are biologically effective. Lysine, which was originally obtained by chemical synthesis, is now produced by a microbiological process (McPherson, 1966). Tryptophan, which may sometimes be required as a supplement, can be synthesized at approximately four times the cost of lysine (Fox, 1963).

D. Plankton

The annual production of organic material on the seas has been estimated to be 10^{10} tons (Borgström, 1970) and approximately one-tenth of this could be protein. It is, however, the huge surface area which accounts for this large production and the product is dispersed at a very low concentration in enormous volumes of water. Harvesting experiments off the Swedish coast have shown that it would be necessary to process 400 tons of water to obtain 10 g of protein (Bigwood, 1966). The possibility of toxic species occurring in the harvest must also be considered (Pirie, 1969b). Due to temperature changes in the water and the flow of ocean currents there are areas of the sea where plankton accumulate in much higher concentrations. Quantities are harvested by the use of fine nets off the coasts of India and Burma and are used for human food (Borgström, 1971). The highest concentration reported occurs in the Antarctic where potential harvests of 100–500 million tons per year have been estimated for the shrimp-like organism (*Euphausia superba*) called krill (Anon, 1971).

The krill is the main food of the Baleen whale and is probably the basic material in the food chains which maintain the wild life of the Antarctic. It is therefore difficult to assess the proportion of the krill which could be regularly harvested. Due to the climatic conditions and the remoteness of the location the large-scale harvesting and preservation of the krill is a difficult technical problem which has yet to be solved. If 10% of the estimated 100 million tons annual production could be regularly harvested, then, at a protein concentration in the krill of 22%, the annual yield of protein would be 2·2 million tons.

E. Fish Protein Products

About one-quarter (11·2 million tons) of the total catch of marine fish in 1963 was used for the manufacture of fish meal for use as animal feed (Lovern, 1966). Some of this meal is made from the by-products of fish processing although most of it is prepared from fish harvested for the specific purpose of processing into meal. It is suggested that stable products suitable for human consumption could be prepared from much of the fish which is currently converted to meal (Lovern, 1969). An alternative is to extract the fat and produce a Fish Protein Concentrate (FPC). Although the sea covers a vast area, the concentration of nutrients is low, and there are considerable losses of the original protein synthesized by the phytoplankton as this protein passes through the food chains to the harvested fish. The maximum potential future catch of fish from the oceans has therefore been assessed at approximately twice that of the present harvest (Borgström, 1970). In 1969 the total world harvest of marine fish was approximately 48 million tons (FAO, 1971). Assuming that one-quarter (24 million tons) of the potential annual harvest is of species which are at present used for fish meal then, at an average protein content of 20%, approximately 4·8 million tons of protein could be diverted to products suitable for human food.

Neither the harvesting of plankton where it occurs in high concentrations, nor the diversion for human use of fish protein which is at present used for animal feed, will require the use of arable land or the appreciable consumption of energy resources.

F. Fish Culture

Fish are dependent for their food on the primary photosynthetic material produced by the growth of aquatic plants or phytoplankton. The yields per unit of surface area can therefore be only one-tenth of those which could be achieved by the growth of plants or algae. However, the culture of fish does have two advantages: they act as harvesters of material which it may be difficult to collect by other methods; and they convert this material to a more nutritious, acceptable food. Under natural conditions in fish ponds in warm climates yields of 500 kg protein/hectare/year are harvested. Higher yields (1800 kg protein/hectare) are obtained in China and Indonesia by introducing vegetation which has been grown on surrounding land and by adding human and animal wastes into the culture ponds (Shapiro, 1968).

Since fish culture requires a minimum of equipment and facilities it need not involve any power input and can therefore be undertaken in large numbers of small units which can be established in even the most remote areas. Neither elaborate storage nor distribution systems are required since production units can be sited to meet local demands for the fresh product. The main limitations on the system are a suitable climate and a sufficient water supply throughout the year. Potential quantities are difficult to estimate. However, there is no doubt that the more widespread adoption of fish culture ponds would make a significant contribution to world protein supplies. From a yield of 500 kg protein/hectare a fish pond one hectare in area would provide 30 g fish protein per day to 466 people.

G. Game Meat

There are some areas of the world where cultivation of the land is not feasible due to the rainfall or the soil conditions. Some of this land is suitable for the grazing of conventional livestock such as cattle or sheep. In other areas, notably in Africa, Central Russia and Australia, it is suggested that larger quantities of biomass can be maintained per unit area by allowing the natural development of the wild animal population. In these areas the wild animal species graze at different levels and do not necessarily consume the same species of herbage. A better balance is therefore maintained with the natural vegetation. The wild animal species are also better adapted to the climate and to adverse conditions such as periods of drought. The highest biomass densities of 200–240 kg/hectare are reported for East Africa (Cloudsley-Thompson, 1969). Studies of the possibilities of harvesting the game as a source of meat have been made. Ledger *et al.* (1967) assume that 10% of the biomass could be harvested each year and estimate a yield of 12 800 tons of meat from the Serengeti, one of the largest (3 million hectares) of the African game parks. The carcasses of most wild game contain a higher proportion of protein than cattle and it can be assumed that 12% of the carcass will be protein (Sachs and Glees, 1967). The annual yield of protein from the 3 million hectares of the Serengeti would therefore be 1500 tons. In Russia harvests of the Saiga antelope yield 7000 tons of meat or approximately 840 tons of protein each year (Maloiy, 1965). The cropping of marsupials in Australia, reindeer in northern latitudes, and the aquatic manatee in fresh waters where water weeds grow profusely, has also been considered. Yields per unit of area will probably be less than those estimated for the African game parks.

Although wild game may provide a nutritious and acceptable protein source in areas where there is a need for improved protein supplies, the total quantities are unlikely to be very significant in terms of world requirements. It is doubtful whether from all sources more than 500 000 tons of protein per year could be produced.

H. Growth of Plants in Controlled Environments

Much higher yields from plants can be obtained if the temperature, humidity, water supply and nutrients are controlled throughout the year at the optimum conditions for growth. Additional carbon dioxide to that present in the air must be provided. Pirie (1969b) has pointed out that carbon dioxide may limit photosynthesis even when plants are growing under natural conditions.

A further increase in the rate and extent of plant growth is obtained if the conditions are adjusted to the optimum for each phase of the plant's growth. This principle of environmental control has been adopted in the tower greenhouse system, where the growing plants move through a series of controlled environments (Bailey *et al.*, 1968). These systems make the maximum use of the potential of photosynthesis and can be sited on land unsuitable for agricultural production.

It is difficult to assess whether the additional food produced would justify the energy input required to supply carbon dioxide and to maintain the controlled environment, since this will vary according to the local climate. The method is particularly suitable for areas where hydro-electric power is available and conventional methods of agriculture are not applicable.

I. Culture of Plant and Animal Tissues

Both plant cells (Nickell, 1962) and animal cells (Merchant and Eidam, 1961) can be cultured by methods similar to those used for micro-organisms and the production of biomass on an industrial scale is a feasible possibility. However, the culture media required are more complex than those which can be used for the production of SCP, and media for the culture of both plant and animal cells may require the presence of amino acids. Wastes such as corn-steep liquor and coconut juice might be used as suitable media and would produce limited quantities of tissue proteins. The upgrading of sources of protein unsuitable for use as human food to animal tissue protein could be a possible application of cell tissue culture in the future.

J. Protein Recovery from Wastes

During the processing of biological materials, including foods, quantities of protein may be separated either as by-products or as wastes that are discarded. In many food processing operations, for example, 10–20% of the food material is removed (Ben-Gera and Kramer, 1969). Most of the by-products are used as sources of protein in animal feedingstuffs. Some of these materials could be converted to protein foods suitable for human consumption. The example of the oilseed protein residues has already been discussed. By-products from the milling of wheat and rice, and from the manufacture of starch from maize are other examples of materials from which protein could be recovered for use in human food.

Wastes which contain protein in low concentration in large volumes of liquid are discarded because of the unfavourable costs of protein recovery. Recent increases in the price of proteins, the need to reduce pollution and the possibilities of applying new techniques have led to renewed interest in the recovery of these proteins. A process for concentrating whey proteins by reverse osmosis has been developed and may make spray drying of the concentrate economically feasible (Fox 1970). The recovery of protein, which is discarded or under-utilized, from by-products or wastes would not require arable land or appreciable quantities of energy.

K. Single Cell Protein

Bacteria, yeasts, fungi and algae have all been investigated as potential sources of food. Biomass containing at least 50% protein can be produced by each of these groups of micro-organisms and the term Single Cell Protein (SCP) has therefore been applied to the products. The composition of fungi, yeasts and algae can however be varied within wide limits by controlling the C : N ratio in the nutrient media and the conditions adopted for growth. Fungal mycelium of the same species, for example, can be produced containing 24·4% fat and 18·6% protein or 4·2% fat and 52·1% protein (Worgan, 1968). A more appropriate term for these products might therefore be Single Cell Food.

Micro-organisms are capable of rapid growth and are efficient in the conversion of sources of energy and inorganic N to biomass containing protein. By the growth of *Fusarium semitectum* 75% of the N supplied as an ammonium salt can be converted to true protein in mycelium (Delaney and Worgan, 1971).

The alternative method of converting inorganic N to protein by conventional agriculture is to apply fertilizer to the soil. Part of this fertilizer is leached away and only a proportion of that which remains is taken up by the plant. When the plant is harvested three-quarters of it may be discarded and only the protein in the remainder is used as food. It is doubtful whether more than 10% of the fertilizer N is converted to edible protein by this procedure.

Bacteria yield biomass containing a higher proportion of protein and in the laboratory grow more rapidly than either fungi or yeasts. The advantage of their high protein content is partially offset by their higher content of nucleic acids. Fungi are frequently reported to be more slow-growing and to yield biomass with lower protein contents. Where protein contents and protein yields are used as the criteria for assessing the optimum conditions for growth, several fungal species will grow as rapidly and give equivalent yields of protein to those of yeasts (Delaney and Worgan, 1970; Worgan, 1971). When the efficiency of the conversion of substrate to protein is taken into consideration, it can be concluded that large-scale processes that use bacteria, fungi or yeasts will all operate at the same rate of growth (Worgan, 1972). Thus the nutritional value of the protein, safety of the product as human food, acceptibility and the ability to use available sources of energy as substrates for growth, are the criteria for the selection of species of micro-organism for the production of SCP.

Food yeast (*Candida utilis*) is the only example of SCP which is currently produced for use in human food. Comparatively small quantities, grown on molasses, are used as a protein supplement in a number of food pro-

TABLE III. Net protein utilization values of various sources of single cell proteins

Micro-organism	n.p.u.	*Micro-organism*	n.p.u.
Aspergillus niger[a]	0·584	*Fusarium semitectum*[e]	0·60
Food Yeast[b]	0·38	*F. semitectum*[f]	0·76
		+ *Methionine*	(t.d. = 0·80;
Spirulina maxima[c]	0·634		b.v. = 0·95)
Yeast[d] (from *n*-paraffins)	0·59		

[a] Mitrakos *et al.*, 1970 [b] Miller, 1963 [c] Bujard *et al.*, 1970
[d] Walker, 1972 [e] Miller, 1968 [f] Palmer and Smith, 1971

ducts (Bressani, 1968). This yeast was originally selected because of its ability to grow on a wider range of substrates than the baker's and brewer's yeast (*Saccharomyces cerevisiae*) and feeding tests were first made more than 50 years ago. In World War II about 15 000 tons per year were used to supplement supplies of human food (Locke *et al.*, 1945). *C. utilis* has therefore aquired an established reputation as a safe food and it is primarily for this reason that it is chosen for production on an industrial

TABLE IV. Essential amino acids in some sources of conventional and unconventional proteins (Values expressed as g amino acid/100 g protein)

Amino acid	*Maize* Seed[a]	*Maize* Leaf[b]	*Peas* Seed[c]	*Peas* Leaf[d]	*SCP*[e] *Fusarium semitectum*	*FAO*[f] *Reference protein*
Isoleucine	3·9	5·2	5·5	4·4	4·2	4·2
Leucine	12·6	10·0	7·0	7·1	6·5	4·8
Lysine	2·4	6·4	6·5	5·6	6·6	4·2
Phenylalanine	4·8	5·6	5·0	5·2	3·9	2·8
Tyrosine	4·1	4·4	2·8	4·3	3·3	2·8
Cystine	1·9	0·6	1·3	1·1	0·5	2·0
Methionine	1·9	1·5	1·3	1·6	1·7	2·2
Threonine	4·7	5·4	3·9	6·3	4·4	2·8
Tryptophan	1·0	1·3	0·8	1·5	—	1·4
Valine	7·1	6·4	5·5	5·9	5·2	4·2

[a] Harvey, 1956 [b] Gerloff *et al.* (Strain 581 d), 1965
[c] Kuppuswamy *et al.*, 1958 [d] Hartman *et al.*, 1967
[e] Smith, 1971 [f] FAO, 1957

scale. The safety of several other species of micro-organisms is currently being tested in long-term feeding trials and the proteins of some of these species have better nutritional values than that of food yeast (Table III). From published information on the amino acid composition of the proteins, cystine and methionine are invariably the limiting amino acids. That cystine and methionine are the first limiting amino acids in *F. semitectum* is confirmed by amino acid analysis of the protein (Delaney and Worgan, 1970; Table IV) and by feeding trials with rats (Palmer and Smith, 1971; Table III).

Bacteria, yeasts and algae grow as individual microscopic cells which have no cohesive properties and therefore no texture. When harvested and dried they form powders which can be added in small quantities as supplements to other foods. Protein isolates from bacteria (Heden *et al.*, 1971) and food yeast (Huang and Rha, 1971) have been spun into fibres, and food products similar to textured soya-bean protein will probably be developed in the future. The hyphae of fungi mat together when the material is harvested and give a product with a texture similar to moist chicken meat, a food which is acceptable in most parts of the world. An acceptable food from fungal mycelium can therefore be produced with a minimum of processing after the material has been harvested.

III. SOURCES OF ENERGY FOR THE PRODUCTION OF SCP

The availability of energy sources for growth is the main factor which will limit the production of micro-organisms as sources of protein.

A. Sunlight

The single-celled algae are the only group of micro-organisms that carry out photosynthesis and are therefore able to utilize the energy from sunlight. The production of algae has therefore an apparent advantage over other methods of producing microbial protein. In practice additional inputs of energy are needed to provide the environment for efficient growth and to harvest the algal cells. Under natural static conditions the cell density is low and because of the small size of the cells simple filtration methods are not applicable. Large volumes of culture have therefore to be centrifuged to harvest the cells. Although agitation and the addition of inorganic nutrients have some influence on cell density, further growth is limited by the supply of carbon dioxide. A large volume of air or air enriched with carbon dioxide has therefore to be introduced into the culture. In most climates temperature control of the culture is necessary. Cell densities even after the provision of these requirements are lower than those obtained by the growth of other micro-organisms. Contaminat-

TABLE V. Substrates for the production of Single Cell Proteins

Substrate	*Comments*	*Yield of protein per 100 g of substrate*[a]
Non-renewable		
Petroleum	Limited resources	50
Natural Gas	Competitive demands	37·5
Coal—distillation and hydrogenation		
Synthetic compounds e.g. methanol	Energy dependent	37·4
$CO_2 + H_2 + O_2$		
Renewable		
Starch and Sucrose	Potential use as human food	25
Cellulosic by-products	Abundant, few competitive demands, resistant to microbial degradation	20
Liquid wastes—Molasses, Sulphite liquor, Food processing wastes	Limited quantities, readily degraded by micro-organism	25

[a] Protein from non-renewable substrates = N × 6·25. From the renewable substrates the yields are of true protein and do not include non-protein N

ing organisms are also a problem and protection of the culture may be needed. As a result of these factors it has been concluded that algal proteins produced by currently available techniques cannot be produced at a cost which compares with conventional sources of protein.

The cells of the blue green algal species *Spirulina maxima* can be separated from the culture by simple filtration methods. This is partly because of the larger size of the cells and partly because the cells tend to agglomerate because of their shape. *Spirulina* grows at a high pH value (9·5–10·0) and this increases the efficiency of the absorption of carbon dioxide into the culture and reduces the problem of contaminating organisms. These advantages improve the economics of production. Yields of 40–45 tons dried algae/hectare/year containing 62% protein (24 800 kg protein/hectare/year) have been reported (Clement *et al.*, 1967).

The production of protein by algal growth does not require the use of agricultural land and it should be worthwhile attempting to improve the efficiency of cultural methods. Pilot plants and small-scale production units to study this problem have been installed in Czechoslovakia and Japan (Enebo, 1969). In laboratory-scale tests simple filtration after the addition of the mycelium of *F. semitectum* to algal cultures has been used as a method for harvesting algal cells (Barlow and Worgan, 1971). The poor digestibility of algal cells may be overcome by the development of mutant strains without cell walls (Davies, 1971).

B. Simple Organic Compounds

Organic compounds, suitable as substrates for the growth of micro-organisms, can be synthesized from carbon, oxygen and water. Coal and petroleum may also be used as raw materials to manufacture compounds such as alcohols which will function as substrates for a wide range of micro-organisms. Certain species of bacteria are able to utilize carbon dioxide as a source of carbon and molecular hydrogen as a source of reducing power and energy. The hydrogen which can theoretically be produced from 1 kWh of electricity by the electrolysis of water is equivalent to 33 g bacterial protein (Schlegel and Lafferty, 1971). Assuming that 1 ton of petroleum is equivalent to 11 332 kWh of electricity (Fleck, 1961) then this quantity would yield 374 kg of protein. If hydrocarbons are used to provide the energy for any of these processes the efficiency of the conversion of the hydrocarbon to protein will be less than that of its direct conversion.

C. Hydrocarbons

Many species of bacteria, fungi and yeasts are capable of utilizing hydrocarbons as sources of carbon and energy for growth. Yeasts have been the main choice for processes which have developed as far as small-scale production units. The presence of potentially toxic aromatic compounds in petroleum requires either a purification step before the hydrocarbons are used or extraction of all residual hydrocarbons from the yeast cells. Both methods are being tested on a production scale by British Petroleum (Llewelyn, 1967; Evans, 1968; Walker, 1972).

Hydrocarbons are not miscible with water and to obtain rapid growth the microbial cells, water, inorganic nutrients, hydrocarbons and oxygen must all be maintained in intimate contact. Because of the highly reduced state of the substrate large quantities of oxygen are required. To provide this oxygen and to ensure thorough mixing the power input needed is therefore greater than that required for growth on carbohydrate substrates. However, the yield of protein is approximately twice that obtained from carbohydrates and on a pilot plant scale 100 tons of hydrocarbon yields 50 tons of yeast protein. Not all of the hydrocarbons in petroleum are suitable for rapid conversion to yeast protein in the process and the average proportion is about 2%. The production of petroleum in 1970 was 2300 million tons and 2% of this quantity used as substrate would yield 23 million tons of yeast protein per year (Walker, 1972).

Only species of bacteria have been reported to grow on methane, the main constituent of natural gas. The yield of protein will be approximately the same as that from liquid hydrocarbons and there are no problems associated with residual toxic factors in the product (Klass *et al.*, 1969). Since the average methane content of natural gas is 75% (Walker, 1972) the yield of protein from 100 tons of natural gas can be estimated at 37·5 tons.

World reserves of natural gas in 1970 were estimated to be equivalent to 28 000 million tons of petroleum and petroleum reserves were estimated to be 84 000 million tons (Walker, 1972). Although these quantities are large the rate of consumption is increasing at a much faster rate than the increase in the population. Even at present rates of consumption supplies will become critical within 30–40 years. It is therefore difficult to estimate the proportion which could be diverted to the production of SCP.

Hydrocarbons suitable as microbial substrates can be manufactured from coal by hydrogenation or low temperature carbonization (Silverman *et al.*, 1966). Because of the intermediate stages involved the overall yield of SCP will be less than that from petroleum, although the process might be justified by the chemical by-products which could be produced from the coal.

D. Carbohydrates

The carbohydrates are the largest replenishable source of carbon compounds that are available for conversion by micro-organisms into biomass containing protein. Several bacteria and most species of fungi are able to utilize a wide range of carbohydrate compounds. Yeasts are less versatile and food yeast (*Candida utilis*), for example, is unable to hydrolyse starch. If growth on a given substrate does occur then the rate of growth and the efficiency of conversion of carbohydrate to protein can be improved by adaptation of the culture. Potential yields will therefore be similar for all micro-organisms grown on a variety of carbohydrate substrates. Calculations indicate that the maximum yield of cell biomass containing 50% protein will be about 60 g/100 g of carbohydrate utilized. The actual yield of 50 g/100 g obtained in the large-scale process for the production of food yeast from molasses is therefore probably near the limits of practical efficiency. Yeasts and fungi can be produced with a true protein content of 50% and bacteria with a content of 70% in the cell biomass. Thus in large-scale processes the maximum yield of true protein will be

TABLE VI. Quantities of some carbohydrate substrates for the production of SCP

Source	Annual world output carbohydrate (×10⁻³, tons)		Estimated conversion to protein (×10⁻³, tons)[g]
	Agricultural by-products	*Processing by-products*	
Wheat straw[a]	286 580		57 000
Wheat bran[b]		57 320	11 460
Maize stover[a]	120 040		24 000
Maize cobs[c]		30 070	6000
Barley straw[a]	52 920		10 060
Sugar cane bagasse[d]		83 000	16 600
Molasses[e]		9300	2300
	Annual USA Output (million gallons)		
Sulphite liquor[f]		12 000	510
Whey[f]		1530	400

[a] Quantities assumed = yields of the grains as listed by FAO, 1971
[b] 20% of the yield of grain
[c] Assumed = 25% grain yield
[d] Ben-Gera and Kramer, 1969
[e] Calculated from data by Peppler, 1968
[f] Data as Peppler, 1968
[g] The conversion of sugars and fibrous sources of carbohydrates to SCP are discussed

25 g/100 g of carbohydrate for yeasts and fungi, and 35 g/100 g for bacteria (Worgan, 1972).

Starch and sucrose are the two carbohydrates that are produced in the largest quantities in the edible portions of crop plants. Both are utilized as energy sources in the human diet. The output of food per unit area of land could be increased by growing a high-yielding starch or sugar crop and converting part of the carbohydrate to SCP. The protein/carbohydrate ratio could be adjusted to that which occurs in a cereal crop. This possibility is illustrated in Table II. The yields per hectare for maize and cassava are the same as those referred to on p. 52. The efficiency of conversion of carbohydrate to SCP by fungi has been discussed above. The total yield of nutritionally balanced food from the cassava–SCP system is nearly three times that obtained from the conventional maize crop.

Quantities of starch, sugars and other compounds which can be utilized as substrates by micro-organisms occur in liquid wastes from the manufacture of cellulose pulp and from many of the operations associated with food processing. Edible material removed during the processing of vegetables, for example, is 5–20% of the food product (Ben-Gera and Kramer, 1969). Relatively small amounts of molasses and waste sulphite liquor, in proportion to the total available, are used for the production of food yeast. World production of molasses in 1966 was 3484 million gallons (Peppler, 1968). This quantity could yield 2 million tons of yeast or fungal protein. Due to the low concentrations of carbohydrates which occur in many liquid wastes their use as substrates has not been considered to be economically worthwhile. The need to reduce the pollution of rivers and lakes into which these wastes have been discharged has renewed interest in the possibility of using them for the production of SCP. Alternative methods to evaporation, such as reverse osmosis, may reduce the energy input required for their concentration and this will improve the economics of their use as substrates. From sources of starch and sugars which are unsuitable for human consumption appreciable quantities of SCP for human use could be added to the supplies of unconventional proteins.

Cellulose (a glucose polymer) and hemicelluloses (polymers of glucose, uronic acids and pentose sugars) are the most abundant sources of carbohydrates. The estimated annual synthesis of cellulose is 10^{11} tons and it comprises approximately one-third of all vegetation on earth (Bellamy, 1969; Han *et al.*, 1971). Although a proportion of this material occurs in inaccessible locations large quantities are produced as by-products of forestry and are harvested inadvertently with many food crops. Further quantities are separated during food processing. Annual world production of sugar cane bagasse, for example, in 1962–3 was 83 million tons (Ben-Gera and Kramer, 1969). A selection of the quantities of some of these by-products is given in Table VI.

The bulk of these materials occurs in the form of ligno-cellulosic plant tissue in which the hemicelluloses are embedded. Due to the protective effect of the ligno-cellulose complex and the partially crystalline structure of cellulose these tissues require pre-treatment before they are suitable as substrates for the production of SCP. Tissue from the crop residues of annual plants are more easily degraded than woody tissue. The natural sequence in the degradation of ligno-cellulose is illustrated in Fig. 1. Few species of bacteria and fungi are capable of reactions L, C1 and C*x*. A larger number are able to start the degradation from native cellulose and a much wider range of species from reactive cellulose. Experimentally neither reactions L nor C1 take place at a rate which would be rapid enough for a large-scale process. Both reactions may be replaced by

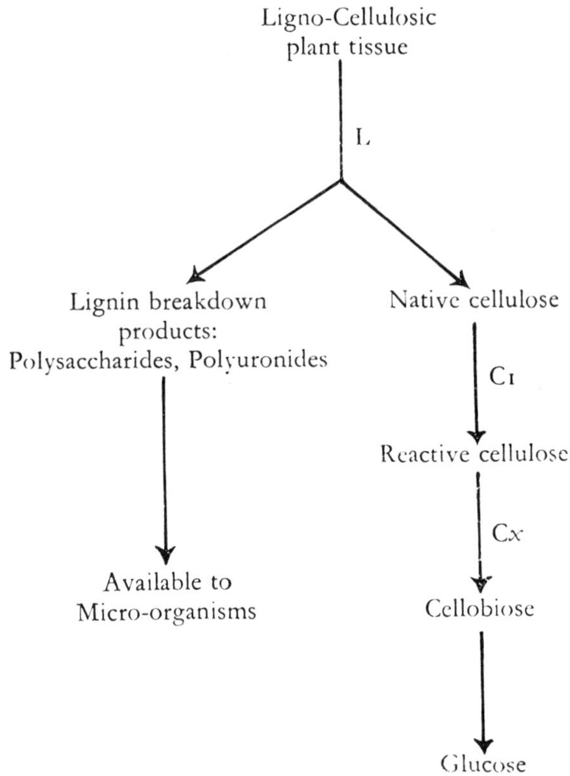

FIG. 1. The degradation of ligno-cellulose

mechanical treatments which require high-energy inputs (Worgan, 1972). Chemical treatments with low-energy inputs can replace reactions L and C1 and rapid growth of fungi is possible on culture media prepared from a variety of agricultural and food industry by-products (Delaney and Worgan, 1970; Worgan, 1971). Alkali treatment of sugar cane bagasse has been used to prepare a suitable substrate for the production of SCP from bacteria (Han *et al.*, 1971).

Reactions L, C1 and C*x* can be replaced by acid hydrolysis of the carbohydrates to sugars. This process is used to produce a suitable substrate for the growth of food yeast. Production units were operated in Germany during World War II and have more recently been established on a large scale in Russia (Bunker, 1968). If a maximum of 20% is assumed for carbohydrate losses during hydrolysis, then the potential yield of yeast or fungal protein from fibrous carbohydrate sources will be no less than 20 g/100 g carbohydrate and for bacterial protein will be 28 g.

Willcox (1959) has estimated that the total quantity of carbohydrate produced per hectare by the growth of sugar cane could be converted to 11 230 kg of yeast protein. In the production of most food crops the material harvested is three to four times greater than that which is eventually used as food. Most of this extraneous material consists of carbohydrates. Thus in the by-products associated with food production there will, therefore, be sufficient carbohydrate for conversion to SCP to ensure that, in relation to total food output, there need never be a shortage of protein. The conversion of this carbohydrate will not require the use of arable land or the consumption of excessive amounts of energy. For the production of 100 lb of yeast about 110 kWh of electricity and 600 lb of steam at 15 lb in^{-2} are needed (US Forest Service, 1964). This requirement is equivalent to approximately 530 kg fuel oil per ton of yeast protein. On the basis of the costs of collection and the lower protein yields from the substrate, SCP from carbohydrates has been estimated to cost more than that from hydrocarbons (President's Science Advisory Committee, 1967). Humphrey (1969) has argued that the greater productivity and higher cell concentration possible with carbohydrate substrates will mean that operating costs with hydrocarbons will be greater and will outweigh the extra yield obtained. In terms of the conservation of resources there would appear to be no doubt that the renewable carbohydrate substrates are preferable to those from petroleum.

IV. COMBINED PRODUCTION SYSTEMS FOR CONVENTIONAL AND UNCONVENTIONAL SOURCES OF PROTEIN

Each of the unconventional sources of protein discussed so far has been treated in isolation. A greater productivity of food and, where necessary, of protein could be achieved by combining several methods in food production systems. Units for the intensive culture of algae, for example, could be combined with the culture of herbivorous fish. During the growth of plants and algae carbon dioxide is required and oxygen is produced. The opposite applies in the case of SCP. Adjacent units with a system for the interchange of gaseous atmospheres would result in a greater overall efficiency.

Probably the most efficient use which could be made of the energy from sunlight would be to grow leguminous plants in a controlled environment and harvest the conventional seed crop. From the leaves and stems of the plant leaf protein could be extracted. The leaf juice and the fibrous residues remaining after protein extraction would be used as substrates for the production of SCP. The nutritional value of the combined harvests could be adjusted to give the required protein/energy ratio and protein quality, by selection of the species of micro-organism and the conditions under which it was grown.

A similar system applied to conventional agricultural production could increase the output of food per unit area of land. This possibility is illustrated for a cereal and a legume crop in Tables VII and VIII. The conventional crop yields and the yields of leaf protein from the same crops are experimental values obtained at the Rothamsted Experimental Station, UK (Arkcoll, 1971). The maize liquor remaining after protein precipitation from the leaf juice was obtained from the same source. The yield of mycelial protein from this liquor is an experimental value obtained

TABLE VII. Nutritional protein quality and protein yields from a combined food production system for a maize crop

	Yield (kg/hectare)						g/100 g *in combined protein*
	Grain	*Leaf*		*SCP*		*Combined protein*	
Dry weight	3300	7500					
		Liquor	*Fibre*	*From liquor*	*From fibre*		
Residues from leaf protein extraction		550	6450				
Conversion to SCP				110	1290		
Maize cobs—conversion to SCP				80			
Total protein	352	300		1480		2132	
Limiting amino acids							
Lysine[a]	8·5	19·2		98		115·7	5·5
Tryptophan	3·5	3·9		20·8		28·2	1·33
Cystine + Methionine	13·4	6·3		32·6		52·3	2·44
	Chemical scores—limiting amino acids						
Lysine[b]	0·57					1·31	
Tryptophan	0·71	0·93				0·95	
Cystine + Methionine		0·50		0·53		0·58	

Calculations of the quantities of amino acids are based on the values given in Table IV

Chemical Scores are based on the FAO (1957) Reference Protein

TABLE VIII. Nutritional protein quality and protein yields from a combined food production system for a pea crop

	Yield (kg/hectare)						g/100 g *in combined protein*
	Seed	*Pods and vines*		*SCP*		*Combined protein*	
Dry weight	1500	8700					
		Liquor	*Fibre*	*From liquor*	*From fibre*		
Residues from leaf protein extraction		625	6830				
Conversion to SCP				125	1366		
Total protein	400	625		1391		2546	
Limiting amino acids							
Tryptophan	3·2	9·9		19·5		32·6	1·3
Cystine + Methionine	10·4	17·7		30·6		58·7	2·3
	Chemical scores—limiting amino acids						
Tryptophan	0·57					0·93	
Cystine + Methionine	0·62	0·64		0·53		0·55	

by the growth of *F. semitectum* (Delaney *et al.*, 1971). Values for the yields of mycelial protein from the fibrous residues and the residual liquor from the pea vines are based on the conversion of 100 g carbohydrate to 20 g protein (p. 63). Yields for the essential amino acids are calculated from the amino acid composition of the proteins listed in Table IV. Since cystine and methionine are the first limiting amino acids in *F. semitectum* the value of 1·4 g/100 g of protein has been assumed for tryptophan. For the essential amino acids which are not listed in Tables VII and VIII the quantities in the proteins are in excess of the FAO (1957) requirements.

In both examples of the combined production system the total yield of protein is approximately six times that of the conventional crop which is still available as food. It is significant that lysine is in excess in both combined harvests and the only deficient amino acids are cystine and methionine. The possibility of varying the protein/energy ratio of these systems has been discussed above. Lignin, which would be a by-product of these systems, would be returned to the soil to maintain the soil structure. As an alternative to its conversion to SCP the fibrous residue could be used as a source of energy for ruminants which were receiving urea as a N source. The efficiency of conversion of starch to protein by ruminants is about 27 : 1 (Worgan, 1972). Assuming that the fibrous residue from maize has a starch equivalent of 50, then the conversion factor to protein will be 54 : 1, and the yield of meat protein from the maize fibre and cobs listed in Table VII would be about 127 kg/hectare.

V. CONCLUSIONS

In considering potential supplies of unconventional proteins on a world-wide basis it is apparent that, in relation to total food output, there need never be a deficiency of protein. Methods can be developed for the conversion of the inedible by-products associated with food production to proteins which are suitable for human consumption. Quantities of proteins may also be produced from other sources, such as the sea, and improvements in the processing of materials which contain under-utilized protein can make further quantities available for human food. Most of these sources of protein do not require the use of arable land or the consumption of excessive quantities of energy for their production.

It is doubtful whether the present proportion of animal protein in the diet can be maintained for the population of 7000 million which it is anticipated will exist in less than 30 years' time. Both the quality and the quantity of unconventional sources of protein are therefore important. In terms of the provision of essential amino acids it is probable that only cystine and methionine would be deficient. Fortunately methionine is one of the simplest of the amino acids to synthesize and it is already being manufactured on an industrial scale.

All systems of agriculture require the input of energy, both directly and in the form of raw materials such as fertilizers which have to be manufactured. This input is liable to increase as the area devoted to agriculture expands and as attempts are made to increase the output of food per unit area of land. Other demands on world energy resources by expanding industrial societies are also increasing. There is therefore a need to conserve world supplies of energy. The present economic system is inadequate to meet this need, since consumption is controlled by price, a factor determined by current demands in relation to current supplies. No account is taken in this system of the possibility that in 20–30 years' time sufficient resources may not be available to meet the fuel requirements for food production and for maintaining essential services. An alternative system of control on a world-wide basis is therefore required. Food production, including the production of unconventional proteins, should obviously have priority in the allocation of resources in any such system of control.

An attempt has been made in this chapter to assess potential sources of unconventional proteins in terms of the energy required for their production. These assessments are only approximate since no account has been taken of transport or of the ancillary services and materials required. It is suggested that a comprehensive survey of the resources needed for the production of unconventional proteins should be made. This information, when taken into account with local conditions, could be applied to the allocation of a system of priorities for protein production.

Almost by definition unconventional sources of protein are not currently available in quantity. Sources for which all the problems of production, acceptability and safety as human foods are solved will require a period of 5–10 years before significant quantities can be produced. Few of the new sources of protein which have been described are in this category. New sources which are still in the stages of development will require a correspondingly longer period before they become available. Confirmation that a new product is safe as a human food is the assessment which may delay their immediate production and use. Further research and development studies on the production of unconventional sources of protein should therefore be encouraged to ensure that, if the need should arise, processes for their production can be put into immediate effect. Where new protein sources do not conform to the rigid safety standards that are laid down for human foods their potential use as animal feedstuffs should be considered.

Palatability is both a physiological and psychological need in the human diet and most of the unconventional sources of protein have still to be converted by economical processes into attractive food products. The functional properties of proteins are an asset in this respect and the development of textured foods from soya-beans is an example of the possibilities. Food products prepared in the future from unconventional proteins need not be colourless, tasteless powders which nobody wants to eat.

REFERENCES

Altschul, A. M. (1970). *In* "Evaluation of Novel Protein Products": proc. symp. 1968 (A. E. Bender, B. Löfqvist, R. Kihlberg and L. Munck eds.), pp. 41–53. Pergamon Press, Oxford.

Anon. (1971). *Fd Technol. Aust.* **23**, 75.

Arkcoll, D. B. (1971a). *In* "Leaf Protein", IBP Handbook no. 20, (N. W. Pirie, ed.) pp. 9–18. Blackwell Scientific Publications, Oxford.

Arkcoll, D. B. (1971b). Personal Communication.

Bailey, W. A., Krizek, D. T. and Klueter, H. H. (1968). *Yb. Agric. U.S. Dep. Agric.* pp. 2–12.

Barlow, C. and Worgan, J. T. (1971). Unpublished results.
Bellamy, W. D. (1969). "Cellulose as a Source of Single Cell Proteins" Report 69-c-335, General Electric, Schenectady, USA.
Ben-Gera, I. and Kramer, A. (1969). *Adv. Fd Res.* **17**, 77–152.
Benjamin, B. (1963). *In* "Food Supplies and Population Growth" (Royal Statistical Society) pp. 13–21. Oliver and Boyd, London.
Bigwood, E. J. (1966). *Int. Congr. Nutr.* 7, Hamburg **4**, 823.
Borgström, G. (1970). *In* "Evaluation of Novel Protein Products" proc. symp. 1968 (A. E. Bender, B. Löfqvist, R. Kihlberg and L. Munck, eds.) pp. 55–76. Pergamon Press, Oxford.
Borgström, G. (1971). "Too Many", p. 275. Collier MacMillan Ltd, London.
Bressani, R. (1968). *In* "Single-Cell Protein" (R. I. Mateles and S. R. Tannenbaum, eds.) pp. 90–121. M.I.T. Press, Cambridge, Mass.
Bujard, E., Bracco, U., Clément, G., Mauron, J., Mottu, F., Nabholz, A. and Wuhrmann, J. J. (1970). *Int. Congr. Fd Sci. Technol.* 3, Washington D.C.
Bunker, H. J. (1968). *In* "Single-Cell Protein" (R. I. Mateles and S. R. Tannenbaum, eds.) pp. 67–78. M.I.T. Press, Cambridge, Mass.
Clément, G., Giddey, C. and Menzi, R. (1967). *J. Sci. Fd Agric.* **18** 497–501.
Cloudsley-Thompson, J. L. (1969). "The Zoology of Tropical Africa", p. 190. Weidenfeld and Nicolson, London.
Davies, D. R. (1971). *Nature, Lond.* **233**, 143–144.
Delaney, R. A. M., Mehta, M. and Worgan, J. T. (1971). Unpublished results.
Delaney, R. A. M. and Worgan, J. T. (1970). *Int. Congr. Fd Sci. Technol.* 3. Washington, D.C. Abstr. p. 113.
Delaney, R. A. M. and Worgan, J. T. (1971). Unpublished results.
Enebo, L. (1969). *In* "Engineering of Unconventional Protein Production" (H. Bieber, ed.). Symposium series 93, Vol. 65, pp. 80–86. American Institute of Chemical Engineers.
Evans, G. H. (1968). *In* "Single-Cell Protein" (R. I. Mateles and S. R. Tannenbaum, eds.) pp. 243–254. M.I.T. Press, Cambridge, Mass.
Ewell, R. (1969). *In* "Engineering of Unconventional Protein Production" (H. Bieber, ed.). Symposium series 93, Vol. 65, pp. 1–4. American Institute of Chemical Engineers.
FAO (1957). "Protein Requirements." *F.A.O. nutr. Stud.* no. 16.
FAO (1971). *St. Fd Agric.*
Fleck, Lord. (1961). *In* "Hunger: Can it be Averted?" (E. J. Russell and N. C. Wright, eds.) pp. 40–48. British Association for the Advancement of Science, London.
Fox, K. K. (1970). *In* "Byproducts from Milk", 2nd ed. (B. H. Webb and E. O. Whittier, eds.) pp. 331–355. Avi, Westport, Conn.
Fox, S. W. (1963). *Fd Technol., Champaign* **17**, 388–392.
Gerloff, E. D., Lima, I. H. and Stahmann, M. A. (1965). *J. agric. Fd Chem.* **13**, 139–143.
Han, Y. W., Dunlap, C. E. and Callihan, C. D. (1971). *Fd Technol., Champaign* **25**, 130–133, 154.

HARTMAN, G. H. Jr, AKESON, W. R. and STAHMANN, M. A. (1967). *J. agric. Fd Chem.* **15**, 74–78.

HARVEY, D. (1956). *Tech. Commun. Commonw. Bur. Anim. Nutr.* no. 19, p. 28 (entry 677).

HÉDEN, C. G., MOLIN, N., OLSSON, U. and RUPPRECHT, A. (1971). *Biotechnol. Bioengng* **13**, 147–150.

HENRY, K. M. and FORD, J. E. (1965). *J. Sci. Fd Agric.* **16**, 425–432.

HOLLO, J. and KOCH, L. (1971). *In* "Leaf Protein", IBP Handbook no. 20 (N. W. Pirie, ed.) pp. 63–68. Blackwell Scientific Publications, Oxford.

HUANG, F. and RHA, C. K. (1971). *J. Fd Sci.* **36**, 1131–1134.

HUMPHREY, A. E. (1969). *In* "Engineering of Unconventional Protein Production" (H. Bieber, ed.). Symposium Series 93, Vol. 65, pp. 60–65. American Institute of Chemical Engineers.

KING-HUBBERT, M. (1971). *Scient. Am.* **224**, 60.

KLASS, D. L., IANDOLO, J. J. and KNABEL, S. J. (1969). *In* "Engineering of Unconventional Protein Production" (H. Bieber, ed.). Symposium Series 93, Vol. 65, pp. 72–79. American Institute of Chemical Engineers.

KOHLER, G. O. and BICKOFF, E. M. (1971). *In* "Leaf Protein", IBP Handbook no. 20 (N. W. Pirie, ed.) pp. 69–77. Blackwell Scientific Publications, Oxford.

KUPPUSWAMY, S., SRINIVASAN, M. and SUBRAHMANYAN, V. (1958). "Proteins in Foods" (Spec. Rep. Ser. no. 33), p. 48. Indian Council of Medical Research, New Delhi.

LEDGER, H. P., SACHS, R. and SMITH, N. S. (1967). *Wld Rev. Anim. Prod.* **3**(11), 13–36.

LLEWELYN, D. A. B. (1968). Symposium on Microbiology, 1967 (P. Hepple, ed.). Institute of Petroleum, London.

LOCKE, E. G., SAEMAN, J. F. and DICKERMAN, G. K. (1945). FIAT Final Report, no. 499. HMSO, London.

LOVERN, J. A. (1966). *In* "World Protein Resources" (R. F. Gould, ed.) pp. 37–51. Advances in Chemistry Series no. 57. American Chemical Society.

LOVERN, J. A. (1969). *Fd Trade Rev.* **39**, 34.

MCPHERSON, A. T. (1966). *In* "World Protein Resources" (R. F. Gould, ed.) pp. 65–74. Advances in Chemistry Series no. 57. American Chemical Society.

MALOIY, G. M. O. (1965). *Nutr. Abstr. Rev.* **35**, 903–908.

MERCHANT, D. J. and EIDAM, C. R. (1961). *Adv. appl. Microbiol.* **3**, 109–130.

MILLER, D. S. (1963). *In* "Recent Advances in Food Science" (J. M. Leitch and D. N. Rhodes, eds.) **3**, 125–132. Butterworth, London.

MILLER, D. S. (1968). Personal Communication.

MITRAKOS, K., SEKERI, K., DROULISKOS, N. and GEORGI, M. (1970). *Int. Congr. Fd Sci. Technol.* 3, Washington, D.C. Abstr. p. 10.

NICHOLLS, L., SINCLAIR, H. M. and JELLIFFE, D. B. (1961). *In* "Tropical Nutrition and Dietetics", 4th ed. p. 246. Baillière, Tindall and Cox, London.

NICKELL, L. G. (1962). *Adv. appl. Microbiol.* **4**, 213–235.

OTTENHEYM, J. H. (1971). *In* "Amino Acid Fortification of Protein Foods" (N. S. Scrimshaw and A. M. Altschul, eds.) pp. 449–466. M.I.T. Press, Cambridge, Mass.

PALMER, R. M. and SMITH, R. H. (1971). Personal Communication.

PEPPLER, H. J. (1968). *In* "Single-Cell Protein" (R. I. Mateles and S. R. Tannenbaum, eds.) pp. 229–242. M.I.T. Press, Cambridge, Mass.

PIRIE, N. W. (1966). *Science, N.Y.* **152**, 1701–1705.

PIRIE, N. W. (1969a). *Int. bot. Congr.* 11 Seattle: All-Congress Symposium on World Food Supply.

PIRIE, N. W. (1969b). "Food Resources, Conventional and Novel." Penguin Books Ltd, Harmondsworth.

PIRIE, N. W. (1971). *In* "Leaf Protein", IBP Handbook no. 20. (N. W. Pirie, ed.) pp. 29–43, 53–62. Blackwell Scientific Publications, Oxford.

PRESIDENT'S SCIENCE ADVISORY COMMITTEE (1967). "The World Food Problem", 2, 364. U.S. Government Printing Office, Washington, D.C.

SACHS, R. and GLEES, A. (1967). Report on the Preservation of Wildlife, Utilization of Mammals and Processing of Game Meat, Tanzania.

SCHLEGEL, H. G. and LAFFERTY, R. M. (1971). *Adv. biochem. Engng* **1**, 143. Springer Verlag, Berlin.

SHAPIRO, S. (1968). *Yb. Agric. U.S. Dep. Agric.* pp. 20–33.

SILVERMAN, M. P., GORDON, J. N. and WENDER, I. (1966). *In* "World Protein Resources" (R. F. Gould, ed.) pp. 269–279. Advances in Chemistry Series no. 57. American Chemical Society.

SMITH, R. H. (1971). Personal Communication.

STAMP, L. D. (1960). "Our Developing World", 2nd ed. Faber and Faber, London.

THODAY, J. M. (1969). *In* "Population and Food Supply" (J. Hutchinson, ed.) pp. 1–10. University Press, Cambridge.

U.S. FOREST SERVICE (1964). Research Note FPL-065, U.S. Department of Agriculture.

WALKER, T. (1972). *In* "The Biological Efficiency of Protein Production" (J. G. W. Jones, ed.). University Press, Cambridge.

WILLCOX, O. W. (1959). *J. agric. Fd Chem.* **7**, 813–822.

WOODHAM, A. A. (1971). *In* "Leaf Protein", IBP Handbook no. 20. (N. W. Pirie, ed.) pp. 115–130. Blackwell Scientific Publications, Oxford.

WORGAN, J. T. (1968). *Prog. ind. Microbiol.* **8**, 73–140.

WORGAN, J. T. (1971). *Int. Congr. Mycology 1, Exeter.* Abstr. p. 106.

WORGAN, J. T. (1972). *In* "The Biological Efficiency of Protein Production" (J. G. W. Jones, ed.). University Press, Cambridge.

CHAPTER 5

The Efficient Use of World Protein Supplies

J. C. ABBOTT

FAO, Rome, Italy

I. INTRODUCTION

In the world of laboratories it is fairly easy to report on new developments: there are generally new experiments being started and a flow of progress reports on those under way. In the world outside—the world of people—progress is less easily distinguished. Improvements in the production and use of proteins for food are great indeed if they show up in national consumption averages. Moreover, we all know that national averages are often misleading. They hide wide inequities in distribution between income groups, between social segments of population at broadly the same income level, and between different members of a family. We can try to examine as indicators of potential lines of progress specific projects designed to correct these inequities in relatively limited areas of distribution. Here there is much the same scope for reporting as on work in the laboratory. It can cover the planning of a project to market a new protein food mix through specific channels, its progress into implementation and the results achieved at various stages. Often it seems that these microprojects come under a magnifying glass at one conference after another. Few, unfortunately, go beyond the equivalent of the laboratory stage in commercial implementation, and one that will change the food protein world is still to come.

A decade ago many such projects were launched without adequate pre-testing on a commercial basis and without much understanding of marketing and promotion. Now pre-testing and promotion are there, but still most of the new products do not catch on.

II. ECONOMIC PRINCIPLES GOVERNING FOOD DISTRIBUTION

A. Protein Food Consumption

The purpose of this chapter is to consider the questions: first, are we using the world's protein resources efficiently and, second, are new and unconventional protein foods being introduced and marketed to the best advantage? In approaching this task the first step is to see clearly the bases on which protein resources are distributed under existing conditions; one may then look at the various measures that are being taken to modify their distribution according to nutritionally desirable criteria. In order to keep this review in a dynamic frame we may also examine the recent FAO Commodity Projections to 1980 for new elements of potential significance.

The first principle to be stated, particularly to those trained in scientific experiment, is that the production and marketing of protein is undertaken not only because techniques have been developed and are available, but to meet evident market demands. It is not difficult to establish that world demand for protein is unsatisfied at present prices, and that it will expand rapidly over the next 20 years from population increase alone, without allowing for any rise in *per caput* income in the developing countries. More difficult is to determine how far this nutritional demand is likely to be effective economically and how large a share of it will go to new forms of food protein. One can assume that the additional population will adopt the tastes and habits of its parents unless these become too costly, or unless specific initiatives are taken to change them. The openings for new food proteins are conditioned, therefore, by the likelihood of existing protein consumption trends being modified by significant changes in price relationships, and/or success in introducing and marketing new competing foods on the basis of their consumer appeal.

Effective demand, i.e. demand that is supported by disposable income and willingness to use it on protein food purchases, is at present directed almost entirely towards the traditional foods. Animal protein foods are preferred by most consumers: demand is limited by price at the current consumer income/production cost equilibrium. Thus the main demand change since before the war has been the shift from grains and pulses to animal protein sources in the better-off countries. Animal protein consumption has risen sharply in Japan, for example, in reflection of expanding consumer income, and demand for the traditional soya-bean products has fallen back.

In recent years widening interest in weight control and concern over cholesterol intake have borne significantly on demand responses with income and there has been a shift away from eggs and milk in North America and in the wealthier parts of Europe. The very high meat consumption levels in Argentina and, to a lesser extent, in Australia, have fallen away somewhat; in these countries income/cost relationships were probably the main factor.

In low-income countries the human desire for protein is great, but the mass of the population has not the means to pay for it. Unskilled workers in India earn two to three rupees per day. Average *per caput* expenditure on food there has been estimated at $36.00 per year—about 10 US cents per day—out of a total income of $63.00. This estimate includes an allowance for home-produced foods. For the mass of the people there can have been little change to date. Sixty per cent of this expenditure was taken up by basic cereals. Under such constraints, proteins are consumed mainly as a natural ingredient of the chief hunger satisfiers—cereals and pulses. The large absolute increases in population forthcoming in such countries will not in themselves affect the nature of the market for protein foods unless income rises more than correspondingly.

As between alternative foods cost is undoubtedly the main demand-limiting factor for the population groups with inadequate diets. It is still important in the competitive servicing of higher-income markets and it remains at the forefront of any appraisal of alternative protein sources. Generally high-protein foods are more expensive than cereals, pulses and vegetables, especially animal proteins, and this sets limits to their use.

The costs of protein foods in wide consumption are compared in Table I. They are based on 1970 or 1971 average quality wholesale purchases at a major source of low-cost supplies of each product. To allow, at least very roughly, for the cost of the energy in each food these have been priced on a par with sugar as a near-pure energy food in wide international demand, and deducted. It is understood, of course, that costs calculated in this way reflect other attributes of these foods as much as protein content; beef steak is not eaten for protein alone. Furthermore, import duties and restrictions, transport costs, distribution margins, and so on, can change radically inter-product cost relationships in a particular country. Account should also be taken of the biological value of the protein which is generally higher in foods of animal origin. Subject to such reservations it is striking how much lower in cost is protein from chick-peas, for example, than is the protein from what are commonly regarded as protein foods. Dried skim milk is the lowest priced animal protein and

TABLE I. Relative cost of protein in major foods

	Price of product (cents per pound)	*Protein content* %	*Price of Protein*[a] (cents per pound)
Chick-peas[b]	5	20	6
Wheat flour[c]	7	11	15
Beans[d]	9	22	24
Skim milk powder[e]	15	36	31
Fish, dried[f]	25	37	64
Cheese[g]	35	25	121
Chicken[h]	27	19	128
Pork[i]	18	10	148
Eggs[j]	23	11	195
Beef[k]	34	15	217
Lamb[l]	32	12	243

[a] Net of energy contribution valued *pro rata* with sugar at 4 cents per pound
[b] Banda, Uttar Pradesh, India, 1971
[c] Toronto, Canada, export price, 1970
[d] Dry, Mexico City, 1971
[e] New Zealand commercial exports July/Sept. 1971
[f] Dried and salted cod exports, Norway, 1970
[g] New Zealand white, London Provision Exchange, 1971
[h] US ready-to-cook broilers, Chicago, 1971
[i] Average all weights, Chicago, 1971
[j] Netherlands export price, 1970
[k] Australia average first and second export quality, 1971
[l] New Zealand frozen carcases, Smithfield, London, 1971

has an established market in India and elsewhere for reconstitution with local milk of high fat content as an acceptable "toned" product.

Patterns of market demand can, of course, be modified considerably by government action. Milk was brought within the reach of the whole population of the United Kingdom during World War II by means of government subsidies. While it is recognized that the developing countries generally lack the means to subsidize consumption of particular foods on any substantial scale, it is appropriate to ask how far they are pursuing policies directed towards securing the highest nutritional dietary levels within their limited means. Most of their governments recognize that malnutrition can prejudice social and economic development significantly through deleterious effects on public health and productivity. While in many cases committing themselves to traditional public health programmes including expenditure of hard currency upon imported drugs, often they find it difficult to implement other measures which would be helpful in reducing protein malnutrition. These include adjustment of agricultural plans and policies to favour food crops against those bringing immediate export earnings, and organizing supplementary distribution of protective foods to children in low-income groups.

B. Consumption of Protein Foods per Head

As a basis for consideration of *per caput* consumption of protein foods the 1963–5 FAO Food Balance Sheets are still relevant. Table II sets out the quantities of protein obtained from various groups of foods in the major regions of the world. Some 70% of the world's protein supply comes from vegetable sources and 30% from animal sources. The penultimate two lines of Table II are a measure of the contrast between the situation in the well-fed parts of the world and the others. Protein supplies through grains are strikingly similar on a *per caput* basis. In contrast, availabilities of protein from meat and dairy products are of the order of 20 g of each daily *per caput* intake, as against 3–4 g in the developing countries, with only a somewhat higher supply from pulses and oilseeds as a partial compensation.

Grains, the staple food in most countries, are also the main source of protein, furnishing almost half the total supply. This proportion ranges from 70% in Pakistan to 17% in the United States. Grains are the main source of protein, except in Argentina, Australia, New Zealand, Canada, the United States and most of North-Western Europe, where it is meat. In Ireland and Sweden dairy products are more important.

Pulses, oilseeds and nuts provide almost 13% of the world's protein supplies. Their contribution is as high as 28% in Brazil and probably of the same order in mainland China. They provide 19% of the protein in Mexico and 18% in India, but in most countries much less.

Fish, too, accounts for only about 3% on a world basis but catches are growing rapidly. It is the main source of animal protein in countries such as Ceylon, Japan, Ghana, the Philippines, Portugal and Taiwan. In Portugal fish supplies 18% of the total protein and in Japan, 17%.

C. Adequacy of Protein Distribution

With the acceptance of the new estimates of individual protein requirements forthcoming from the FAO/WHO Expert Committee of April 1971, most countries with adequate energy intakes appear to have more than enough protein. Still more strategic than before is the point that more protein food than needed to cover average requirements must be available if all of the population is to get enough. Food consumption surveys

TABLE II. Protein supplies *per caput* (g/day) by major food groups and regions[a]

	VEGETABLE PROTEIN				ANIMAL PROTEIN				
	Grains	*Starchy roots*	*Pulses, oilseeds and nuts*	*Vegetables and fruit*	*Meat and poultry*	*Eggs*	*Fish*	*Milk and milk products*	*Total*
North America	15·7	2·3	4·7	4·6	31·9	6·0	2·5	25·3	93
Australia and New Zealand	24·3	2·4	2·1	3·1	36·8	3·5	2·2	19·5	94
Western Europe	30·5	4·4	5·0	4·1	16·2	3·1	2·4	17·3	83
Eastern Europe and USSR	48·3	8·2	2·0	2·5	12·9	2·2	1·9	16·1	94
Latin America	26·5	2·7	10·7	2·8	13·8	1·2	1·5	7·4	67
Far East	32·2	1·8	12·0	1·7	3·0	0·4	2·2	2·2	56
Near East	48·5	0·7	9·5	3·6	4·6	0·5	1·1	7·4	76
Africa	32·2	7·1	9·0	1·7	5·8	0·4	1·3	3·5	61
Europe, North America, Australia, New Zealand, Argentina, Paraguay, Uruguay	33·4	5·2	3·8	3·6	19·8	3·3	2·4	18·5	90
Far East, Near East, Africa, Latin America, (except Argentina, Paraguay and Uruguay)	33·2	2·3	11·6	1·8	3·8	0·4	1·9	2·9	58
World	33·4	3·2	9·0	2·4	8·8	1·2	2·3	7·7	68

[a] Source: Food Balance Sheets, 1963–5, FAO, Rome

demonstrate that during seasonal food shortages, not only do these inequities in distribution become more acute but the number of families that are undernourished also increases. *Per caput* levels of consumption decline significantly with rising sizes of family, so there is a high statistical probability that children in large families are undernourished. This is supported by specific survey information that the available food is very often distributed disproportionately between the various members of a family. The adults satisfy their needs at the expense of the children, who are inclined to eat more slowly. Yet children's protein needs are proportionately greater than adults' because both maintenance and growth must be covered. Surveys carried out in Nigeria, Ghana, Central America, Colombia and a number of other countries showed that even where family supplies were satisfactory children were receiving only 70–80% of their requirements. This is confirmed by a study of Indian household data which showed that the addition of a child to the family is associated with relatively small increases in the consumption of animal and total proteins in both urban and rural areas. It is clear from the evidence available that the present distribution of proteins both among and within families is likely to lead to malnutrition in children rather than in adults. Bornstein and Morgan (1971) have shown how religious influences can militate against an adequate share of protein for women and small children, and how a figure for average meat consumption can be made up of lavish supplies at certain feast times and paucity for long periods in between.

Protein deficits appear to be most probable in the maize-eating countries of Latin America, in Equatorial Africa because of the predominance of starchy foods there, and in the rice-eating countries of South-East Asia. In these areas there is a protein/energy imbalance. Energy requirements are met but the protein intake is low. In the wheat-eating countries of the Mediterranean basin and the Near East and in the millet- and sorghum-consuming zones of the African savannah, the protein/energy balance is better. The cereals which constitute the largest part of the protein supply provide more protein for the same amount of energy.

The people who do not get enough protein usually receive inadequate diets as a whole. Thus, in practice, any programme to improve the food situation of low-income groups would have to concentrate very largely on basic foods already in wide use, such as grains and pulses, and much of their protein deficit would be met by the protein in such basic foods.

D. Projections to 1980

What changes in the protein supply/demand relationship can be expected from the continuation of present trends over the next decade? The FAO Agricultural Commodity Projections 1970–80 (1971) provide some dimensions for this (Table III). They originate with current demand data. Adjustments are then made to reflect expected growth in population and income and the impact of the estimated elasticity of demand with respect to income for different foods. Thus these projections refer to market demand only, not to nutritional requirements. They show that, assuming prices remain constant, *per caput* food demand in developing countries would grow by 8% in terms of value over the 1970's, with an annual rate of a little under 1%. The daily energy intake per person implied by the projected demand would rise from 9176 kJ to 9652 kJ and

TABLE III. *Per caput* daily food requirements and levels of demand in 1980

	PER CAPUT REQUIREMENTS[a]		PERCENTAGE OF REQUIREMENTS			
			1970 *consumption*		1980 *demand*	
	Energy (kJ/day)	*Protein*[b] (g/day)	*Energy*	*Protein*	*Energy*	*Protein*
WORLD	9979	38·7	101	173	105	178
HIGH-INCOME COUNTRIES	10 711	39·5	121	229	123	237
Developed market economies	10 690	39·2	119	228	122	237
USSR and Eastern Europe	10 753	40·0	124	232	126	238
DEVELOPING COUNTRIES	9556	38·4	96	147	101	155
Asia and Far East	9301	36·6	93	141	99	150
Africa	9770	41·5	93	141	98	149
Latin America	9970	37·7	106	172	110	179
Near East	10 276	45·5	97	147	101	153

[a] Revised standards
[b] Expressed in local proteins

the daily protein demand from 56·4 g to 59·5 g, in both cases an annual increase of 0·5%. The satisfaction of these demands would thus mean a modest but definite rise in the quantity and quality of food intake on a national *per caput* average basis. However, the rise in *per caput* demand for animal proteins is likely to be much larger in high-income than in developing countries and the gap between the two groups of countries would widen.

There are areas where national average demand for energy is projected to remain distinctly below the level of requirements—in West and North-West Africa and in Asia, for example. The projections show that in 1980,

42 developing countries with a total population of 1400 million would, even if market demand is fully met, have average energy intakes below requirements. Because of the projected population increase over the decade of about 750 million people in the lower-income countries, the absolute number of underfed people would not fall much over the 1970s. However, the rise in the national average energy intake implies that the average extent of undernourishment of such people would be lessened over the period. Protein deficiency is hard to judge from these projections because they bear only indirectly on the main consideration which is the distribution of protein foods within particular population groups.

III. TRADE MOVEMENTS OF FOOD PROTEIN

Per caput availabilities of protein foods in particular countries are affected substantially by trade movements in response to international market incentives. Most of the existing international trade in protein-rich products is directed towards the developed countries, either from other developed countries and "semi-developed" countries like Argentina—mainly animal products—or, from the developing countries, speciality products such as frozen shrimps, and oilseeds, oilcake and fish meal in bulk.

The developing countries are constrained by economic necessities to export such of their production as finds a more remunerative market in the developed countries. Little foreign exchange is available to pay for food movements in the opposite direction. Processed and other speciality food items are imported in small quantities for the limited number of consumers who can afford them. Where food imports are needed on a large scale they are necessarily the cheapest available or what can be obtained on concessional terms.

In, for example, Brazil and some African countries livestock and meat are exported from some zones while in others large segments of the population subsist on diets very low in protein because they cannot afford to buy more of the meat which is produced in the country. Such "perverse" movements are generally founded, however, on solid economics. Recently the government of Guatemala sensed criticism that beef was being exported from that country to the USA while a large part of the domestic population could buy hardly any because the price was too high. In an effort to remedy this it set a lower price for beef by administrative edict. The result was a sharp drop in production because of lack of incentive to the farmer. More than 100 000 tons of rice are exported annually from Nepal yet in the mountain villages people are said to be starving. To divert exports to them the government has both to forgo foreign exchange earnings and provide subsidies that will bring down the price to a level they can afford. It has not the means to do this except on a very small scale.

Another subject of nutritionally motivated criticism is the large-scale shipment of potential human protein food supplies such as oilseeds, oil-cake, and fish meal out of the developing countries to meet a steadily growing market demand in Europe, North America and Japan for live-stock feed (Table IV).

Anchovy fishing in Peru for fish meal production has grown remarkably in recent years. Attracting international investment and management, the industry emerged from obscurity to first place among the world's fish meal producers in less than a decade. Concurrently, it became the country's principal earner of foreign exchange.

TABLE IV. Exports of potential protein food from developing countries[a] (in million tons)

	PRODUCTS[b]			PROTEIN EQUIVALENT[c]		
	1967	1968	1969	1967	1968	1969
Fish meal	1·82	2·38	2·01	1·09	1·43	1·21
Soya-bean	0·40	0·33	0·56	0·18	0·15	0·25
Groundnut	2·05	2·26	1·78	0·94	1·04	0·82
Cottonseed	1·17	1·15	1·27	0·48	0·47	0·52
Copra	0·85	0·87	0·83	0·17	0·17	0·17
Rapeseed	0·05	0·04	0·05	0·01	0·01	0·01
Sunflower seed	0·53	0·48	0·39	0·19	0·17	0·14
Sesame seed	0·07	0·07	0·09	0·03	0·03	0·04
TOTAL				3·09	3·47	3·16

[a] Including minor exports to other developing countries
[b] Oilseeds and cakes, meal, etc., in terms of cake equivalent
[c] Protein percentages: fish meal 60; soya-bean 44; groundnut 46; cottonseed 41; copra 20; rapeseed 28; sunflower seed 36; sesame 39

From many developing countries the bulk of such crops as coconuts, peanuts, soya-beans and sesame seed has long been exported in the form of whole oilseeds or oilcakes. In those few countries where a significant amount of these crops is processed locally to meet the growing domestic demand for fats and oils, the protein-rich press-cake is generally used as fertilizer, animal feed or fuel, or even wasted altogether. Processing for human nutrition is technically quite feasible; it awaits favourable economic conditions and the necessary initiatives.

Would an increase in the use of oilseed protein concentrates to fortify cereal foods significantly affect world trade in these commodities or the availability of oilcakes for animal feeding? The diversion of oilseeds for use as human food in developing countries can in practice only be gradual. Its effect on world trade patterns or on food supplies in the developed countries could normally be discounted against the additional incentive to growers to expand production. However, should the production response in a particular country be inelastic, there might be a perceptible effect upon export earnings. An increase of only 1 g per person per day in coconut protein intake in the Philippines, for example, would be at the expense of a reduction in exports of some 50 000 tons of copra cake. This would mean a loss in export earnings of about US $3 million annually, or about 1½% of the country's annual earnings from coconut products.

IV. OBSTACLES TO DISTRIBUTION OF INCREASED QUANTITIES OF PROTEIN FOODS WITHIN LOWER-INCOME COUNTRIES

An efficient marketing system must adapt the seasonal outflow of produce from the farm to a relatively stable and continuous demand from consumers. This is done by the mobilization of transport and storage facilities, skilled handling and processing, detailed knowledge of supply and demand conditions and sources, the provision of adequate credit, and willingness to accept risks and responsibilities. Limitations of capital, equipment, management and skilled operating staff all bear heavily on the ability of protein food distribution systems in the developing countries to serve lower-income consumers. Animal protein foods require fairly elaborate production and marketing systems if they are to be provided in large quantities and to maintain their quality through to the consumer. Transport is often a limiting factor in the distribution of food products and a major element in its cost. For example, a wholesale price of beef in Accra or Kinshasa of 32 cents per pound corresponds to 14 cents in Fort Lamy in Chad, since it must be brought over more than 600 miles from the savannah regions either as live animals driven on foot or as carcases by air. Many of the agricultural products containing the most valuable protein are highly perishable, and their marketing calls for special handling, treatment and storage arrangements, especially in tropical climates. The Masai cattle raisers in East Africa, for example, consume large quantities of milk *per caput* in relation to their income; but their production capacity is limited and the cost of marketing small surpluses to distant consumers is too great to support a continuing supply channel.

Fish are fairly abundant in consuming areas of developing countries closely adjacent to sea coasts, rivers and lakes, but integrated large-scale organization of fishing and marketing is rare. Thus in West Africa fresh fish are plentiful up to a distance of about ten miles from the coast. Only in a few countries, such as Ghana, Ivory Coast and Liberia has there been a full-scale attempt in recent years to develop a deep-sea fishing fleet, and the cold storage and distribution chain that would enable fish to become a major contributor of protein to the national diet. Dried fish are traded widely in Africa because of relative ease of handling, but losses due to insects and quality deterioration are considerable. These add substantially to the cost of the protein actually reaching the consumer and restrict distribution among lower-income consumers accordingly.

The long-standing absence of a marketing system for fish, either fresh or dried, lies behind what might seem a striking nutritional anomaly—the massive exports of fish meal from Peru while large parts of its 12 million population remain on a low-protein diet. Anchovetta, the main raw material for fish meal, are not suitable for human consumption. In addition, because there has been no system of bringing other acceptable fish to the inland population, especially on the Sierra, there is little familiarity with fish—except for salted sardines in limited quantity—as a normal ingredient of the diet. There is still a carry-over effect on consumption when people from the Sierra move to Lima and come within easy access of fresh fish at relatively low prices. A comparable situation prevails in the areas adjacent to the various parts in developing countries such as Egypt, India, Mexico and Pakistan where profitable industries exporting frozen shrimps and prawns have grown up in recent years, and in Mexico as regards sardines. Inadequate internal marketing arrangements interrelated with lack of consumer interest have effectively limited domestic utilization. In some cases religious or other taboos play a role, particularly regarding flat fish and Crustacea.

It is, of course, sound economics from both the private enterprise and national point of view to direct saleable produce to the markets where it will bring the greatest return. Development of a strong preference for certain species amongst consumers with the financial means to make it effective has opened the way to such returns. It is to be hoped, however, that the opening of profitable export markets for certain products and qualities would provide the initial economic basis for associated distribution to less affluent local markets of lower-valued species and quality items forthcoming as a joint product of the primary enterprise.

Proteins of vegetable origin often require quite elaborate processing, as for instance the fermentation and related treatment of soya-beans in East Asia and the washing of protein out of wheat in India. Centralized industrial processing faces the cost of packaging and distributing such oilseed protein products in consumer-sized lots. In practice this may figure more largely in the final price than either raw material or processing costs. Particular problems are those of ensuring that the product reaches the consumer in unimpaired condition and is presented in a package of convenient size and adequate sales-appeal. Unfamiliarity with such processed products and the difficulty of fitting them into established eating habits and preferences, particularly of the lower-income groups, means that intense promotional efforts will usually be needed, with only limited prospects of a market large enough to repay development costs.

V. IMPROVEMENT OF PROTEIN FOOD DISTRIBUTION

A. Government Action

Governments can take direct measures to improve protein nutrition which open up defined markets for protein products adapted to such programmes. Such measures may be designed to raise overall purchasing power in lower-income groups or they may be specific to the distribution of nutritionally desirable food products. Projections of demand which assumed changes in the distribution of incomes in developing countries would also result in higher growth rates for food. Preliminary analyses of a number of Latin American countries show that a moderate change in income distribution would result, in the circumstances of those countries, in a direct rise of some 9–9·5% in total food demand over 1970–80 or about 13–14% in the case of a "drastic" change in income distribution (FAO, 1971b). A "drastic" change in income distribution has been carried through in Cuba, for example. Here, distribution of a new food could be automatically assumed to be successful because the redistribution of income and rationing of many other foods leaves ample purchasing power available.

Another approach for governments is to make it compulsory that a protein product be included in certain basic processed foods and in institutional diets, wherever such measures can be enforced. The government of Israel requires that all flour for bread includes 2·5% soya-bean flour. Similarly, lysine fortification of cereal products might be undertaken by government action. However, while the governments of developing countries may have the desire and authority to introduce such programmes, they may well not possess the means to subsidize the cost. Individual consumers are unlikely to buy protein-fortified products selectively if they are going to cost more.

Mass protein fortification in the developing countries would, of course, be greatly facilitated if there were a supplement which could be added to established basic foods without involving any significant price increase.

This implies an ingredient cost around 5 cents per pound in the case of wheat flour, perhaps 7 cents for rice. On these terms, even the poorest government could introduce compulsory supplementation. Regrettably, some of our recent hopes for low-cost protein seem still very distant. This seems to be the case with fish protein concentrate (FPC) which still costs too much with present technology. According to the 1971 Tropical Products Institute survey, FPC, to compete on the world market, would have to be produced at an opportunity cost of only 15 cents per pound. As the lowest estimate for FPC production at that time was 25 cents per pound, it seemed unlikely that it could be competitive with other protein concentrates. Comparative prices for other protein sources were soya-bean flour (50% protein), 10·2 cents per pound; skim milk powder (36% protein), 11·7 cents per pound (Halliday and Disney, 1971). It also appears that petroleum-based protein suitable for human consumption will be more expensive than was first expected, around 23 cents per pound of pure protein from a plant of 10 000 tons per year capacity. Breeding cereal varieties with a higher protein content is another possibility which has aroused considerable expectations. Production cost and consumer-appeal issues have still to be settled (Penstrup–Andersen 1971).

B. Marketing Requirements

What are the requirements that must be met to give the best chance of success for a new protein food launched on a free market? These are now well known following the detailed analysis prepared for the UN Protein Advisory Group by Wickstrom (1971). Such a food should have a competitive advantage in price or in some attribute such as quality, convenience, flavour or functional properties that is specifically recognized by processor or consumer, and there must be effective presentation, distribution and promotion.

If the protein-fortified product must inevitably cost more than the basic foods already available then it should be offered for sale in the most attractive and palatable form possible within existing economic limitations. It cannot be too strongly emphasized that protein or protein concentrates by themselves are not attractive products to the majority of consumers. Much more attention is needed to the flavour and texture of new protein products.

The obstacles to be overcome in attaining wide commercial use of protein-enriched cereal foods lie not only in their preparation in a safe, nutritious, palatable and sufficiently inexpensive form, but in effective distribution and promotion. In the developing countries the introduction of a cheap packaged food must surmount inefficient distribution systems and high mark-ups, low, scattered consumer purchasing power and great attachment to traditional foods. The slow purchasing response to some oilseed protein products put on to the market in India, Nigeria and elsewhere, and the long gestation and high promotion outlay relative to retail sales of "Pronutro" in South Africa, illustrate the costs and risks to be faced. Because of the difficulty in obtaining commercial acceptance of new foods, something which can be incorporated into standard items of existing diets may offer the best immediate prospect of distribution in volume. The vehicle would be institutional meals, bread flours, chapatty and porridge mixes and so on, coupled with publicity for its much higher food value and low cost. The initial success of "filled milk" (imported non-fat dried milk and domestic coconut oil) sales in the Philippines, which climbed from 1 to 43 million litres in 4 years, is attributed to its similarity to an established product and lower cost.

The trend towards greater consumption of processed foods and prepared meals, even in the developing countries, constitutes an opening for products such as soya-beans and cottonseed which have adverse market attributes because of wartime and livestock feed connotations, and negative or at best passive colour, flavour and consistency. This also facilitates greater emphasis on brand names, and separation of high- and low-income markets permitting a commercial enterprise to sell at lower prices to the poorer market than would otherwise be possible.

Setting up a plant in a developing country where most of the ingredients are available locally solves the foreign exchange problem and would seem to offer the best prospects of sales to the population groups most needing additional protein. Although there have been a number of such ventures it is difficult to point to many that have taken root and flourished. "Incaparina" goes on in Central America and Colombia. In India the Tata Company is reported to be expanding its daily production for food uses of protein isolate from groundnuts from 2 tons to 6 tons. The Gujerat Agro-Industries Corporation is sponsoring a plant to process cottonseed for protein food uses. Modern Bakeries is about to open new branches in several Indian cities. Its managers claim that a part of their amino acid fortified product is bought by protein-deficient groups.

There are government-sponsored projects to launch oilseed-based protein foods for vulnerable groups in a number of North African and Near Eastern countries. "Superamine"—utilizing oilseed and chick-pea protein sources—went well initially in Algeria, but consumer demand has probably been overestimated. It has been commented that the substantial promotional investment helped over the longer run competing products aimed at a higher-income market.

The weaning food "Faffa" (57% wheat flour, 18% defatted soya-bean flour, 10% pea flour, 8% sugar, 5% defatted skim milk, 1% salt and 1% additives) has been marketed now for several years in South-Western Ethiopia. Sales reached 700 tons over the two years 1970–1. In one area investigated 16% of all the children in the correct age group were Faffa consumers, consuming about 20 kg per year of Faffa or 4 kg of proteins. Whether this means a net supplementation of the diet with the quantity stated was not determined. According to Gedda (1971) these results are a basis for cautious optimism.

VI. CONCLUSIONS

1. Economic forces tend to attract the production of protein food materials and direct them into the most profitable uses. Important determinants are production and processing techniques and costs, consumer attitudes and spending power and initiatives in marketing. Present world use patterns for protein reflect these factors in the main. They result in such nutritional anomalies as fish protein exports from Peru and oilseed protein from India while many people in those countries have diets that are protein-deficient.

2. Redistribution of income to permit purchase of desirable amounts of protein at free market prices by such groups is hardly practicable within the overall resources of the countries concerned. More specific measures to make increased protein food supplies available to groups with deficient diets are feasible, but would involve major international financial and organizational assistance. Approaches include direct provision of protein foods free or at subsidized prices to children at schools, and to mothers and pre-school children through designated shops or mobile units, sale of protein-fortified foods or cereals combined with educational and sales-promotion campaigns to shift consumption expenditure towards them, and similar measures to modify free market purchases.

3. There is still a long way to go before the needs of the population groups presently suffering from a nutritional maldistribution of protein food are met. The scale of the problem calls for major inputs of capital, organizing ability, and technical and promotional training.

4. The need for specific marketing efforts to compensate for income inequalities and consumption preferences that are nutritionally perverse is likely to increase rather than diminish.

REFERENCES

Bornstein, A. and Morgan, T. B. (1971). "Socio-Cultural Factors in Relation to Food and Nutrition with Reference to the Near East Region". Paper presented at the FAO/SIDA Inter-Regional Seminar on Food Promotion, Turkey, Oct. 1971.

FAO (1971a). "Agricultural Commodity Projections, 1970–1980." Vols I and II. Food and Agriculture Organization of the United Nations, Rome.

FAO (1971b). "The Impact on Demand of Changes in Income Distribution," CCP 72 WP.2. Food and Agriculture Organization of the United Nations, Rome.

GEDDA, O. (1971). "Marketing of the Weaning Food 'FAFFA'." Paper presented at the FAO/UNICEF Eastern Africa Regional Seminar on the Production, Utilization and Marketing of Soya-beans, Kampala, February 1971.

HALLIDAY, D. and DISNEY, J. G. (1971). "Fish Protein Concentrate: a Review." Tropical Products Institute, London.

PENSTRUP-ANDERSEN, P. (1971). "The Feasibility of Introducing Opaque-2 Maize for Human Consumption in Colombia." Centro Internacional de Agricultura Tropical, Cali.

WICKSTROM, B. (1971). "Marketing of Protein-rich Foods in Developing Countries." FAO-WHO-UNICEF Protein Advisory Group, United Nations, New York.

CHAPTER 6

Protein–Energy Interrelationships

D. S. MILLER

Queen Elizabeth College, London, England

I. INTRODUCTION

Implicit in the title of this symposium is the concept that the biological value of protein depends on its chemical and physical properties. However, all of the participants may be presumed to be in nitrogen balance; that is to say that all the protein N that they consume, no doubt excessive, can be recovered in their urine. This implies, of course, that the eventual fate of all the essential amino acids they have eaten was to be burnt for energy purposes. It does not follow from this that man does not have a minimum requirement for essential amino acids to replace endogenous losses, but it does underline the role of protein as an energy source.

Some of us have spent much of our professional lives evaluating protein quality; this study has been both intellectually rewarding and academically useful in establishing minimum protein and amino acid requirements. However, it is dangerous to confuse academic with pragmatic objectives. In particular, it is of little practical value to study protein in isolation from the rest of the diet—especially in isolation from the energy component. The efficiency of utilization of dietary protein is in practice less influenced by its amino acid composition than by the energy value of the diet. This arises because protein can act both as an energy source and as a nutrient; the proportion burnt to meet the energy needs of the body is increased when protein is in surfeit or when food is limited. Both these factors apply almost without exception in human nutrition.

II. METHODS OF PROTEIN EVALUATION

It has been known for a long time that one could "spare protein", i.e. reduce losses in both man and the rat, by the addition of various energy sources to the diet. It should be noted that this dietary manipulation not only increases the energy intake but also lowers the protein–energy ratio. It took much work subsequently to establish that both these factors influence N balance and that their effects, although related, are separate. I should like to illustrate this by reference to three types of experimental procedures that have been used in protein evaluation (Table I).

TABLE I. Some experimental procedures for protein evaluation

		Variable factors	
	Constant factor	*Experimental*	*Consequential*
Mitchell (1923–4)	Protein %	*Ad lib.*	E & N intake
Allison and Anderson (1945)	E intake	N intake	Protein %
Munro (1951)	N intake	E intake	Protein %

A. Constant Protein Concentration in Diets

In the classic work of Osborne *et al.* (1919) and of Mitchell (1923–4), the influence of protein concentration on the values obtained for Protein Efficiency Ratio (PER) and biological value, respectively, was investigated. Both groups of workers fed their rats *ad libitum* and were aware that the amount of food consumed was influenced positively by both protein concentration and quality. Mitchell showed that different groups of animals consuming different amounts of the same diet (i.e. same concentration) gave substantially the same biological value. Osborne *et al.* (1919) showed that maximum values for PER were obtained at different protein concentrations depending upon the quality of protein examined. Their recommendation for bioassays was that this maximum value should be estimated for each protein, a recommendation that was ignored by subsequent workers, notably by the Association of Official Agricultural Chemists (1960) who stipulated that the protein concentration should be 9·09% (why such precision?). It should be noted that in the assay of PER and of biological value, neither the N intake nor the energy intake is controlled since the animals are fed *ad libitum*, despite the fact that these have a major effect on growth. Here we are abandoned to the whim of the individual rat.

B. Constant Energy Content in Diets

Allison, who worked principally with dogs and established the Nitrogen Balance Index (NBI) as a measure of protein quality, controlled the energy intake of his animals and studied the influence of N intake on N balance. He showed that this relationship was curvilinear and recommended that the slope of the curve at or around maintenance should be taken as the index of protein quality. His experiments again demonstrated that the efficiency of protein utilization was not a constant but depended upon N intake. However, by holding energy intake constant and varying the quantity of protein consumed, he concomitantly varied the protein concentration.

C. Constant N Intake from Diets

In 1951 Munro reviewed his own work and relevant literature concerning the protein-sparing action of dietary energy sources. He demonstrated that the N losses following a protein meal are reduced by supplementation with increasing quantities of carbohydrate and/or fats. Calloway and Spector (1955) attempted to quantify this phenomenon and have calculated that 1·6 mg N is spared per kJ. However, Munro has observed that at high energy intakes this value is lower, and that an acceptable explanation of the phenomenon should include both situations. In this group of experiments it should be noted that dietary protein concentration is not controlled but will fall as energy supplementation increases, and that high figures for N utilization are obtained only when the protein concentration is low.

This early work clearly demonstrated that N balance depends upon the concentration of protein, the N intake, and the energy intake. Since these are interrelated it is only necessary—and more convenient—to consider the influence of two of them, the amount and the quality of the diet. The latter has been expressed by us (Platt and Miller, 1959) as Net Dietary-protein and is calculated by multiplying protein concentration by its efficiency of utilization: that is, it is the concentration of utilizable protein. This proposal, however, forced us to distinguish between two kinds of net protein utilization (n.p.u.). Standardized values, $\text{n.p.u.}_{\text{st}}$, when the protein concentration is fixed for assay purposes at an arbitrary figure, and operative values, $\text{n.p.u.}_{\text{op}}$, when the protein concentration is some other value—in particular that of a human diet as consumed by man. Net Dietary-protein values determined with the rat are thus intended as estimates of the potential value of diets for man, and are expressed in terms equivalent to a completely utilizable protein, that is in the same terms employed by most authorities stating protein requirements. Such values depend, of course, upon the amino acid composition, but this chapter is concerned only with the effect of varying protein concentration and energy intake.

III. PROTEIN CONCENTRATION

The early work established unequivocally that the efficiency of utilization of the protein fell as the concentration in the diet increased, but the algebraic relationship between these factors is still under dispute. Forbes *et al.* (1958) proposed a linear model with rats, and Summers and Fisher (1961) supported this conclusion from their work with chicks. Miller and Payne (1961a) further demonstrated that the slopes of the lines depended upon which protein was used. However, the linear models would all indicate that the efficiency of utilization would be zero at some concentration between 50 and 60%, and subsequent workers have objected that this does not agree with observation. Morrison *et al.* (1963) proposed a logarithmic model which fits the observations better at high concentrations but is less satisfactory at the other end of the range. Subsequently, Payne (1972) has suggested a parabolic model which is probably the most satisfactory to date. However, it should be pointed out that none of these models differs significantly over the range of concentrations found in diets as consumed by man and farm animals (see Fig. 1). Both the n.p.u.$_{op}$ and

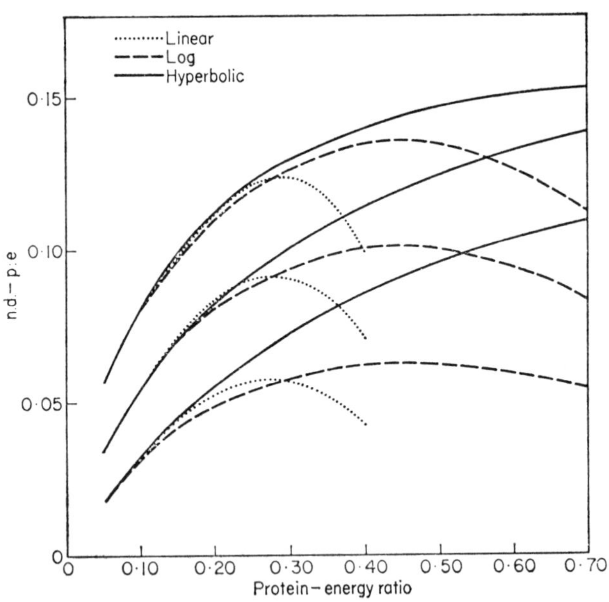

FIG. 1. Models relating efficiency of utilization of a protein with its dietary concentration

the net dietary protein of human diets may be predicted with reasonable accuracy from the results of chemical analyses and one of these models. Nomograms are available to simplify the calculation.

IV. ENERGY INTAKE

As early as 1958, Allison observed that animals given restricted amounts of food burn increasing amounts of protein for energy purposes. As one might expect in the life process, the demand for energy has precedence over all other requirements. In our work (Miller and Payne, 1961b) with diets from the developing countries, we have found that N balance in many cases depends simply upon food intake rather than protein quality. Diets with apparently excellent amino acid composition and protein concentration are unable to support growth when fed in restricted amounts. If the food intake is reduced to meet only the needs for basal metabolism then the efficiency of protein utilization is zero (Fig. 2).

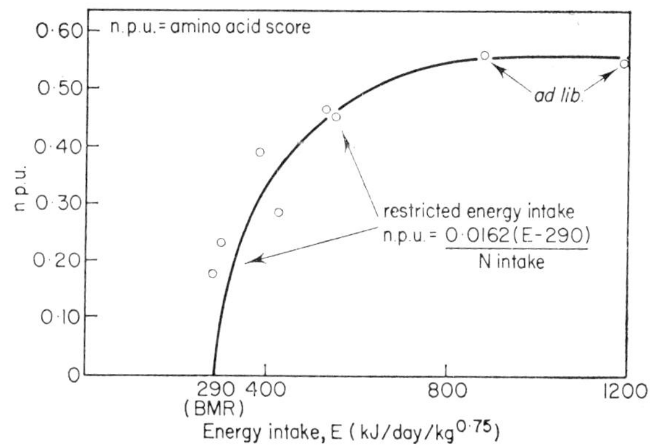

FIG. 2. Dependence of efficiency of utilization of protein on energy intake

A model has been proposed to account for this phenomenon (Miller and Payne, 1961c). From the above it is clear that even with good diets there is a minimum energy intake required for maintenance of N balance and we have shown this to be 448 kJ/$W^{0 \cdot 75}$ for the rat and the pig (Miller and Payne, 1962). Such a diet at that energy intake would have a n.d.–p : e of 0·06. Diets of lower protein value need to be consumed in larger amounts to produce N balance. This is shown diagrammatically in Fig. 3. Above the line growth is possible, and below it animals go into negative N balance. The diagram illustrates that maintenance may be achieved over a very wide range of energy intakes and we have demonstrated that this can be achieved by the pig (Miller and Payne, 1962), but the range is smaller

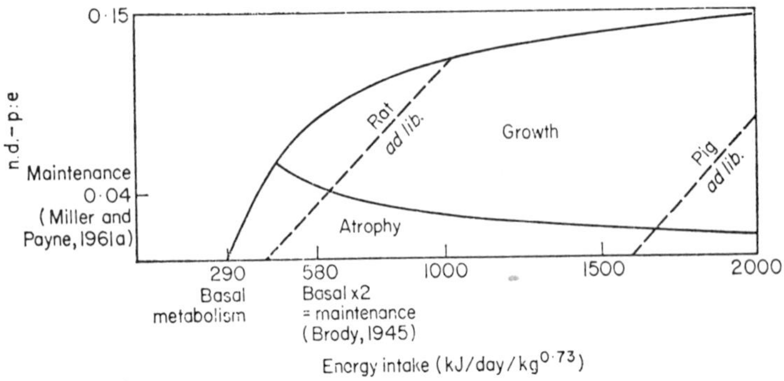

FIG. 3. Maintenance and energy intake

for the rat because it will not eat excessive amounts of low-protein diets. However, man can also maintain N balance on incredibly low protein intakes if the energy intake is excessive (Table II). There are a number of cases in the literature of adults maintaining N balance on daily intakes of less than 20 g of protein, but these have only been possible where the energy intake was in the region of 17 000 kJ/day in order to ensure maximum protein utilization. In man there is evidence that in long-term

TABLE II. Levels of net dietary-protein and energy intake that have supported N balance in man

	Subjects	*Weeks*	*Net dietary-protein*[a] (g)	*Energy density* (kJ/kg)
Bricker *et al.* (1949)	9	10	19	190–210
Rose and Wixom (1955)	38	1	20	230
Miller and Mumford (1964)	2	6	18	210
Miller and Mumford (1967)	6	4	19	240

[a] Cf. requirements = 32 g

undernutrition some individuals can adapt by reducing N losses, but this observation is not inconsistent with the above, since such individuals also reduce their basal metabolic rate.

V. INTEGRATION

There are two situations where energy intake affects the protein value of diets. The first may be explained by reference to the well-established relationship between protein concentration and protein utilization, a sort of law of diminishing returns. The second is best understood if one considers the energy requirements of basal metabolism and those for protein synthesis. In practical terms the second is the more important. Most mammals burn a major proportion of their dietary protein, the young because growth is fundamentally an inefficient process, and the adults because they inevitably consume a plethora of protein if they meet their energy needs. In man this situation is most marked because of his slow growth rate compared with animals, and because of the economic division of the world's resources. Thus an undernourished child in a developing country is burning protein because he is energy-deprived, whereas a child in our affluent society is doing the same thing because he is eating a high protein diet. Similarly, adults in N equilibrium are by definition using all their protein for energy purposes. In none of these cases is the biological value of the protein of much significance to the individual. It is apparent from FAO (1971) statistics that low energy intakes play a major role in causing protein deficiency and that the best use of protein supplies can only be effected in the presence of an adequate energy intake. Since most human diets have an adequate protein–energy ratio, the most practical solution to the world food problem seems to be to supply more of the foods already consumed. This ratio is about 10% (Autret and Perisse, 1968) and there is much to be said for assaying new proteins at this level (n.p.u.$_{10}$) as proposed by Mitchell (1923–4)—long, long ago.

During the next 30 years the world's population will double, and so will mankind's total nutrient requirements. In order to meet this growing demand it is essential to realize that the need is to supply increased amounts of nutrients in much the same proportions as are consumed at present. An examination of staple foods (see Table III) currently consumed shows that all but three have sufficient protein to meet the needs of man. The three exceptions are cassava, sago and plantain. However, when one examines diets, even those based on cassava, one finds that the staple is never eaten alone, but with sufficient supplements to fill the protein gap, except for the new-born who would receive breast milk.

Thus if protein deficiency exists at the present time it is associated with an inadequate intake of food. Such low food intakes imply a concomitant low protein intake, but also as mentioned earlier a lower efficiency of utilization of the protein. Hence the protein deficiency is an indirect result of the energy deficiency and could not be corrected by the addition of extra protein to the diet. This principle has been recognized by WHO, who refer to the deficiency syndrome as protein–energy malnutrition.

A complete scientific evaluation of nutrient requirements does not, however, provide a recipe for a satisfying diet, however economical. We eat food because we like it and it may be that a varied diet is essential for the consumption of enough food. It cannot be denied that most of the diets of the world are monotonous and frequently made up of only a few foods. Morever, a varied diet is more likely to meet the requirements for vitamins and minerals. In the future it is to be hoped that the food technologist will provide cheap, appetizing foods which are also nutritionally

TABLE III. Net dietary protein–energy ratios of a number of staples and diets based on them[a]

	n.d.–p : e ratios	
Staple	*Alone*	*Diets*[b]
Sago	0·003	—
Cassava	0·009	0·040 (7)
Plantain	0·016	—
Yam	0·046	0·046 (2)
Maize	0·047	0·062 (3)
Rice	0·049	0·064 (9)
Sorghum	0·049	0·080 (5)
Millet	0·053	0·115 (1)
Potato	0·059	0·096 (4)
Wheat	0·059	0·092 (7)

[a] Cf. requirement for adult man = 0·04
[b] The figures in parentheses are the numbers of diets assayed

balanced, especially with regard to protein and energy. Judging from the trends in food consumption taken by developed countries, these will contain not only more protein but also more sugar and more fat. These low bulk, easily digested, energy-rich foods are universally prized by man; whether their excessive consumption is responsible for the "diseases of civilization" is another matter.

REFERENCES

ALLISON, J. B. (1958). *Ann. N.Y. Acad. Sci.* **69**, 1009–1024.

ALLISON, J. B. and ANDERSON, J. A. (1945). *J. Nutr.* **29**, 413–420.

ASSOCIATION OF OFFICIAL AGRICULTURAL CHEMISTS (1960). "Official Methods of Analysis", 9th edition.

AUTRET, M. and PERISSE, G. (1968). *F.A.O. Newsletter.*

BRICKER, M. L., SHIVELEY, R. F., SMITH, J. M., MITCHELL, H. H. and HAMILTON, T. S. (1949). *J. Nutr.* **37**, 163–183.

BRODY, S. (1945). "Bioenergetics and Growth." Hafner, New York.
CALLOWAY, D. H. and SPECTOR, H. (1955). *J. Nutr.* **56**, 533–544.
FAO (1971). *St. Fd Agric.*
FORBES, R. M., VAUGHAN, L. and YOHE, M. (1958). *J. Nutr.* **64**, 291–302.
MILLER, D. S. and MUMFORD, P. M. (1964). *Proc. Nutr. Soc.* **23**, xliii.
MILLER, D. S. and MUMFORD, P. M. (1967). *Am. J. clin. Nutr.* **20**, 1212–1222.
MILLER, D. S. and PAYNE, P. R. (1961a). *Br. J. Nutr.* **15**, 11–19.
MILLER, D. S. and PAYNE, P. R. (1961b). *J. Nutr.* **74**, 413–419.
MILLER, D. S. and PAYNE, P. R. (1961c). *J. Nutr.* **75**, 225–230.
MILLER, D. S. and PAYNE, P. R. (1962). *J. Nutr.* **78**, 255–262.
MITCHELL, H. H. (1923–4). *J. biol. Chem.* **58**, 905–929.
MORRISON, A. B., SABRY, Z. I., GRIDGEMAN, N. T. and CAMPBELL, J. A. (1963). *Can. J. Biochem. Physiol.* **41**, 275–281.
MUNRO, H. N. (1951). *Physiol. Rev.* **31**, 449–488.
OSBORNE, T. B., MENDEL, L. B. and FERRY, E. L. (1919). *J. biol. Chem.* **37**, 223–229.
PAYNE, P. R. (1972). *In* "Protein and Amino Acid Functions" (E. J. Bigwood, ed.) pp. 259–306. International Encyclopaedia of Food and Nutrition, vol. 11. Pergamon Press, Oxford.
PLATT, B. S. and MILLER, D. S. (1959). *Proc. Nutr. Soc.* **18**, vii–viii.
ROSE, W. C. and WIXOM, R. L. (1955). *J. biol. Chem.* **217**, 997–1004.
SUMMERS, J. D. and FISHER, H. (1961). *J. Nutr.* **75**, 435–442.

CHAPTER 7

The Protein Needs of Malnourished Children

R. G. WHITEHEAD

Medical Research Council Child Nutrition Unit, Kampala, Uganda

I. THE NEED FOR INFORMED NUTRITIONAL THERAPY

Until relatively recently, the requirements of even healthy children for protein and other nutrients have been regarded as something of a mystery; a corresponding absence of precise knowledge concerning the dietary requirements of the malnourished child is therefore not really surprising. This manifests itself in a variety of ways, the charitable but often haphazard dietary therapy of some child welfare clinics, the not infrequently rather wild computation of foods by food technologists for the prevention of malnutrition and, most seriously of all, in the ineffective efforts of many otherwise well-qualified "aid" teams sent to help developing countries.

It is one of the natural hazards of nutritional science that practically everybody can claim some degree of competence in dealing with matters of nutrition; we are all concerned, in one way or another, with the daily preparation of nutritionally quite acceptable foods. Understandably, therefore, it is often considered unnecessary to seek the scientific advice of a nutritionist both in connection with one's own food and in the planning of diets for malnourished children. But effective and economic, preventive or curative nutritional therapy is not really such a simple matter. In an attempt to formulate a balanced concept concerning the protein needs of malnourished children and the desirability of different degrees of protein supplementation of traditional diets, I have combined the results of practical experience gained in our wards and outpatient clinics in Uganda with estimates based on recent scientific and mathematical theories concerning nutritional requirements. I hope to show that dietary therapy is both capable of and deserves the same precise considerations which are normally reserved for the quantitative aspects of drug therapy.

II. THE NON-MALNOURISHED CHILD

Before discussing the needs of a malnourished child, it is first necessary to look at the more normal individual and to clear up one or two commonly held misconceptions which have a bearing on the planning of dietary therapy.

TABLE I. Changes, during the past 30 years, in the minimum amounts of protein (g/kg body-wt/day) and energy (kJ/kg body-wt/day) which have been considered satisfactory for the health and growth of young children

Year	*Weight* (kg)	*Energy*	*Protein*	*Protein–energy ratio*	*Reference*
1941, 1945, 1948	12	420	3·3	0·132	NRC (1948)
1963	13	420	2·5	0·100	NRC (1963)
1965	(1–3 year)	—	1·5[a]	—	FAO (1965)
1968	12	385	2·1	0·091	NRC (1968)
1969	11·4	440	1·7	0·065	DHSS (1969)

[a] If $\text{n.p.u.}_{\text{op}} = 0{\cdot}70$

Table I shows the changes which have occurred during the past few years on our ideas of minimum requirements for protein and energy of 1–2-year-old children. The protein values have been falling steadily and it is no longer considered essential to have 10–15% of the total energy coming from protein.

This realization has had a profound effect on the interpretation of data from dietary surveys; Table II provides an example from Uganda. Using the NRC (1948) values for reference, primary protein malnutrition would seem clear-cut but this conclusion could not be reached so readily on the basis of the more recent interpretation guide-lines of either FAO (1965) or DHSS (1969). It would now have to be concluded that, if the children were able to eat more of the traditional diet to satisfy fully their energy requirements, they would be quite adequately protected from protein malnutrition. Similar conclusions are now being made by a variety of nutritionists in different parts of the world; notable examples can be found in the results of Sukhatme (1970) who was working in India.

TABLE II. The interpretation of dietary data from Uganda on the basis of NRC (1948) and DHSS (1969) minimum requirement values

NUTRIENT INTAKE	*Ugandan children* (mean)	*NRC* (1948)			*DHSS* (1969)		
		Recommended	*Adequacy* (%)	*Limiting factor*	*Recommended*	*Adequacy* (%)	*Limiting factor*
Protein (g/kg/day)	1·5[a]	4·5[b]	33	+++	2·1[c]	71	—
Energy (kJ/kg/day)	280[a]	420	67	—	420	67	+

[a] From data of Rutishauser and Whitehead (1972), protein–energy ratio of largely vegetable diet 0·09; $n.p.u._{op}$ 0·55 (assumed)

[b] NRC value recalculated for a diet of $n.p.u._{op}$ 0·55 assuming US diet to be $n.p.u._{op}$ 0·75

[c] For a diet $n.p.u._{op}$ 0·55

Can children really live and grow on these low protein intakes? The answer is a qualified yes; provided the child *can* eat enough of the often very bulky food to obtain sufficient energy for the protein to be fully utilized. Figure 1 summarizes the results of feeding a wholly vegetable diet to a young Ugandan child who was at risk to malnutrition. During the second and third weeks of feeding, the child was eating on average 525 kJ/kg body-wt/day and 2·4 g/kg body-wt/day of protein, a diet with

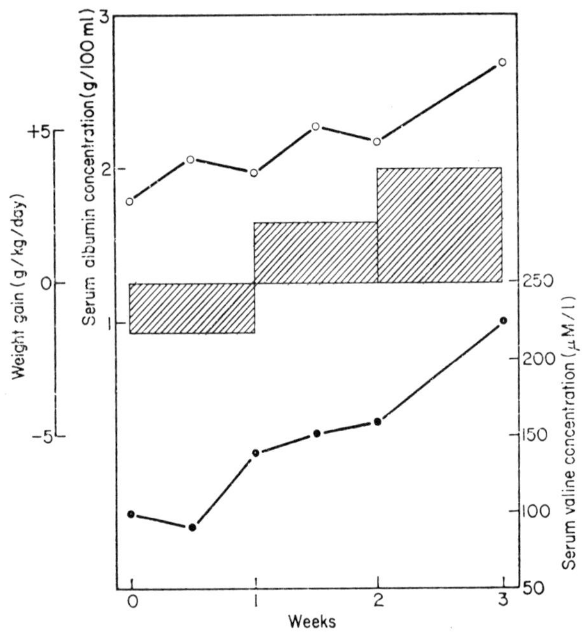

FIG. 1. The effect of feeding a vegetable diet (protein–energy ratio 0·078) on weight gain, serum albumin and valine concentration in a child at risk to kwashiorkor

a protein–energy ratio of only 0·078. In spite of this low protein concentration, there was steady, if somewhat slow, catch-up growth as well as gradual restoration of fasting serum valine and albumin concentrations. In practice, however, a child is often physically unable to eat enough of such diets because of their bulk, a topic to which I shall refer again later in greater detail.

Another point needs clarification. Although we now know that it is by no means essential to have diets routinely containing higher concentrations of protein, this does not diminish the desirability of introducing such foods if this is economically possible and if, and this is important, there is a corresponding rise in the availability of total dietary energy.

TABLE III. Basis of the calculation of protein requirements for malnourished babies and young children. The principle used is the incremental method of DHSS (1969)

Increment	*Nitrogen requirement*	*Incremental factor*	*Reference*
Maintenance	Endogenous urinary loss	8·37 mg N/basal kJ	FAO (1965)
	Metabolic faecal loss	2·39 mg N/basal kJ	DHSS (1969)
	Skin loss	0·34 mg N/basal kJ	Sirbu *et al.* (1967)
	Total nitrogen loss (NL)	11·1 mg N/basal kJ	—
Growth	Nitrogen for growth (NG)	23·4 mg N/g weight gain/ day	Fomon (1967)[a]
	Total nitrogen requirement (N)	NL + NG	—
Reference protein (RP)	—	N × 6·25	
Protein in therapeutic diet (TP)	—	RP/n.p.u.$_{op}$	
Provision for individual variation	—	TP + 20%	DHSS (1969)

[a] It is assumed that the chemical composition of the growth increment is similar to that of a one-year-old child.

Under special circumstances, moderately high protein foods do have certain advantages; this will become more apparent after the problems of the malnourished child have been discussed.

III. THE MALNOURISHED CHILD

A. Protein Requirements

A different set of factors from those affecting the protein requirements of the normal child must come in for consideration when one is dealing with malnourished children. The crucial aim of dietary therapy is to achieve as rapid a rate of recovery as possible both in terms of weight gain and of the correction of biochemical abnormalities such as hypoalbuminaemia. It is important to know the optimum levels of nutrients for this to be achieved.

It is possible to calculate theoretical protein needs on an incremental basis and Table III shows such a system based on the one used by DHSS (1969) for the requirements of normal children. Allowances are made for the nitrogen needed to replace obligatory losses and also for that required

TABLE IV. Theoretical milk protein requirements for different rates of growth[a] during recovery from protein-energy malnutrition

	Rate of growth (g/day)			
	10	30	50	70
NITROGEN REQUIREMENT (g/day)				
Maintenance[b]	1·09	1·09	1·09	1·09
Growth	0·23	0·70	1·17	1·64
	1·32	1·79	2·26	2·73
PROTEIN REQUIREMENTS				
Ref. protein (g/day)	8·3	11·2	14·1	17·1
Dietary protein[c] (g/kg/day)	1·59	2·13	2·69	3·26
Cover for individual variation	1·90	2·56	3·23	3·96

[a] The calculation is based on a child weighing 7 kg

[b] The basal metabolic rate used was $397 \times 7^{0.75}$ kJ/day, the value obtained for children living in the tropical environment of Uganda (Ablett and McCance, 1971)

[c] It has been assumed that the milk protein is supported by sufficient energy to support an n.p.u. of 0·75

during growth. From these nitrogen figures, average protein requirements can then be calculated, taking into account the utilization efficiency (n.p.u.) of the dietary protein. It is also usual to add an extra increment to cover individual variation. In Table IV this principle has been used for calculating the amounts of milk protein, when the n.p.u. is 0·75, needed to support different rates of catch-up growth in a 7 kg malnourished child. Tissue growth, with a normal composition, of 50 g/day would theoretically be covered by an intake of 3·2 g protein/kg body-wt/day.

The *average* rate of growth in our ward is 6 g/kg/day, 42 g/day for a

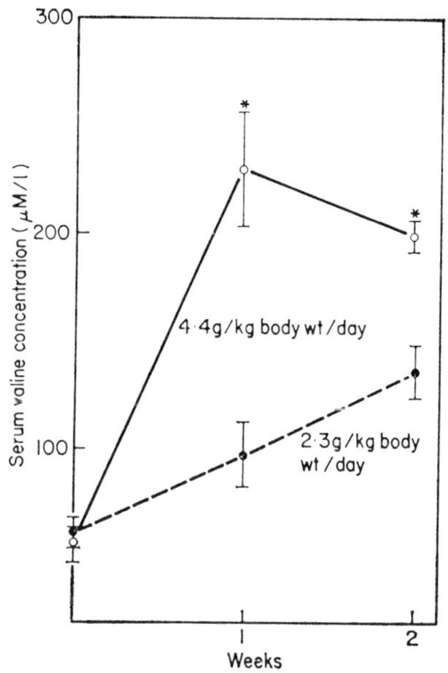

FIG. 2. The effect on serum valine concentrations of feeding different levels of protein, under isoenergetic conditions, to two groups of children with kwashiorkor. Values, mean ± SE, *values significantly different $P<0{\cdot}01$

7 kg child, and this is normally achieved by feeding about 4·4 g protein/kg body-wt/day. The fact that a relatively high protein intake, at least 3 g protein/kg body-wt/day, is desirable for the rapid therapy of such children is illustrated by the results in Figs 2 and 3. A special group of children was treated with, on average, only 2·3 g protein/kg body-wt/day and 573 kJ/kg body-wt/day and their progress was compared with another group receiving essentially the same energy intake but 4·4 g protein/kg body-wt/day. Although restoration of serum valine (Fig. 2) and albumin concentration (Fig. 3) did take place with both levels of protein, the response was significantly faster with the higher protein

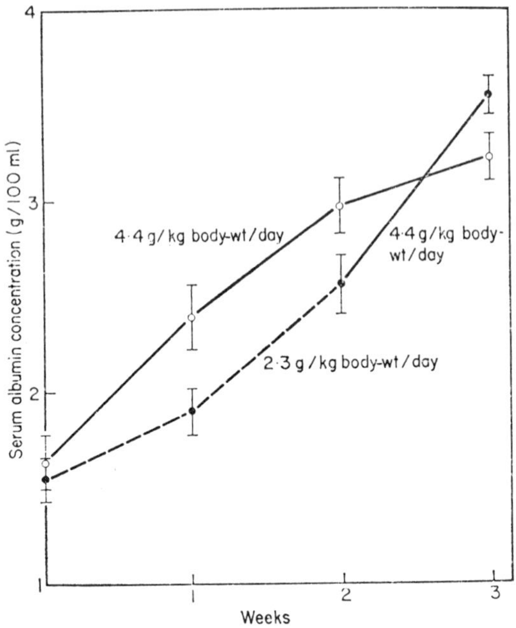

FIG. 3. The effect on serum albumin concentrations of feeding two levels of protein, under isoenergetic conditions, to two groups of children with kwashiorkor. Values, mean ± SE

intake. Hospitals are notoriously unhealthy places, especially when the immune response to infection may be impaired; the more rapidly a child can be prepared for discharge the better. We recommend a milk diet which is fed to provide 4 g milk protein/kg body-wt/day. This allows a generous safety margin for biological variation among individuals and for what can most politely be called "administrative losses" from the food kitchen.

B. Energy Requirements

It cannot be over-emphasized that these higher protein intakes are effective only if they are supported with sufficient dietary energy. This point has been well substantiated by the work of Ashworth *et al.* (1968). As with protein, it is possible to calculate, on an incremental basis, the energy needed to support different rates of growth. The principle, derived from the work of Payne (1971) is shown in Table V and the resultant energy requirements for catch-up growth in a 7 kg malnourished child are given in Table VI. It will be seen that calculated energy needs are about 50% greater than normal during recovery from malnutrition.

These theoretical requirements for a high energy intake are well borne out by practical experience. The formula for the therapeutic milk diet

TABLE V. Basis of the calculation for energy requirements of malnourished babies and young children

Increment	*Incremental factor*	*Reference*
Energy for Nitrogen balance	1·5 × BMR	Payne (1971)
Energy for growth	100 kJ/g protein deposited together with other cellular components	Payne (1971)
Energy expenditure	Dependent on activity	

TABLE VI. Theoretical energy requirements (kJ/day) for different rates of growth[a] during recovery from protein–energy malnutrition

	Rate of growth (g/day)			
	10	30	50	70
Nitrogen balance[b]	2573	2573	2573	2573
Growth[c, d]	0	293	586	877
Activity[e]	732	732	732	732
TOTAL (kJ/kg body-wt/day)	472	514	556	597

[a] The calculation is based on a child weighing 7 kg
[b] The basal metabolic rate used was $397 \times 7^{0\cdot75}$ kJ/day (see Table IV)
[c] It is assumed that the BMR measurement probably includes a component for normal growth, extra energy is only included for catch-up growth
[d] It is assumed that the N content of the growth increment is 2·34 g% (Fomon, 1967)
[e] An activity allowance of 105 kJ/kg body-wt/day is included to cover active playing after initial recovery

used in Uganda (CADSU) is given in Table VII; it is fed to provide 4 g protein/kg body-wt/day, but by itself the diet is relatively ineffective. In spite of the fact that the dried skim milk has been supplemented with sucrose and oil, the diet still contains too little energy; the n.p.u.$_{op}$ can be as low as 0·31 (McCance *et al.*, 1970). The extra energy needed for better protein utilization is supplied by the culturally important local plantain staple, matooke, which is given at every meal, after the milk, *ad libitum*.

TABLE VII. The ingredients and nutrient content of the routine Casilan[a]-dried skim milk-sucrose diet CADSU used in Uganda for the treatment of kwashiorkor (Staff, 1968).

Ingredients of the "dry" mixture (g)		*Nutrient content per 100 g of reconstituted diet*	
Casilan	33	Protein, g	4·0
Dried skim milk	30	Fat, g	6·1
Sucrose	30	Carbohydrate, g	4·6
Cottonseed oil	60	Energy, kJ	377
Potassium chloride	2·7	Potassium, mequiv	4·7
Magnesium hydroxide	0·3	Magnesium, mequiv	1·3
Sodium chloride	None	Sodium, mequiv	0·9

Note: The effectiveness of this diet depends on the provision of extra energy from local staple foods eaten *ad libitum* (see Fig. 5).
[a] A proprietary roller-dried whole protein (casein) powder

Figure 4 illustrates the energy contribution of the voluntary intake of extra matooke; the energy of the diet as a whole is boosted into the range of the theoretical needs, about 630 kJ/kg body-wt/day. The effect on growth rate is seen in Fig. 5; rapid catch-up is obviously dependent on the provision of extra energy.

An even more dramatic example of the importance of high energy intakes is provided by results from an individual child shown in Fig. 6. During the first 20 days on CADSU, although oedema was lost, no

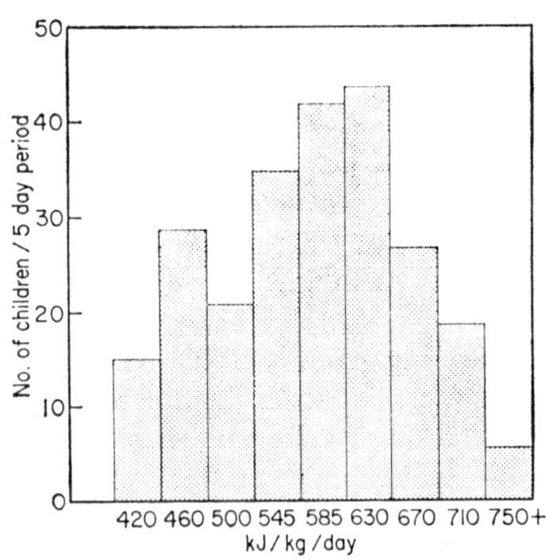

FIG. 4. Voluntary energy intake in children during recovery from kwashiorkor

weight gain occurred; the child was too feeble to eat any extra matooke. The introduction of a new diet containing extra fat, supplying 840 kJ/kg, immediately initiated a steady and rapid rate of catch-up growth and serum albumin levels also regenerated more quickly.

From a combination of the data in Tables IV and VI it is possible to

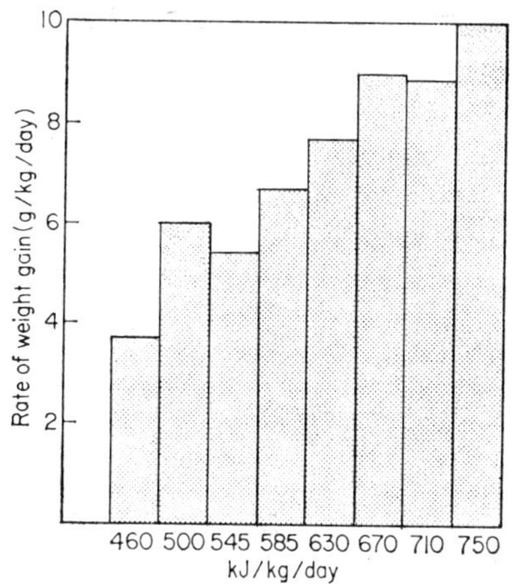

FIG. 5. The effect of energy intake on weight gain on diets supplying 4·2–4·8 g protein kg body-wt/day

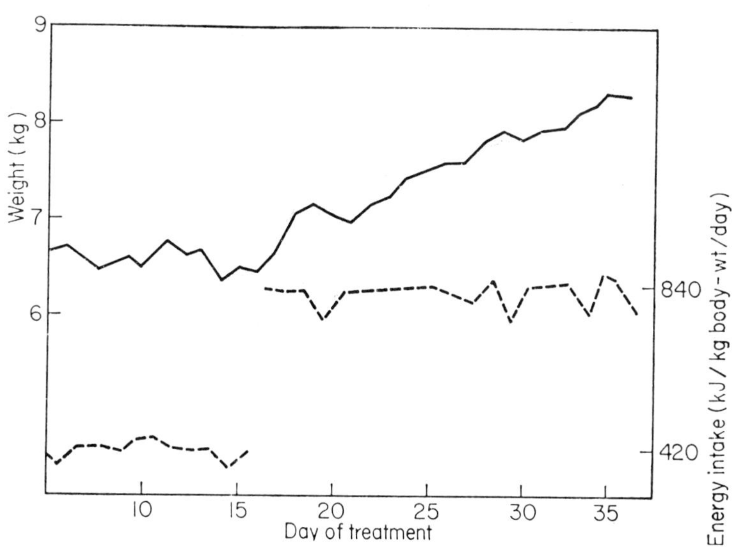

FIG. 6. The effect of changing the energy intake on the rate of growth of a malnourished child receiving 4 g milk protein/kg body-wt/day

obtain an estimate of the concentration of protein, relative to energy, that it would be advisable to recommend for diets designed to allow for rapid growth (Table VIII). A level of protein giving n.d.–p : e 0·05 would be adequate for the growth of a normal 1–2-year-old child, but the accelerated rates of catch-up growth of which the malnourished child is potentially capable would probably be achieved more readily on moderately higher levels of protein, up to n.d.–p : e 0·083. These theoretical considerations tie in quite well with those which are effective in practice.

TABLE VIII. Protein concentrations, relative to theoretical energy requirements, in therapeutic diets (n.p.u.$_{op}$ 0·75), needed to support different rates of catch-up growth in a young child

	Theoretical[a] *Rate of growth* (g/day)			
	10	30	50	70
Protein–energy ratio	0·067	0·086	0·097	0·111
n.d.–p : e	0·050	0·065	0·073	0·083

Practical

1. Minimum n.d.–p : e requirement for normal growth of 6·6–9·5 kg child (13 g/day) (DHSS, 1969) 0·045–0·052
2. n.d.–p : e of human milk, supporting growth of 30 g/day in young infant (if n.p.u.$_{op}$ 0·95) 0·065
3. n.d.–p : e of CADSU diet plus staple eaten *ad libitum* supporting growth of 60 g/day (if n.p.u.$_{op}$ 0·75) 0·086
4. n.d.–p : e of UK children's diet, assuming n.p.u.$_{op}$ 0·75 (Widdowson, 1947) 0·090

[a] Based on Tables IV and VI

One advantage of the apparently excessive levels of protein normally found in the English child's diet is that any reduction in protein-sparing action by carbohydrate resulting from a fall in total food intake is partially mitigated as long as there is a corresponding fall in energy expenditure; during infections this is usually the case. However, recommendation of dietary supplementation in developing countries to n.d.–p : e values of greater than 0·083 (a protein–energy ratio of 0·11 if n.p.u.$_{op}$ is 0·75) would almost certainly be wasteful as well as ineffective in producing faster rates of growth.

C. Protein Supplementation and Dietary Bulk

Once the need for extra energy to support protein supplementation has been appreciated, one is left with a practical problem of some magnitude. Technically, it is relatively simple to enrich traditional diets with protein but it is not so easy to supply the necessary extra energy without the diet becoming too bulky. For the child in hospital given CADSU and matooke the problem of bulk is overcome by feeding five times a day and, in special circumstances, even eight times a day. This is possible because of our trained nursing staff but the solution is not so easy for mothers looking after their children at home using modified local diets. Table IX shows the type of dietary modification routinely recommended in Uganda. The protein content of the traditional diet has been supplemented with meat and protein-rich vegetables to a value well above the minimum requirements. However, to get enough energy, even for normal growth, the child must eat 1000 g/day of solid food. This contrasts with the child living on the English type of diet, also demonstrated in Table IX; he has only to eat 244 g.

The question of excessive dietary bulk is one of the biggest problems which faces nutritionists in the developing countries, a fact which has been masterfully highlighted in a recent review article by Nicol (1971), the deputy director for nutrition, FAO. It is one of the reasons why the nutritional progress of a child is so often prone to the anorexic effects of even minor bouts of infections (Frood *et al.*, 1971; Poskitt, 1971). It also explains the slow rate of catch-up growth after these infections. The European child can and does achieve energy intakes of up to 630 kJ/kg body-wt/day after an infection by eating only 400 g solid food plus milky drinks but the young Ugandan child would need to eat 1·5 kg food, even the protein-supplemented variety.

Food technologists need to extend their efforts into devising not just high-protein diets but high-protein, high-energy, low-bulk diets which, at the same time, are fully acceptable to young children. The diets routinely given to European children offer clues as to how this can be done. These diets contain a good proportion of fat and many items have a relatively low water content (bread, biscuits, cake, etc.). The liquid foods are also very important, especially during illness. The introduction of similar changes into the diets of children in developing countries would be an important contribution but this will need the full co-operation of agriculturalists and food technologists, taking into account modern ideas on nutrient requirements as recommended by nutritionists. Biologically significant improvements to traditional diets will not be achieved by the fragmented efforts of these three groups of scientists working in isolation from each other.

TABLE IX. A comparison of the bulkiness of two nutritionally satisfactory daily diets[a] as eaten by 1–2-year-old healthy Ugandan and European children

Meal	*Weight* (g)	*Volume* (ml)	*Energy* (kJ)	*Protein* (g)
UGANDAN				
Breakfast				
Plantain	100	—	380	1
Sweet tea	—	225	270	—
Midday				
Plantain	300	—	1130	3
Groundnut stew	100	—	630	7
Sweet tea	—	225	270	—
Evening				
Plantain	300	—	1130	3
Meat and vegetable stew	200	—	1050	16
Sweet tea	—	225	270	—
	1000	775	5130	30

Meal	*Weight* (g)	*Volume* (ml)	*Energy* (kJ)	*Protein* (g)
EUROPEAN				
Breakfast				
Boiled egg	46	—	315	6
Bread, butter, marmalade	25	—	465	2
Cocoa	—	225	985	10
Break				
Biscuits	50	—	1090	6
Milk	—	225	690	9
Lunch				
Corned beef	30	—	250	7
Potato	50	—	170	1
Baked beans	43	—	170	2
Supper				
Cocoa	—	225	985	10
	244	775	5120	53

[a] DHSS (1969) minimum requirement values are 5020 kJ and 19 g protein (n.p.u.$_{op}$ 0·70)

REFERENCES

ABLETT, J. G. and MCCANCE, R. A. (1971). *Lancet* **ii**, 517–519.

ASHWORTH, A., BELL, R., JAMES, W. P. T. and WATERLOW, J. C. (1968). *Lancet* **ii**, 600–603.

DEPARTMENT OF HEALTH AND SOCIAL SECURITY (1969). "Recommended Intakes of Nutrients for the United Kingdom." *Rep. publ. Hlth med. Subj., Lond.* No. 120, HMSO, London.

FAO/WHO(1965). "Protein Requirements." *F.A.O. Nutr. Mtg Rep. Ser.* no. 37.

FOMON, S. J. (1967). "Infant Nutrition." W. B. Saunders, Philadelphia.

FROOD, J. D. L., WHITEHEAD, R. G. and COWARD, W. A. (1971). *Lancet* **ii**, 1047–1049.

MCCANCE, R. A., RUTISHAUSER, I. H. E. and BOOZER, C. N. (1970). *Archs Dis. Childh.* **45**, 410–416.

NATIONAL RESEARCH COUNCIL (1948). *Publs natn. Res. Coun., Wash.* no. 129.

NATIONAL RESEARCH COUNCIL (1963). *Publs natn. Res. Coun., Wash.* no. 1146.

NATIONAL RESEARCH COUNCIL (1968). *Publs natn. Res. Coun., Wash.* no. 1694.

NICOL, B. M. (1971). *Nutr. Rev.* **29**, 83–88.

PAYNE, P. R. (1971). *In* "The First Asian Congress of Nutrition". Heidelberg. (In press.)

POSKITT, E. M. E. (1971). *Lancet* **ii**, 68–70.

RUTISHAUSER, I. H. E. and WHITEHEAD, R. G. (1972). *Br. J. Nutr.* **28**, 145–152.

SIRBU, E. R., MARGEN, S. and CALLOWAY, D. H. (1967). *Am. J. clin. Nutr.* **20**, 1158–1165.

STAFF, T. H. (1968). *E. Afr. med. J.* **45**, 399–406.

SUKHATME, P. V. (1970). *Br. J. Nutr.* **24**, 477–487.

WIDDOWSON, E. M. (1947). "A Study of Individual Children's Diets." *Spec. Rep. Ser. med. Res. Coun.* no. 257. HMSO, London.

CHAPTER 8 DISCUSSION

Are World Supplies of Protein Foods Adequate?

I. SOME OBSERVATIONS ON THE USE OF PROTEIN FOODS IN NUTRITION

It is evident that there are many different views as to the nature of the "protein problem". In particular, two aspects have always led to confusion. One concerns the social and cultural factors which influence the protein content of freely selected diets, such that as income rises from a low level, so protein intake also rises, especially protein of animal origin. The other concerns the fulfilment of physiological needs, specifically the maintenance of nitrogen balance in the adult, and achievement of reasonable standards of growth in children.

It is instructive to outline these two aspects, and to examine briefly the nature and magnitude of the problems they indicate, and also to try to identify areas for discussion.

A. Social and Cultural Factors

Most of the estimates of the so-called "protein gap" of the developing countries are based upon projections into the future of demand, i.e. purchasing power, matched against predictions of food production. Obviously any deficit of supply in relation to demand can be described as a nutrient gap, though it is often forgotten that in most cases there is a total food, i.e. energy, gap which would, if closed by provision of more of the existing types of foods, automatically reduce the protein deficit. It is perfectly reasonable to say that as personal income rises, people tend to spend more money on enriching the variety of their diet, and in most societies, though by no means in all, this implies the consumption of more animal protein foods. However, it cannot be too strongly emphasized that the need in this case is not for protein *per se*, but for the kind of protein-containing foods that people like to eat. It is a measure of the confusion that exists in people's minds about this very simple distinction that the protein gap is often expressed in terms of millions of tons of pure protein, or of skim milk powder. This kind of analysis tends to give the impression that there is a large and growing demand for protein sources which might perhaps be filled by the provision of a tasteless, odourless, colourless product of high nutritive value and low cost. There is, however, no need to elaborate upon the total failure in the past of attempts to increase the consumption of fish flours, dried skim milk and other protein isolates. In the absence of any appreciable sales of such products, there have been various attempts to include them in diets more or less surreptitiously, by incorporating them in bread or biscuits, on the grounds, presumably, that if people don't know what is good for them, they should somehow be induced to eat it. At the moment, fortunately, most of these schemes are in decline, since the more developed countries are finding a use for their agricultural surpluses in their own animal feed industries.

What are the aspects of this problem to which food scientists and nutritionists can contribute? Firstly, I think we need to know very much more in quantitative terms about the organoleptic properties of protein foods and, in particular, how these are related, if at all, to our more conventional ideas about nutritive value, involving tests for N balance, growth or amino acid composition, for example. Does man crave for high-protein foods? Or for foods containing proteins of high biological value? Or does he simply seek to increase the variety of his diet?

Secondly, the economic aspects of production and consumption must not be forgotten. This is particularly so in relation to unconventional food sources. The production of these must be seen in relation to the whole economy of a developing country. What is the relevance of a petroleum-grown yeast plant employing perhaps 20 men to the economic development of a predominantly subsistence-farming community with a very high unemployment rate? Perhaps the level of capital investment per job created is much more important than the cost per kg of the product.

B. Physiological Requirements

Let us now turn to the problems connected with meeting basic physiological needs for protein. Is there widespread protein deficiency in the developing world? Let us first pose this question as precisely as possible. Are their many people whose health status is limited specifically by their intake of protein, i.e., whose diets contain too low a proportion of protein in relation to energy and other nutrients?

Until fairly recently, many nutritionists would have answered emphatically, "yes, there are many people in the third world of whom this is true". However, as Dr Whitehead has shown, the situation is now seen to be much more complex. Firstly, over the past 20 years estimates of requirements have fallen drastically, so much so that if current estimates of the needs of infants had been available during the early 1950s, the syndrome known as kwashiorkor would probably never have been associated with a specific lack of dietary protein. Incidentally, another consequence of these reduced requirement estimates is that it is no longer possible to demonstrate a "physiological protein gap" (i.e. between requirements and consumption) for any country as a whole.

Secondly, there is a great volume of evidence available, in particular from India, to the effect that many children remain in good health while others develop the symptoms of either marasmus or kwashiorkor on diets of the same composition and quality. The only differences are in the total amounts eaten. Both types of syndrome are associated with a low intake of energy, which in that part of the world at least seems to be the primary deficiency.

Thirdly, much research in recent years into signs, symptoms and biochemical measures which might be indices of specific protein deficiency has served only to underline the fact that in most instances there is not one single factor limiting health, but many. In addition, attempts to improve growth and reduce infant mortality rates by dietary means alone have been remarkably unsuccessful, and we are forced to conclude that only a concerted effort to improve public health, eradicate infectious disease and increase the quantity and quality of food consumed will be of any value at all. Thus the lessons to be learned from the past few years are:

1. At the physiological level, probably no country has an overall shortage of protein, so that the problem, if any, is one of unequal distribution and is not basically one of supply.
2. Doubt has been cast both upon the accuracy of current estimates of minimum requirements for protein and on the criteria used in establishing them. It is, however, essential to realize that nutrition policies can be formulated only on the basis of detailed studies of the food and general health background of different sections of the community in order to establish, firstly, who are poorly nourished and, secondly, if there is a

specific deficiency in the diet of one single nutrient, rather than a low intake of energy.

Establishing high target figures for recommended intakes of protein or of any other nutrient, serves only to distort the planning of food supplies, and to impede the establishment of correct priorities for the deployment of resources in health programmes. Just as in diagnosing the nutritional situation in a country, comparison of average intakes with recommended allowances gives little or no information about the prevalence of deficiency, so the achievement of some stated national target for average *per caput* consumption may, and often does, still leave the less privileged sections of the community in want.

3. Nutrition programmes in general, and protein foods programmes in particular, cannot be seen either as cheap substitutes for overall community health development, or as a means of salving the consciences of the developed countries. Providing free skim milk or lysine to put in the tea in India does nothing to reduce the need for social progress and for a more equitable division of wealth between the developed and developing countries.

II. PROTEIN AND NUTRITION POLICY

A. Introduction

This book is the product of the co-operation of specialists in a number of related and overlapping fields. In the first group are those concerned with experimental work on biochemical and physiological aspects of nutrition; within this group we can distinguish between work on farm animals, on the white rat and other laboratory animals, and on man. A second group is concerned with physical and chemical aspects of proteins. The third group covers agricultural production and utilization, the newer non-agricultural methods of synthesis, and aspects of food research and development.

The present discussion is concerned with *human* nutrition and my task is to examine how far different approaches can lead to a better knowledge of the food requirements of man, and of the utilization of foods by man, and how far and in what ways they can help in guiding national and international policies.

Debates have taken place for nearly 100 years on the role of protein in the human diet; in particular on the daily quantities of protein required, and on the relative merits of plant and animal proteins. These debates in Europe and North America have been extended in recent years to include the nutrition problems of tropical and semitropical countries where daily intakes of protein are usually low and where kwashiorkor and other disorders classified as protein-energy deficiency diseases are common.

The recent report of the FAO/WHO Joint Expert Committees on Nutrition (FAO/WHO, 1971) provides a critical review of present knowledge of protein-energy disorders and attempts to place them in perspective by affirming (i) that we are concerned in any one country first and foremost with the *general* nutrition picture: the need for balanced diets, adequate in quality and quantity, and (ii) that within this framework special attention should be given to protein. This philosophy will be followed here.

Von Muralt (1969) has examined protein needs in terms of the principles of homeostasis elaborated by Cannon in his "Wisdom of the Body" and other publications. These concepts go back to pioneer studies in nutrition, and I am indebted to Tremolieres (1971) for drawing attention to the words of Atwater and Benedict (1902):

> "One principle which thus far has not received adequate recognition in dietary standards may perhaps be expressed by saying that the standards must vary not only with the conditions of activity and environment, but also with the nutritive plane at which the body is maintained.
>
> "A man may live and work and maintain bodily equilibrium on either a higher or lower nitrogen level or energy level. One essential question is what level is most advantageous?
>
> "The answer to this must be sought not simply in metabolism experiments and dietary studies, but also in broader observations regarding bodily and mental efficiency and general health, strength, and welfare."

In the light of this statement these remarks are divided into two main sections, to examine first some problems of the countries of Europe and North America and countries on other continents which have followed the path of industrialization and urbanization, and then to make some comparisons with the developing or low-income world comprising tropical, semitropical and other countries, mainly in Africa, Asia and South America. These two groups of countries are distinguished by many indices used by economists, but there is no rigid line of demarcation; some writers prefer to add a third intermediate group of countries in a transitional stage of development.

B. Industrialized Countries

1. *Applied Nutrition*

Many of the most significant investigations and discoveries in human nutrition have come from the laboratories and clinics of Europe and North America and over the past 70 years nutritional ideas have been gradually accepted by people and governments.

The application of nutritional knowledge to man has taken place through the physician and dietician in the hospital and outpatient clinic, and through many other channels—through national and local public health authorities, catering officers of schools and residential institutions, the quartermaster or victualling officers of national defence services, scientific bodies and health-promotion groups, and general educational programmes reaching the public at large. As a consequence, many once-prevalent deficiency diseases have been virtually eradicated in temperate-zone countries over the past half-century (Davidson and Passmore, 1969; Aykroyd, 1970). In such countries, deficiency diseases may be almost unknown except when brought about in limited sections of the population by a combination of poverty and other factors—as with the geriatric problems of elderly people living alone on a food pattern limited in range and in quality.

2. *Experiences in World War II*

The validity of nutritional principles as applied to large populations was demonstrated in several countries during World War II when many of the nations involved had to implement food and nutrition policies as a condition of national survival. The methods employed in the United Kingdom are of special importance because of the magnitude of the problems faced in the supply of food for some 50 million people on an island which had for a long period imported 50% or more of its food, and the success achieved—the recognition that the health of the people was in many respects better at the end of the war than at the beginning. This success was recognized in 1947 by the Lasker Awards Committee of the American Medical Association which recommended "Awards for scientific and administrative achievements to the British Ministries of Food and Health and to the four great leaders in this historic enterprise Lord Woolton, Sir Jack Drummond, Sir Wilson Jameson and Sir John Orr". The committee believed that "this has been one of the greatest demonstrations of public health administration that the world has ever seen".

Some details of UK wartime programmes are given in various publications including Hollingsworth (1958), Baines *et al.* (1963), and Hollingsworth and Greaves (1970). It is accepted that the key success lay in the "successful collaboration between food scientists and the statisticians engaged in drawing up programmes; the first application of nutritional principles to a piece of economic planning" (Hammond, 1951).

Within a relatively rigid framework of wartime rationing, efforts were made: (i) to maintain the maximum freedom of choice; (ii) to ensure that extra food supplies were available for special groups, for example those engaged in heavy manual labour; (iii) to provide supplies of welfare foods for children and other groups; (iv) to apply fortification procedures to a limited number of staple commodities to ensure a minimum intake of nutrients from these sources (especially cereal products and margarine).

3. *National Policies*

Few countries can continue rationing and other wartime policies in time of peace, for throughout history it has been recognized that food supplies and food prices represent a sensitive area which can quickly affect—and produce reactions from—all sections of a population. In general, all European countries (including those in Eastern Europe with centralized economies) aim at providing the conditions under which people have the greatest freedom of choice of food. State action—in Europe, North America and elsewhere—has usually been through efforts (i) to maintain supplies through agricultural production policies with incentives to farmers to produce particular types of products; (ii) to control prices through agricultural and other subsidies; and through control of imports. Other lines of policy in many countries include (iii) the provision for limited groups in a population of free or subsidized meals or welfare foods; (iv) regulations for food hygiene, food safety (including the control of additives), food standards and fortification (cf. FAO/WHO 1971), and (v) the encouragement of food and nutrition education and research.

Many of the agencies concerned with the formation of public opinion about food are, in normal circumstances, *non-governmental*: medical and scientific organizations, universities and research centres; industrial bodies that sponsor educational and research programmes; and voluntary bodies of different types including those concerned with "health" programmes. To these we must add the press, radio and television used as media on the one hand for advertising, and on the other for the dissemination of factual information or opinions on topics related to food, nutrition and health. Within the formal education systems, concepts of nutrition are now introduced in some programmes of health education and in other syllabuses in schools, colleges and universities, although much remains to be done in this respect in Britain and other countries.

In looking at the formation of food and nutrition policy we cannot ignore the importance of individuals who have attempted, often with some success, to transmit laboratory and clinical findings, first to scientific bodies and then to the general public; in the United Kingdom nutrition workers such as Gowland Hopkins, McCarrison, Boyd Orr and Drummond have each made a contribution over the past 40 years both to the formation of public opinion and to government policy.

4. *National Trends*

Food choice is influenced over the course of time by a complex of social and economic factors (Anon., 1969a; Aylward, 1970a; Booher, 1948; Burgess and Dean, 1962; Yudkin and McKenzie, 1964). One lesson to be learned from European and North American experience is that good standards of nutrition depend on continuous vigilance; there are no permanent mathematical expressions that can be used to define either food composition or personal habits. Changes in food preservation and processing methods can alter the supplies of available nutrients from any one commodity, and fluctuations in general or personal economic standards can and do affect levels of intake, especially among the poor and the old. The recent White House Conference (Anon., 1969a) revealed some of the current problems in the United States, as also do geriatric investigations from several countries and reports on child health such as those on the re-emergence of rickets in some urban populations in Britain. Such reports in no way conflict with the widely-held opinions that over-nutrition in both children and adults is a major problem in many high-income countries.

With regard to protein supplies in such countries, three areas of current investigation and controversy are of special importance: (i) the relative values of plant and animal protein; (ii) the introduction of new sources of protein; and (iii) the protein requirements of children.

5. *Proteins from Plant and Animal Sources*

The newer analytical techniques as well as biological experimentation have led to the rejection of the older concepts that animal proteins were to be regarded as first class and that plant proteins were necessarily in an inferior category; research has confirmed the importance of mixed plant proteins as important components of the diet (Booher, 1948; Dean, 1953; Bender *et al.*, 1970). In most high-income countries a large proportion of the food protein comes from plant sources; for example, in Britain some 30% of protein is derived from bread and other cereal foods.

Important practical implications arose from the discovery of vitamin B_{12} (present in animal foods, but absent from most plant foods) namely that the virtues of animal products must be considered, not only in terms of the protein component but also in relation to minor constituents, which can include vitamin B_{12}, polyunsaturated lipids, and, no doubt, other nutrients not yet identified. Work on vegans (i.e. complete vegetarians) has confirmed both the value of plant protein and the importance of accessory factors. (Davidson and Passmore, 1969.)

6. *New Sources of Proteins*

Reports on the preparation and use of new sources of protein have often been given in the context of low-income countries; many such reports have tended to obscure the changes that have taken place in *industrialized* countries. Over the past 5 years there has been a notable increase in the use of protein isolates in textured and other forms in the American diet as is shown by the US Government publication on substitutes for agricultural products (Anon, 1969b) and by the establishment by the US Food and Drug Administration of standards of identity with provision for fortification.

Most of the major food firms in North America and several in Europe are now involved in research and development work on proteins from soya-bean or other oilseeds (such as groundnut, cottonseed, sesame or rapeseed), or from other plant sources (e.g. the broad bean or leaves). In addition there is active research on protein supplies from micro-organisms.

7. *Optimum Growth Rates*

In many nutritional studies with experimental animals and with man growth rates have been used as indices of the adequacy of a diet. Growth rate statistics have had a wide influence in relation to the formulation of infant and weaning foods and to welfare programmes for supplementary milk and meals for school children.

Over the past few years scientific workers in different countries have questioned some of the older assumptions and have then linked together current lines of research on the ageing process and studies on the rate of attainment of puberty. Attention has been drawn to the investigations of McCay (carried out over the 1930–50 period); he showed that with rats and other experimental animals given diets nutritionally complete, but restricted in quantity, a slowing down of the growth rate took place with a corresponding increase of the life span (McCay, 1955). These results, confirmed by several other workers, lead to questions fundamental to experimental work on animal and human nutrition. Is the *maximum* growth rate the *optimum* rate? Is the maximum diet the optimum diet?

These life span studies have been linked (cf. Aylward, 1972) with surveys carried out in North America and Western Europe which have shown that the age of puberty for girls (and probably also for boys) has been falling in recent decades. American workers have suggested that, in some populations, the age of maturity in girls may have declined by 3 or 4 months in each decade in this century and that the actual age may be linked to weight (Frisch and Revelle, 1971).

From these and other more recent studies it is clear that there are many unanswered questions. Is the lowered age of puberty desirable? What are the causes? How far is diet involved and, if so, do proteins or other nutrients play a direct role? These questions concern not only physiologists concerned with growth studies; they have implications in many different fields—in education, sociology and politics and in nutrition and public health policy.

With farm animals, the objectives of feeding practices can be largely defined in terms of the economic production of a given type of meat (or milk or eggs) at a given age. No such criteria can be applied to man. Cathcart (1947), a British pioneer in nutritional science, expressed his misgivings about certain trends in dietary practices when he stated "any diet can be regarded as defective if you put your so-called standard high enough". These misgivings are confirmed by physicians who regard obesity as the major nutritional disease in high-income countries.

C. Low-income Countries

1. *Protein–energy Deficiency Diseases*

Throughout the present century, parallel to nutritional studies in Europe and North America, important nutritional investigations were carried out in Asia and elsewhere. In many tropical and semitropical countries the extent of nutritional deficiencies was masked by the much more striking effects of malaria and other parasitic diseases. Such diseases are still endemic in many regions, but over the past twenty years public health authorities, with the aid of the newer chemotherapeutic agents and other techniques, have been able to reduce the incidence of many once-common disorders. Thus the food factor in health has become more evident, and its importance to individuals, families and communities has been recognized.

There is extensive literature on the nutritional problems of low-income countries and many reports issued by the World Health Organization, the Food and Agriculture Organization and the United Nations Children's Fund review the nutritional position in different countries or regions. Other reports deal with different aspects of malnutrition including kwashiorkor and related protein–energy deficiency diseases.

The WHO/FAO publication by Brock and Autret (1952) provided evidence for the widespread occurrence of conditions related to kwashiorkor throughout the tropical world and evidence also that these conditions led to high mortality rates among children in many countries. The term protein–energy malnutrition was adopted to cover a spectrum of disorders (see FAO/WHO 1962) and has been the subject of many reviews including those of Waterlow (1955), Latham (1965), von Muralt (1969) and McLaren and Pellett (1970). Whitehead has treated clinical and related aspects fully in Chapter 7. The recently published Report of the Joint FAO/WHO Expert Committee on Nutrition (FAO/WHO 1971) provides a detailed statement of current information with policy proposals.

2. *Current Controversies*

Over the past few years a number of writers have questioned the emphasis given to protein in UN and other aid programmes and some have gone further, to the point of suggesting that there are no protein shortages and that the major deficiencies are of energy.

These are serious questions which concern all who are responsible in any way for national policies in low-income countries and for technical assistance policies through national or international agencies. The problem may be examined from two different angles (i) clinical and other observations and associated health statistics (ii) statistical and other information about food production and distribution.

3. *The Public Health Picture*

Physicians and public health workers with experience in tropical countries are agreed that the high mortality rates among children in low-income countries are in part the result of malnutrition and, as Aykroyd (1961) said, "the most important evidence comes from direct observations, i.e. from what doctors have seen with their own eyes". He noted the "impressive volume of information coming from many parts of the world, about the prevalence of malnutrition in children attending hospitals and outpatient departments in the tropics and sub-tropics".

Although it is well recognized that nutritional problems may well arise in many areas because of shortage of energy the FAO/WHO (1971) report concludes that there is ample clinical evidence of widespread deficiencies which are caused in part by low protein intake and that these deficiencies occur not only among children but also among adults. Attention is drawn to the relationships between food intakes and infections and the importance of assuring intakes of protein and other nutrients above the physiological minimum for individuals who are suffering from parasitic and other disorders still common in tropical communities. The report may, therefore, be summarized in terms of:

(a) the importance of an adequate intake of food to supply energy.
(b) the importance of minimum supplies of all nutrients.
(c) the importance of extra intakes of protein and other nutrients required to meet conditions of stress.

4. *Food Production and Distribution*

Much of the recent controversy has centred round agricultural and food statistics. It is well recognized that in most low-income countries the intake of total protein is much lower than in high-income countries. It is also accepted that in many areas the intake of animal protein is very low indeed. Nevertheless when national figures are examined in terms of the current levels of protein requirements as proposed by the joint FAO/WHO Expert Committee (FAO/WHO, 1965), it appears that in many countries the protein produced from agriculture (and fisheries) should, on a *per caput* basis, supply *minimum* requirements.

This picture must be qualified in several ways. Agricultural statistics in many regions are far from accurate, more especially when crops (and animals) are used in large measure for home or local consumption. The extent of waste in many countries is unknown, but it may be considerable. Food distribution among the population may be very uneven, in part because of seasonal variations and transport problems, in part because of different income levels and poor purchasing habits. Further inequalities occur within the family either because of traditional patterns whereby men have first choice or because of taboos or other traditions that may affect women and children. Many of those who use statistics of low-income countries do not appear to appreciate the many possible errors which may give excessively high or excessively low figures for the intakes of any one individual or family. Detailed surveys of actual consumption are still few in number.

5. *Food Patterns*

In practice a distinction must be made between three groups of countries depending on whether the major staple is (a) wheat or millet; (b) sorghum, rice or maize; (c) starchy roots, tubers or plantain. In the first group there is a reasonable chance that if energy needs are met then protein intakes will also be adequate; in the second group protein intakes may be marginal; in the third group the protein intakes may be markedly deficient. Within any one pattern of staples much may depend on the availability and use of supplementary foods (for example the consumption of legumes, cheese or eggs).

One factor to be considered is the bulk of many vegetarian diets. This may be unimportant for the adult, but may present a real problem to growing children, more particularly if the local tradition is based on one main meal per day. The ordinary vegetarian staples usually have two disadvantages, the concentration of protein and other nutrients may be too low and the content of fibre too high. It is for these reasons that there are difficulties in so many regions where milk is not available as a component of weaning foods and where there is no readily available cheap protein equivalent.

6. *Protein Supplies*

In spite of the unsatisfactory nature of many agricultural statistics and the legitimate criticisms of the interpretation of statistics, there is little reason to dispute the importance of programmes to improve protein supplies and to ensure a better distribution. Over and above debates on current statistics is the shadow of the population increase which is a characteristic of most low-income countries. Food, including protein supplies, must be considered, not only in terms of existing populations but in relation to the likely expansion over the next few decades.

The three UN Agencies (WHO, FAO and UNICEF) primarily concerned with nutrition and protein matters established in 1958 a Protein Advisory Group to provide a forum for joint discussions and action. More recently the membership of the group has been broadened to include other bodies associated with the United Nations, and protein problems have been examined by various special committees such as the UN Advisory Committee on the Application of Science and Technology to Development. The publications of these bodies (United Nations, 1968a,b) and of other groups (e.g. President's Science Advisory Committee, 1967) have drawn world-wide attention to protein questions and have played a part in stimulating governments in both low-income and industrialized countries to examine ways and means of increasing protein and other food supplies and of improving distribution and utilization.

Many of the lines of research and development are described elsewhere in this book; they include efforts to increase the production of agricultural crops including legumes, methods for the fractionation of produce to give materials more rich in proteins and methods for the production of protein-rich infant and weaning foods.

7. *National Food and Nutrition Policies*

Whatever advice is provided by expatriate specialists from UN or other technical assistance agencies, national food policies must by their nature be worked out in the country concerned by the responsible governments. Policies, if they are to be successful on a long-term basis, must be implemented by local people familiar with local traditions and local food patterns.

Methods for the formulation and examination of national policies have been discussed in publications sponsored by UN Agencies (FAO/WHO, 1962; Johnston and Greaves, 1969). In most countries at least four ministries or departments of government are involved: Agriculture, Health, Education, Finance and Economic Development. The UN surveys stress the importance of food and nutrition officers (or units) in *each* of the ministries concerned with provision for inter-departmental co-operation through national food and nutrition councils or similar bodies.

The primary initial task of a national food and nutrition council is to secure accurate information about the nutritional situation in the country concerned, as a prelude to decisions about methods of improvement. Economics and balance of trade considerations often limit the possibility of supplies of protein foods through imports; the first stage towards a national policy is therefore the examination of existing local agricultural sources of plant and animal proteins and the preparation of a plan for increasing production and utilization.

Utilization involves the chain of operations from farm to consumer and may involve programmes for (a) reducing waste; (b) better preservation and processing; (c) the improvement of existing food products and the introduction of new ones; (d) provision for special groups, e.g. infants and school children (Aylward, 1971). In relation to (c) and (d) it is necessary to make available foods that are acceptable to individuals and groups. Various food components (e.g. lipids, vitamins and minerals) are clearly important as well as protein; protein supplies cannot be divorced from the question of general food supplies.

In many countries there are barriers to the increased production of agricultural products because of the absence of an established chemical industry (to produce fertilizers) and there are similar barriers to the use of microbiological syntheses in the absence of local production of ammonia or its equivalent.

A key point of policy is the training of local personnel at all levels (from the craftsman and technician to the graduate) able to deal with food (as distinct from agricultural) problems. The shortage of local personnel, trained in food science or some aspect of food processing, is often even more acute than the shortage of physicians or agricultural scientists (Aylward, 1971). Many governments are now taking steps to encourage the establishment of food and nutrition teaching centres at both university and sub-university levels.

It is now widely recognized that, parallel to public health and agricultural programmes, there should be active efforts to promote the diffusion of knowledge of nutrition with a view to the modification, when necessary, of local food habits. In this connection studies of food acceptability become of great importance; protein and other nutrients are of little use unless they are incorporated in foods readily acceptable by people in need and available at a sufficiently low price.

D. Some Conclusions

In industrialized countries there are still many questions of nutrition policy to be solved. One of the most important is that relating to the ideal requirements to secure optimum growth rates of children and to the criteria to be used for determining optimum nutrition. More information is required on this subject to form the background to decisions on welfare programmes such as school milk distribution. A second important question relates to the use of the newer protein sources from agricultural produce and from micro-organisms. Such products are likely to come into more common use for economic reasons, because of the rising costs of animal produce.

Low-income countries have a far wider range of policy matters to be determined. More detailed information is required on optimum levels of protein, as well as of other nutrients, to ensure adequate health of children and adults exposed to infections or other forms of stress. The relation of protein and other nutrients to the development of the brain and nervous system and to the learning process, is now to be regarded as a central area for research of great potential social importance (Elliot and Knight, 1972). There is increasing recognition of the importance of good nutrition as one of the keys to economic development (Vahlquist, 1972).

Many of the present food and nutrition problems of low-income countries have parallels in Europe during World War II. Some of the wartime programmes used in the UK and elsewhere can be studied, therefore, with advantage and applied with appropriate modifications. This is especially true in those low-income countries where two obvious recent changes are population growth with the concentration of populations in urban and industrial centres (Aylward 1970b).

REFERENCES

Anon. (1969a). "White House Conference on Food, Nutrition and Health: Final Report." U.S. Government Printing Office, Washington, D.C.

Anon. (1969b). *Misc. Publs Econ. Res. Serv. U.S. Dep. Agric.* no. 1141.

Atwater, W. O. and Benedict, F. G. (1902). *Bull. Off. Exp. Stns U.S. Dep. Agric.* no. 109. (Quoted by Tremolieres, 1971.)

Aykroyd, W. R. (1961). *Proc. Nutr. Soc.* **20**, 91–93.

Aykroyd, W. R. (1970). *F.F.H.C. Basic Study* no. 24. WHO, Geneva.

Aylward, F. (1963). *In* "The Better Use of the World's Fauna for Food" (J. D. Ovington, ed.), pp. 1–15. Institute of Biology, London.

Aylward, F. (1970a). *In* "Chemistry and Industry in the 1990s" (J. G. Gregory, ed.), pp. 73–83. Society of Chemical Industry, London.

Aylward, F. (1970b). *Proc. Nutr. Soc.* **29**, 169–175.

Aylward, F. (1971). *In* "Progress in Human Nutrition" (S. Margen, ed.), pp. 53–67. Avi Publ. Co., Westport, Conn.

Aylward, F. (1972). *Science Policy*, January.

Baines, A. H. J., Hollingsworth, D. F. and Leitch, I. (1963). *Nutr. Abstr. Rev.* **33**, 653.

Bender, A. E., Kihlberg, R., Lofqvist, B. and Munck, L. (eds.) (1970). "Evaluation of Novel Protein Products" proc. symp. 1968. Pergamon Press, Oxford.

Booher, L. E. (1948). *In* "Proteins and Amino Acids in Nutrition" (M. Sahyun, ed.), pp. 132–198. Reinhold Publishing Corp., New York.

Brock, J. F. and Autret, M. (1952). *Monograph Ser. WHO* no. 8.

Burgess, A. and Dean, R. F. A. (eds.) (1962). "Malnutrition and Food Habits" rep. conf. Cuernavaca 1960. Tavistock, London.

Cathcart, E. P. (1947). *Proc. Nutr. Soc.* **5**, 45–52.

Davidson, S. and Passmore, R. (1969). "Human Nutrition and Dietetics", 4th ed. E. S. Livingstone, Edinburgh.

Dean, R. F. A. (1953). *Spec. Rep. Ser. med. Res. Coun.* no. 279.

Elliot, K. and Knight, J. (eds.) (1972). "Lipids, Malnutrition and the Developing Brain" Ciba Foundation Symposium. Elsevier, Amsterdam.

FAO/WHO (1962). Joint FAO/WHO Expert Committee on Nutrition, Sixth Report. *F.A.O. Nutr. Mtg Rep. Ser.* no. 32.

FAO/WHO (1965). "Protein Requirements." *F.A.O. Nutr. Mtg Rep. Ser.* no. 37.

FAO/WHO (1971). Joint FAO/WHO Expert Committee on Nutrition, Eighth Report. *F.A.O. Nutr. Mtg Rep. Ser.* no. 49.

Frisch, R. E. and Revelle, R. (1971). *Archs Dis. Childh.* **46**, 695.

Hammond, R. J. (1951). "Food. Vol. 1, The Growth of Policy." HMSO and Longmans, London.

Hollingsworth, D. F. (1958). *In* "The Englishman's Food", 4th ed. (J. C. Drummond and A. Wilbraham), ch. 24. Cape, London.

Hollingsworth, D. F. and Greaves, J. P. (1970). *In* "Proteins as Human Food" (R. A. Lawrie, ed.), pp. 32–45. *Proc. Easter Sch. agric. Sci. Univ. Nott.* no. 16, 1969. Butterworths, London.

Johnston, B. F. and Greaves, J. P. (1969). Manual on Food and Nutrition Policy. *F.A.O. nutr. Stud.* no. 22.

Latham, M. (1965). Human Nutrition in Tropical Africa. FAO, Rome.

McCay, C. M. (1955). *Ciba Fdn Colloq. Ageing* **1**, 173–185.

McLaren, D. S. and Pellett, P. L. (1970). *Wld Rev. Nutr. Diet.* **12**, 43–127.

President's Science Advisory Committee (1967). "The World Food Problem." 3 vols. US Government Printing Office, Washington, D.C.

Tremolieres, J. (1971). *In* "Progress in Human Nutrition" (S. Margen, ed.), pp. 1–28. Avi Publ. Co., Westport, Conn.

United Nations (1968a). "Feeding the Expanding World Population: International Action to Avert Impending Protein Crisis." United Nations, New York.

United Nations (1968b). "The Protein Problem." Report Secretary-General no. E/4592. United Nations, New York.

VAHLQUIST, B. (ed.) (1972). "Nutrition as a priority in African Development" proc. 1971 seminar. Dag Hammarskjold Foundation, Uppsala.
VON MURALT, A. (ed.) (1969). "Protein-calorie Malnutrition" Nestlé Foundation symposium. Springer, New York.
WATERLOW, J. C. (ed.) (1955). "Protein Malnutrition" proc. conf. Jamaica, 1953. University Press, Cambridge, for FAO, WHO and Josiah Macey Jr Fdn.
YUDKIN, J. and MCKENZIE, J. C. (1964). "Changing Food Habits." MacGibbon and Kee, London.

III. GENERAL DISCUSSION

Opening the discussion, Professor A. Spicer drew attention to some of the points which he thought should be clarified. He pointed out that the question of whether there is an actual world shortage of food or of protein had been answered in many different ways by different authors who always based their answers on selected statistics.

He thought that the following points made by Dr Mauron deserved further amplification. (1) Even if the supply of food were adequate, lack of distribution would mean that it would not be available at the critical time and in the critical areas. (2) The economic conditions in many parts of the world did not allow people to buy what was available. (3) There were areas in which energy and protein needs were satisfied statistically but millions of people were forced to consume a monotonous diet and for that reason they stayed underfed.

He thought that consideration should be given to Dr Mauron's view that supplies in all areas would be adequate only if more food than was needed were available.

Several speakers had stressed the wide discrepancy between developed and underdeveloped countries. The expectation that time would even out the inequalities of wealth had not materialized. While the developed countries had gained further economic strength and material wealth, uncontrolled population growth had resulted in most of the poorer countries becoming still poorer. Was there any sign of a rational approach to population control in developing countries?

Although food production in the industrialized nations had kept pace with population increases this was not so in some developing nations and it had not risen at all in Africa. Was the "green revolution" being held back by poor irrigation facilities? Was there hope in the introduction of new varieties of cereals and legumes or were we looking for entirely new agronomical systems?

Neither the green revolution on its own, nor the improvements of protein quality by synthetic amino acid fortification or by the production of single cell proteins, and protein isolates from oilseeds and legumes, could provide the answer in isolation. Each would have to be examined on its own merits with regard to the needs of the areas concerned. What then were the criteria by which we were going to judge the suitability of one or another as a means of resolving the protein or energy shortage?

Dr R. G. Whitehead said that there was a need to determine the causes of malnutrition in various parts of the world. For example, the concentration of protein in the Ugandan diet was not too inadequate, but frequent infection toppled the precarious balance attained. An attack of measles could lead to a weight loss of 1 kg, and to replace this loss a pint of milk per day for 15 days would be needed. It would be cheaper and more practical to immunize against infection.

Mr P. R. Payne commented on the poor distribution of food. If it were true, as had been suggested, that 20–25% of Americans could be described as malnourished, then there could be no conceivable problem of supply, although certainly a severe problem of economics and social pattern. Dr D. M. Hegsted doubted this figure of 20–25%, for which there was no medical or other evidence.

Professor A. E. Bender suggested that there was a need to look at the problem as a whole. A test for malnourishment brought up the question of requirements, and here it was important to distinguish between adults and children. For adults a physiological minimum could be calculated on the basis of protein turnover, but one would not *recommend* such a diet, since it would be unpleasant. In animals, dietary protein levels which preserved balance in the liver, musculature and so on had been determined. Yet even here there was another factor. A minor stress had been inflicted on the test rats in the form of a single Nembutal injection. Those on high protein diets slept for about 2h, whereas those on a maintenance (5% protein) diet all died. Babies represented a special case, since even in hygienic Western societies they suffered an average of six bouts of mild infection in a year. Professor Bender further asked whether there was any evidence to show that animal proteins were necessary as such, since the n.p.u. of diets in advanced countries were about 0·70 and those in underdeveloped countries 0·60, on the face of it not a startling difference.

Dr B. R. Stillings asked whether, having estimated the total population's diets' n.p.u. on a national or regional basis, there was any method of estimating the adequacy or inadequacy of such a diet.

Dr B. M. Nicol recalled that he had remarked at a previous meeting that solely vegetable diets could be made quite adequate, but subsequent discussion suggested that it was cheaper to add a small amount of animal protein to ensure adequacy. He also remarked that figures for total protein production do not include items such as the African snail and the pangolin which nevertheless make an important contribution to the diet in some areas.

Dr D. S. Miller knew of no benefit from protein additional to the allowances, although he conceded that the infant was a special case. He questioned whether there really was a protein gap, since the requirement levels were so low, or whether there was simply a shortage of food. Was there any justification for producing protein rather than food?

Dr B. M. Nicol replied that FAO's recently published (1971) Commodity Projections, 1970–80 indicate that at the present time the protein available at *world production* level, using the "safe level of intake" recommended by the 1971 FAO/WHO Expert Committee on Energy and Protein Requirements, would meet 169% of human needs. However, some of this protein is diverted to animal feeds, fertilizers, and other non-food uses. In spite of the fact that there does not appear to be an overall protein *gap* there is an important protein *problem*, or rather a protein food problem, due to inequalities of food distribution between developed and developing countries and between socio-economic groups within regions and communities. Such inequalities are closely connected with employment and purchasing power, as Professor A. Spicer also indicated, since the consumer must be capable of influencing distribution. Another important factor in the protein problem is a lack of dietary energy (or food) in many developing countries which impairs protein utilization, particularly in the case of infants and young children.

Dr J. T. Worgan thought that the specific production of protein as such could be justified on the grounds that more energy could easily be produced from the same area of land in this way. He questioned whether too much protein was at present given to animals.

Dr R. G. Whitehead asked whether the reasons for protein–energy malnutrition were insufficient food or insufficient protein, or too low a dietary n.p.u., and how protein–energy malnutrition could be defined.

Dr B. M. Nicol said that the WHO/FAO definition would not be clinical; they would say that such malnutrition would be likely to occur where population intake was below requirements.

Dr K. J. Carpenter suggested that the data used by FAO was often economic, so that the protein gap could be defined as the gap between what people may want to buy in the future and what is available now. He thought that distribution problems were responsible for this gap.

Professor A. E. Bender asked whether, if one excepted babies, there were any people in the world of whom it was true to say that despite this 169% supply of protein, they were eating enough energy-containing food but insufficient protein. If not, there would be no protein gap, for at worst people need more food. Studies have shown that with greater prosperity, people buy more of the staple (e.g. rice), then more of the second staple (e.g. wheat) and only then meat. This would seem to show that people feel the lack of food most acutely.

Dr A. Uzel suggested that the greatest problem was with pre-school children. Yet what was the exact nature of the problem; was it lack of food, lack of protein, the ignorance of the mother of which foods to give the baby? She felt that perhaps an improvement in education might prove an important factor.

Mr J. C. Abbott stressed that the FAO multiprojection was a prediction based on trends in population and food production and demand. Its assumptions were general; no individual tests were included and it was not a measure of whether people will have enough protein.

Dr B. M. Nicol and Dr K. J. Carpenter urged that the discussion in this context should not be about proteins. Proteins occur in foodstuffs. The problem is a maldistribution of food, and in particular of expensive, attractive, high-quality, protein-rich foods.

Dr B. R. Stillings expressed the hope that the current confusion over malnutrition and the protein gap would be clarified and stressed that one's aim should be not merely to avoid the symptoms of clinical malnutrition but to produce a positive state of well-being.

Dr J. T. Worgan said that it was also his view that the protein problem was one of economics and distribution. He thought that in the future developing countries would face even greater problems as they now export protein to developed countries to obtain much-needed foreign exchange.

Professor H. Zucker stated that people do not buy "protein", they buy food, preferably food which they enjoy eating. Since in most cases this means animal products we should examine carefully any suggestion that we cannot "afford" animal agriculture.

Professor F. X. Aylward thought that it would be well to bear the nitrogen cycle in mind; except with legumes, it was necessary to supply nitrogen as well as minerals to the growing crops, and without an organized chemical industry there was no prospect of cheap and readily available fertilizers. He also stressed that critical examination of published figures was essential. The figures published in FAO documents did not reveal the assumptions, guesses and approximations made in the various stages of calculation. Despite such calculations, he thought that the evidence for protein–energy malnutrition was actual experience, what the physician actually saw in the field.

CHAPTER 9

The Analysis of Food Proteins, Amino Acid Composition and Nutritive Value

J. MAURON

Nestlé Products Technical Assistance Co. Ltd, La Tour de Peilz, Switzerland

I. INTRODUCTION

The central dogma of protein nutrition is that the nutritive value of a protein is defined by its essential amino acid composition. It is implied, of course, that the protein contains sufficient non-essential amino acids to minimize metabolic diversion of the essential amino acids to cover unspecific N needs. Although this central dogma is now challenged by some, we still have to rely on this working hypothesis for all practical purposes of protein evaluation. It is true that the latter is accomplished most accurately *in vivo*, but it should be borne in mind that the nutritive value of a protein food as sole protein source does not give any information about the supplementary value of such a protein in a mixed diet. The basis for such information can be given only by amino acid composition data, corrected, whenever possible, for availability and by application of the balanced aminogram concept to these data.

In essence, then, the problem lies in deciding how far amino acid data allow a prediction of protein value. Most of this discussion will be devoted to this problem. First, however, a few comments on methodology are necessary.

II. METHODOLOGY

A. Analysis of Nitrogen and Amino Acids in Foods

1. *Protein and Other Nitrogen Components*

First, we should be aware that we do not really determine protein in foodstuffs but that conventionally protein content is estimated from the N content as determined by the Kjeldahl procedure. For comparison of different materials the 6·25 factor has proved satisfactory, but with the advent of Single Cell Protein (SCP) containing high amounts of non-amino acid N in the form of nucleic acids and, to a smaller extent, amino-sugars, the controversy is again relevant. In SCP nucleic acid content must be estimated separately by extraction with perchloric acid and spectrophotometric determination at 260 nm. (For a review of nucleic acid determination see Munro and Fleck, 1966.) The nucleic acid content may then be deducted from the conventional protein value obtained from N × 6·25 in order to get an estimate of "true" protein. Another way would be to take the sum of the amino acids determined by column chromatography as an estimate of "true" protein. A distinction between conventional and "true" protein is justified only if it can be shown that the nucleic acids do not contribute to the N economy of the organism. We have found in our laboratory that nucleic acids are completely digested and absorbed, mostly as nucleosides, and that the pyrimidine nucleosides are partly incorporated into nucleic acids and partly metabolized, making their N available. We can therefore tentatively admit that about 50% of the N in nucleic acids is available, namely that of the pyrimidine bases. Since in most average diets unspecific N enhances the utilizable protein content (Kofranyi and Jekat, 1964; Kies *et al.*, 1965), nucleic acids should tentatively be included in the conventional protein figure.

A definitive settlement of the question must await precise N balance studies of the protein-sparing effect of nucleic acids.

In contrast, the N contained in the cell-wall substance of SCP is probably unavailable.

2. *Individual Amino Acids*

Automated column chromatography is nowadays the method of choice for amino acid determination and has attained a high degree of sophistication and accuracy (Light and Smith, 1963; Jacobs, 1970). There are, however, still some problems of variability when different systems are used (Porter *et al.*, 1968). In spite of these achievements, the nutritionist is still confronted with the fundamental shortcoming of amino acid analyses in foodstuffs, namely the destruction of amino acids during acid hydrolysis (Light and Smith, 1963).

In order to reduce amino acid destruction in foodstuffs the hydrolysis should be carried out in a large volume of HCl (12 mg N or less in 300 ml 6N HCl) and under N_2 (Dustin *et al.*, 1953). Twenty-four-hour hydrolysis is most commonly used. Some destruction of serine and threonine occurs and the branched-chain amino acids are not always completely liberated. The best way to overcome these difficulties is to use two hydrolysis times, 24 h and 72 h, for instance, and to extrapolate to zero and infinite times (Light and Smith, 1963). However, these precautions do not prevent the complete loss of tryptophan and the partial loss of cystine. Because of their importance tryptophan and the sulphur amino acids should always be determined independently. The sulphur amino acids should be determined routinely after performic acid oxidation of the protein, as cysteic acid and methionine sulphone (Moore, 1963). For tryptophan, no method is yet completely satisfactory, as is demonstrated by the fact that every year sees new methods appearing in the analytical market-place. A convenient method with some foodstuffs is the colorimetric determination of Spies and Chambers (1949) after predigestion with papain (Mauron *et al.*, 1960) or pronase (Procedure W of Spies, 1967).

A special separation problem arises with SCP of bacterial origin. In the ordinary chromatographic run, the diaminopimelic acid present in bacteria overlaps with methionine, resulting in greatly exaggerated methionine values and giving rise to high hopes among manufacturers of SCP. Separation of diaminopimelic acid from methionine is easily achieved by increasing the pH of the buffer by a few hundredths of a pH unit, so that cystine is moved towards alanine. It should also be noted that in the acid hydrolysates of heat-treated proteins containing reducing sugars, two basic amino acids derived from lysine appear in the chromatogram, furosine and pyridosine (Finot *et al.*, 1968, 1969). They can be used as "markers" for heat treatments. The possibility of using them for a quantitative evaluation of lysine deterioration is discussed by Finot in Chapter 34.

3. *Available Amino Acids*

Amino acid levels determined after acid hydrolysis of foods predict their *potential* value in nutrition. For some materials, and some methods of preparation, the effective value is significantly less. Despite progress in developing procedures to study how far individual amino acids are reduced in availability, the problem is far from solved.

Chemical, microbiological and enzymic methods as well as bioassays are used to estimate availability.

(*a*) *Chemical methods*. The most used chemical method is that of

Carpenter for available lysine (Carpenter, 1960; Booth, 1971). In spite of some theoretical drawbacks (discussed in Chapter 34) it certainly remains the most appropriate laboratory method with which rapidly to evaluate heat-damage to proteins.

No chemical methods are available for the determination of the availability of the other individual amino acids with the possible exception of methionine. There are some indications that methionine sulphoxide represents a form of unavailable methionine (Smith, 1972). It is found in protein isolates and in some SCP material, especially yeast. Methionine can now be distinguished from the sulphoxide by gas–liquid chromatography according to Ellinger and Smith (1971), a method that is specific for free methionine.

(*b*) *Microbiological methods*. A great advance in the determination of available amino acids was achieved by the introduction by Ford (1960) of microbiological methods using *Streptococcus zymogenes*.

The availability of seven amino acids can be determined in this way: methionine, leucine, isoleucine, arginine, histidine, valine and tryptophan (Ford, 1962). When the conditions of predigestion with papain are properly standardized, the results are quite reproducible. The method has been used most extensively for the determination of methionine. The ultimate validity of the method rests upon its confirmation by biological assays *in vivo*. For methionine good correlation with the results *in vivo* have been obtained (Carpenter *et al*., 1972). The advantage of *Streptococcus zymogenes* is that the same organism may be used to determine amino acid content in the acid hydrolysates, so that the same test series provides a comparison between amino acid content and availability. An assay for threonine, using *Streptococcus durans*, is being developed in our laboratory by Anantharaman.

(*c*) *Enzymic methods*. These have been used with success with some materials, especially milk products, to evaluate heat-damage (Mauron, 1961). The digestion is generally performed with pepsin, followed by pancreatin (Mauron *et al*., 1955). The separation of the undigested material from the amino acids and small peptides is carried out either by dialysis (Mauron *et al*., 1955), gel filtration (Ford and Salter, 1966) or membrane filtration (Prahl and Täufel, 1966). The amino acid determinations in the dialysate or filtrate are made by column chromatography or microbiological assay. For available lysine, high correlation was obtained between the enzymic *in vitro* digestion test of Mauron *et al* (1955) and the FDNB method of Carpenter (1960) with a series of milk samples (Bujard *et al*., 1967).

Enzymic digestion methods have played an important role in exposing the problem of availability and in helping to uncover some of the mechanisms involved. They have been much less successful, however, in the routine determination of available amino acids. The main reason for this is that enzymic *in vitro* digestion is never complete, so that a standard of reference represented by the unheated material is always necessary.

(*d*) *Bioassays*. The ultimate standards for the *in vitro* methods of measuring amino acid availability are bioassays with animals. Procedures using the rat or the chick have been developed for several amino acids: lysine, methionine, isoleucine and tryptophan (Pellett, 1963). Care should be taken in designing such bioassays that they are amenable to statistical analysis, such as by the slope-ratio technique described by Finney (1964). Expressing the response as "g gain/g food eaten" seems less open to error caused by appetite effects. From a recent collaborative study on the bioassay of available methionine using chicks (Carpenter *et al.*, 1972) it is concluded that materials can now be ranked consistently, but that absolute estimates of methionine availability still vary between assays and further improvements are therefore desirable if bioassays are to be used for the calibration of the *in vitro* procedures.

A completely different type of bioassay using as parameter not growth but the response of tyrosine transaminase has been proposed (Nadeem Chaudry and Evans, 1971). Since the principal factor controlling the concentration of this enzyme appears to be dietary tryptophan, its availability could be measured in this way. The first results are encouraging, but need confirmation, especially in view of the fact that tryptophan might not be the sole "regulating" amino acid.

B. Biological Assay Methods for Protein Evaluation

Methods such as the determination of PER, b.v., d., and n.p.u. are considered in other chapters, but it is appropriate to mention the use of these biological methods with intact animals for the detection of heat-damage. It is quite clear that none of these methods will detect any heat-damage involving amino acids that are not limiting in the particular protein food. In other words, essential amino acids in excess of the requirements can be damaged up to the point where they become limiting without modification of the protein value as measured by these tests. Multiple assays with various combinations of supplementary amino acids, such as have been proposed by Bender (1954), can, however, overcome this difficulty and give information on all essential amino acids.

It should also be noted that PER determination has the great advantage of disclosing possible toxic effects in protein foods, since growth is extremely sensitive to toxic factors. Whenever growth retardation persists, even after supplementation with the limiting amino acids, there is a strong suspicion of the presence of a toxic substance.

III. CORRELATION BETWEEN IN VITRO AND IN VIVO METHODS OF PROTEIN EVALUATION

A. The Chemical Score and Amino Acid Indices

1. *Chemical Scores* (c.s.)

Mitchell and Block (1946) were the first to provide a reasonably successful method for the chemical evaluation of proteins based on amino acid content. They used whole egg protein as a reference. The ratio of the quantity of each essential amino acid in a test protein to the quantity of that amino acid in whole egg protein was computed and stated as a percentage value. The chemical score of the protein was taken as the lowest egg ratio. [Under the recently-agreed system of nomenclature, values of chemical score (c.s.) are expressed relative to whole egg protein = 1·0.] The lower the lowest egg ratio, the poorer the protein as a source of amino acids; the higher the chemical score the better was the protein. Block and Mitchell (1946–7) found a good correlation between their chemical score and biological value, in spite of many imperfections, but a systematic bias was found in the sense that the chemical score underestimated biological value.

An important point in the chemical scoring method is obviously the choice of the reference protein. Thus, an alternative method for scoring proteins was proposed by the Joint FAO/WHO Expert Group in 1963, based on the provisional pattern of amino acid requirements proposed by the FAO Committee on Protein Requirements in 1957. Other possible reference proteins are human milk and cow's milk protein. In a very thorough study, Cresta *et al.* (1971) calculated the chemical scores of 339 diets from food composition tables, using egg, human milk, cow's milk and the FAO reference pattern (1957) as standards. They correlated the scores with biological value (87 cases), PER (187 cases) and n.p.u. (65 cases). They found the best correlation with n.p.u. was with egg as the standard reference. The poorest correlation was always found with the FAO reference pattern. The tendency to revert to the egg reference pattern therefore seems justified.

Bender (1961), on the other hand, found that egg had a surplus of all essential amino acids for the rat, when n.p.u. was used as the parameter. He determined the extent of the excess of each amino acid using mixtures of synthetic amino acids and arrived at target figures that can be used to calculate an alternative chemical score.

The critical part of all c.s./b.v. correlations is the lower range, where the theoretical line differs from the experimental findings. Bender showed that this part of the correlation depends on the limiting amino acid. Only when the sulphur amino acids or valine are limiting is the theoretical correlation observed; in all other cases c.s. is lower than biological value. The discrepancy is most pronounced when lysine is limiting.

We found in our laboratory that, when rat growth (PER) was taken as the parameter, egg protein could not be diluted with non-essential amino acids without loss of protein efficiency (Mauron and Mottu, 1970).

2. *Integrated Amino Acid Indices*

Because of the many discrepancies of the "score" methods, and because the concept of the "limiting amino acid" appears to be an oversimplification, not fully confirmed by experiment (see the lysine–threonine interaction reported by Rosenberg and Eckert, 1961), it was found necessary to consider additional factors. For instance, amino acids are used in metabolic processes other than the synthesis of proteins. The full complement of amino acids is not always required for these other processes, so that the utilization of a protein is not entirely limited by deficiency in a single amino acid. For tissue protein synthesis, on the other hand, all the necessary amino acids must be available at the site and at the time of synthesis. Oser (1951) therefore developed an integrated index where he used the geometric mean of the egg ratios to estimate the biological value of a protein. Another feature of Oser's index is that the assumption is made that a small amount of even the missing essential amino acid will be present in the tissue of the animal due to re-use of the products of tissue catabolism and coprophagy during the relatively short test periods used. The minimum egg ratio possible is therefore not 0 but 0·01. On the other hand egg ratios greater than 1·00 are reduced to 1·00. Mitchell (1954) modified Oser's index slightly by eliminating arginine from the calculation. The essential amino acid index according to Mitchell (MEAA) is then simply the geometric mean of the egg ratios of the essential amino acids (+ histidine).

The correlation of this index with biological values was found to be superior to that found with the original chemical score of Block and Mitchell (1946–7). However, here again a certain bias was found, but this time the computed values of the MEAA index tended to overestimate biological value. This index therefore predicts the maximum potential value of a protein.

B. Integrated Indices Based on in vitro Digestion

1. *The Pepsin Digest-Residue (PDR) Amino Acid Index*

The overestimation of biological value by the integrated indices based on total amino acids has been attributed by Sheffner (1967) to the influence of the digestive processes which modify the biological potential of the protein. He therefore studied the relationship between the pattern of amino acids released by digestive enzymes and the biological value of food proteins. Amino acid patterns resulting from *in vitro* pepsin digestion revealed differences between proteins that were not apparent from their total essential amino acid content. Consequently, an amino acid index was devised that combined the pattern of essential amino acids released by *in vitro* pepsin digestion with the amino acid pattern of the remainder of the protein, to produce an integrated index, the pepsin digest-residue (PDR) amino acid index (Sheffner *et al.*, 1956).

The PDR index correlated well with n.p.u. for a number of representative proteins and was especially valuable in detecting the effects of heat-damage (Sheffner, 1967).

However, because of its limitation to pepsin digestion, the liberated amino acids can be determined only by microbiological assay.

A modification of the PDR index that involved digestion with pepsin followed by pancreatin was therefore introduced by Akeson and Stahmann (1964).

2. *The Pepsin–Pancreatin Digest–Dialysate* (*PPDD*) *Index*

Taking advantage of our *in vitro* digestion procedure with simultaneous dialysis for the determination of amino acid availability, we combined the results of our *in vitro* digestion with Sheffner's method of calculation to establish an integrated index of protein quality, the PPDD index.

(*a*) *Description of the method.* An amount of sample corresponding to 4 g protein is first dialysed against tap water and subsequently against 0·1 M HCl. This step is not essential and can be omitted with foods containing no low molecular weight sugars. The sample is then incubated under stirring with 50 mg pepsin at a pH of about 2 and at 30°C for 16 h. After neutralization to pH 7·4 with sodium hydroxide, 100 mg pancreatin are added and the sample is transferred into a dialysis bag. Toluene and iodine are added to prevent growth of micro-organisms. The digestion mixture is incubated for 24 h at 50°C in an apparatus which incorporates automatic adjustment of the pH, stirring, heating and means of taking sample portions of dialysate at regular intervals; twenty-seven samples are taken in 24 h. Aliquots of each dialysate sample are pooled and acidified to pH 4·5. The volume of the final pool is reduced to one-sixth by concentration in a rotary evaporator at 40°C. An aliquot of this concentrated pool is taken for the determination of amino acids by automatic column chromatography according to Moore *et al.* (1958).

Determinations are also made of the total amino acid content of the material after acid hydrolysis.

(*b*) *Principle of calculation:*

(1) The essential amino acids in the protein are divided into two fractions:
 (a) The quantity of amino acids liberated by pepsin and pancreatin digestion;
 (b) the remainder of these amino acids in the protein, i.e. the residue.

(2) The patterns of amino acids in these two fractions of the protein to be tested are then compared with the respective fractions of standard egg protein, without consideration of the amount of amino acids in the fractions.

(3) A correction is made for the total quantity of essential amino acids in the fraction relative to the respective fraction of egg protein. In other words, a value is determined for the quality of the pattern and multiplied by how much of that pattern is present.

(4) Since the standard egg protein fractions are divided into about one-third of the protein in the pepsin and pancreatin digest fraction and about two-thirds in the residue fraction, when the biological value of the two fractions (the corrected geometric means) are integrated, the values are weighted accordingly.

Consequently the formula as constituted is based upon the assumption that the two most important factors which determine the efficiency of utilization of a protein are:

(a) the pattern of essential amino acids in the pepsin-pancreatin and residue stages; and

(b) the amount of amino acids as a group containing the particular pattern.

The calculations are performed exactly as described by Sheffner *et al.* (1956).

C. Correlation Between Chemical, Enzymic and Biological Protein Evaluation

In order to establish the relative merits of the different laboratory procedures in estimating protein quality, we started systematically to determine amino acid content and enzymic amino acid release in a series of conventional and unconventional proteins, protein foods and whole dishes. The aim was to have the same samples analysed in the same laboratory with the same methods in order to avoid reliance on food composition tables and published figures for nutritive value, because samples with identical names sometimes differ enormously and are really not comparable.

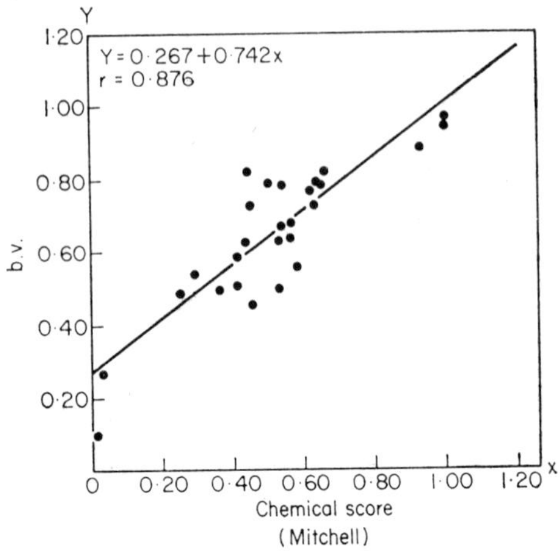

(A)

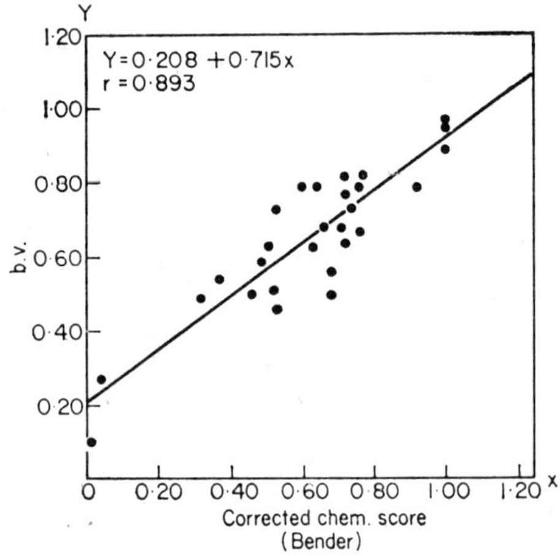

(B)

Methods used:

Amino acid content was determined in 24 h acid hydrolysates, according to Moore *et al.* (1958).

Sulphur amino acids were determined after performic oxidation of the protein (Moore, 1963). Tryptophan was measured colorimetrically according to Spies and Chambers (1949), after papain predigestion (Mauron *et al.*, 1960).

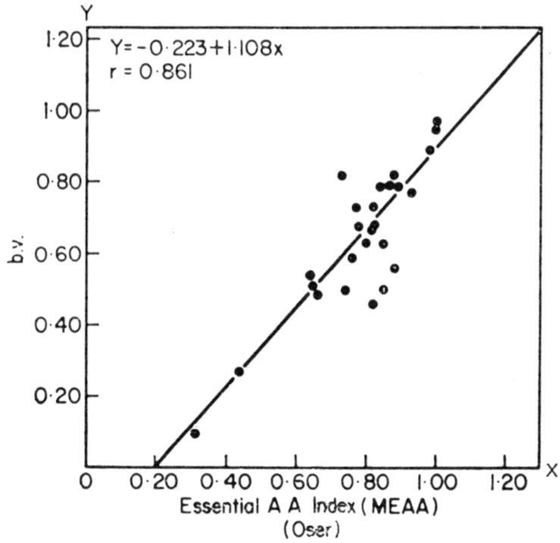

(C)

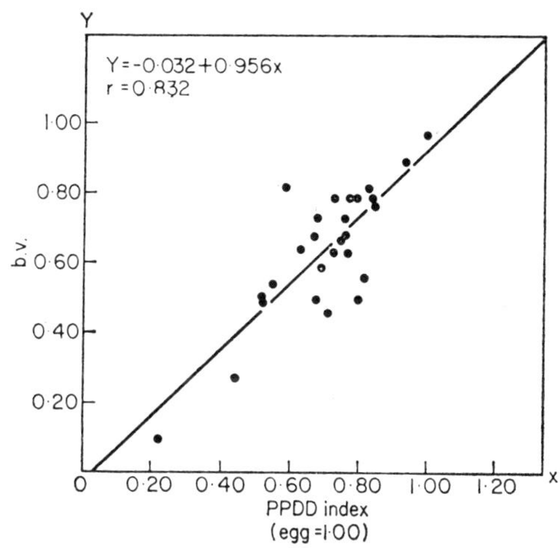

(D)

FIG. 1. The relationships between biological value and (A) chemical score; (B) corrected chemical score; (C) MEAA index and (C) PPDD index

The PPDD index was determined from enzymic *in vitro* digestion as just described.

Biological value, digestibility and n.p.u. were determined with the classic N balance method of Mitchell (1923–4) using an adaptive period of 6 days. The test diet was fed at the 10% protein level and a 2·7% egg protein diet was used for the determination of endogenous N.

The preliminary results are given in Table I.

TABLE I. Relationship between PPDD index, chemical scores and biological evaluation

Protein	*PPDD index*	*Biological value* (b.v.)	*Digestibility* (d.)	*Net protein utilization* (n.p.u.)	*Chemical score* (Mitchell)	*Corrected chemical score* (Bender)	*Essential A.A. index* (Oser) *MEEA*
Whole egg lyophilized	1·00	0·97	0·99	0·96	1·00	1·00	1·00
Whole egg defatted and lyophilized	1·03	0·95	0·96	0·91	1·00	1·00	1·00
Whole egg solids NBC	0·94	0·89	0·96	0·86	0·93	1·00	0·98
Spray-dried milk	0·85	0·77	0·93	0·71	0·62	0·72	0·93
Roller-dried milk	0·77	0·63	0·83	0·52	0·53	0·63	0·85
Beef meat	0·83	0·82	0·96	0·78	0·66	0·77	0·88
Fish protein meal	0·80	0·50	0·81	0·40	0·53	0·68	0·85
Fish protein isolate meal	0·79	0·79	0·97	0·77	0·50	0·60	0·84
Soya-bean isolate	0·71	0·46	0·97	0·44	0·45	0·53	0·82
Green pea flour	0·69	0·59	0·80	0·48	0·41	0·49	0·76
Yellow pea flour	0·73	0·63	0·89	0·56	0·43	0·51	0·80
Bean flour	0·82	0·56	0·85	0·48	0·58	0·68	0·88
Mashed potatoes	0·67	0·68	0·80	0·55	0·56	0·66	0·78
Wheat gluten	0·52	0·49	0·99	0·48	0·25	0·32	0·66

Protein	*PPDD index*	*Biological value* (b.v.)	*Digestibility* (d.)	*Net protein utilization* (n.p.u.)	*Chemical score* (Mitchell)	*Corrected chemical score* (Bender)	*Essential A.A. index* (Oser) *MEEA*
White bread (dried)	0·55	0·54	0·91	0·49	0·29	0·37	0·64
Rye flour	0·59	0·82	0·76	0·63	0·44	0·72	0·73
Zein	0·44	0·27	0·48	0·13	0·03	0·04	0·44
Maize (cooked)	0·68	0·50	0·91	0·45	0·36	0·46	0·74
Rice (cooked)	0·75	0·67	0·94	0·63	0·54	0·76	0·82
Yeast (*Candida Krusei*)	0·68	0·73	0·85	0·62	0·45	0·53	0·77
Spirulina (Maxima)	0·76	0·73	0·83	0·61	0·63	0·74	0·82
Green algae (Scenedesmus)	0·76	0·68	0·83	0·57	0·56	0·66	0·82
Gelatin (Merck)	0·22	0·10	0·89	0·09	0	0	0·31
European breakfast	0·63	0·64	0·96	0·62	0·56	0·72	0·77
Anglo-Saxon breakfast	0·78	0·79	0·97	0·77	0·65	0·92	0·87
Complete meal	0·73	0·79	0·93	0·73	0·54	0·64	0·84
Protein-enriched cereals	0·84	0.79	0·91	0·72	0·64	0·76	0·89
Chilean diet	0·52	0·51	0·98	0·50	0·41	0·52	0·65

So far twenty-eight samples have been tested. Some figures still need confirmation by repetition. Nevertheless, the general trend of the correlations is quite obvious from Fig. 1. As expected, the two chemical scores underestimate b.v., so that for a score of 0 the b.v. is still 0·20 or more but, apart from this, the correlation is satisfactory. The score according to Bender (1961) appears to give slightly better estimates than the score according to Mitchell and Block (1946).

Oser's integrated essential amino acid index, as modified by Mitchell (1954) (MEAA), overestimates b.v. to about the same extent as the chemical score underestimates it.

The best estimate of b.v. is given by the PPDD index in the sense that the regression line now goes through the origin, so that there is no longer any systematic bias. The correlation itself is, however, no better than that obtained with the estimates based only on amino acid content, because the dispersion of the experimental points is not reduced.

IV. CONCLUSIONS

From the theoretical point of view it is interesting to note that an index based on the geometric mean of the egg ratios corrected for enzymic release of the essential amino acids gives the postulated 1 : 1 relationship with biological value. This could imply that the theoretical considerations upon which this index is founded have a certain validity.

From a practical point of view one may still question the benefit of the extra work involved in performing enzymic digestion of the sample instead of relying exclusively upon the chemical amino acid analysis. This depends on each particular case. Certainly, the MEAA index gives a fair, although slightly exaggerated, estimate of the nutritive potential of a protein, but it fails to show to what extent this potential is actually realized *in vivo*. In raw legumes or in severely heat-processed foods only a small part of this potential may be realized, and the MEAA index may therefore give very erroneous estimates of the nutritive value. Performing an enzymic *in vitro* digestion of the sample in addition to the chemical analysis is a safeguard against such wrong conclusions.

This enzymic method of evaluation will not only yield a PPDD index as an estimate of the biological value, but it will also supply data on amino acid availability. In many cases the latter information is even more useful than the former.

It is generally agreed that the methods of last resort for the biological evaluation of proteins are assays *in vivo*. Animal tests are, however, expensive and time- and material-consuming and yield valid information only in the hands of the expert. Even so, the results are open to a wide range of interpretations. Animal assays are generally too slow to follow the different steps of a new industrial operation or to guide a genetic screening. For these reasons *in vitro* methods, be they chemical, microbiological or enzymic, are here to stay, in spite of all their imperfections. When used with discrimination they are of great help to the nutritionist and represent an indispensable complement to the animal assays.

REFERENCES

Akeson, W. R. and Stahmann, M. A. (1964). *J. Nutr.* **83**, 257–261.

Bender, A. E. (1954). *J. Sci. Fd Agric.* **5**, 305–318.

Bender, A. E. (1961). *In* "Progress in Meeting Protein Needs of Infants and Pre-school Children" proc. symp. 1960 (L. Voris, ed.) pp. 407–424. *Publs natn. Res. Coun., Wash.* no. 843.

Block, R. J. and Mitchell, H. H. (1946–7). *Nutr. Abstr. Rev.* **16**, 249–278.

Booth, V. H. (1971). *J. Sci. Fd Agric.* **22**, 658–665.

Bujard, E., Handwerck, V. and Mauron, J. (1967). *J. Sci. Fd Agric.* **18**, 52–57.

Carpenter, K. J. (1960). *Biochem. J.* **77**, 604–610.

Carpenter, K. J., McDonald, I. and Miller, W. S. (1972). *Br. J. Nutr.* **27**, 7–17.

Cresta, M., Périssé, J., Autret, M. and Lombardo, E. (1971). *Annls Nutr. Aliment.* **25**, 61–76.

Dustin, J. P., Czajkowska, C., Moore, S. and Bigwood, E. J. (1953). *Analytica chim. Acta* **9**, 256–262.

Ellinger, G. M. and Smith, R. H. (1971). *Biochem. J.* **124**, 15P.

FAO (1957). "Protein Requirements." *F.A.O. nutr. Stud.* no. 16.

Finney, D. J. (1964). "Statistical Methods in Biological Assay", 2nd ed. Griffin, London.

Finot, P. A., Bricout, J., Viani, R. and Mauron, J. (1968). *Experientia* **24**, 1097–1099; (1969) *Experientia* **25**, 134–135.

Ford, J. E. (1960). *Br. J. Nutr.* **14**, 485–497; (1962). *Br. J. Nutr.* **16**, 409–425.

Ford, J. E. and Salter, D. N. (1966). *Br. J. Nutr.* **20**, 843–860.

Jacobs, S. (1970). *Analyst. Lond.* **95**, 370–378.

Kies, C., Williams, E. and Fox, H. M. (1965). *J. Nutr.* **86**, 357–361.

Kofranyi, E. and Jekat, F. (1964). *Hoppe-Seyler's Z. physiol. Chem.* **338**, 154–158.

Light, A. and Smith, E. L. (1963). *In* "The Proteins". 2nd ed. (H. Neurath, ed.) Vol. 1, pp. 1–44. Academic Press, New York.

Mauron, J. (1961). *In* "Progress in Meeting Protein Needs of Infants and Pre-school Children" proc. symp. 1960 (L. Voris, ed.) pp. 425–442. *Publs natn. Res. Coun., Wash.* no. 843.

Mauron, J. and Mottu, F. (1970). Unpublished results.

Mauron, J., Mottu, F. and Egli, R. H. (1960). *Annls Nutr. Aliment.* **14**, 135–150.

Mauron, J., Mottu, F., Bujard, E. and Egli, R. H. (1955). *Archs Biochem. Biophys.* **59**, 433–451.

Mitchell, H. H. (1923–4). *J. biol. Chem.* **58**, 873–903.

Mitchell, H. H. (1954). *In* "Symposium on Methods for Evaluation of Nutritional Adequacy and Status" (H. Spector *et al.*, eds.) pp. 13–28. National Research Council, Washington, D.C.

Mitchell, H. H. and Block, R. J. (1946). *J. biol. Chem.* **163**, 599–620.

Moore, S. (1963). *J. biol. Chem.* **238**, 235–237.

Moore, S., Spackman, D. H. and Stein, W. H. (1958). *Analyt. Chem.* **30**, 1185–1190.

Munro, H. N. and Fleck, A. (1966). *Meth. biochem. Analysis* **14**, 113–176.

Nadeem Chaudry, M. T. and Evans, R. A. (1971). *Proc. Nutr. Soc.* **30**, 69A–70A.

Oser, B. L. (1951). *J. Am. diet. Ass.* **27**, 396–402.

Pellett, P. L. (ed.) (1963). "Evaluation of Protein Quality." *Publs natn. Res. Coun., Wash.* no. 1100.

Porter, J. W. G., Westgarth, D. R. and Williams, A. P. (1968). *Br. J. Nutr.* **22**, 437–450.

Prahl, L. and Täufel, K. (1966). *Z. Lebensmittelunters. u. -Forsch.* **133**, 73–78.

Rosenberg, H. R. and Eckert, R. E. (1961). *In* "Progress in Meeting Protein Needs of Infants and Pre-school Children": proc. symp. 1960 (L. Voris, ed.) pp. 451–467. *Publs natn. Res. Coun., Wash.* no. 843.

Sheffner, A. L. (1967). *In* "Newer Methods of Nutritional Biochemistry" (A. A. Albanese, ed.) Vol. 3, pp. 125–195. Academic Press, New York.

Sheffner, A. L., Eckfeldt, G. A. and Spector, H. (1956). *J. Nutr.* **60**, 105–120.

Smith, R. C. (1972). *Biochim. biophys. Acta* **261**, 304–309.

Spies, J. R. (1967). *Analyt. Chem.* **39**, 1412–1416.

Spies, J. R. and Chambers, D. C. (1949). *Analyt. Chem.* **21**, 1249–1266.

CHAPTER 10

Ion-Exchange Chromatography for Amino Acid Assay: Application for Determining Amino Acid Requirements of the Rat

JOHN B. LONGENECKER

University of Texas, Austin, USA

Experimental work in our laboratory has utilized *in vivo* plasma amino acid techniques to assess the adequacy of the dietary amino acid intake (Longenecker and Hause, 1959; Longenecker and Hause, 1961; Thirumurthi and Longenecker, 1966) and the metabolism of amino acids under various stress conditions, particularly those relating to inborn errors in metabolism (Longenecker *et al.*, 1970). For many of our studies with newborn or young adult rats ion-exchange chromatography for amino acid analyses at micro-levels are required. Several systems used in our laboratory for the micro-analysis of amino acids by ion-exchange chromatography are described and results are presented that illustrate the use of these micro-techniques in adapting to the rat our Plasma Amino Acid ratio procedure, originally developed with man or dog as the test subject, to determine amino acid requirements. This adaptation to the rat will make it possible to carry out long-term growth studies to determine the validity of the procedure. If the findings are satisfactory a rapid, *in vivo* procedure will be available for the first time to assess amino acid requirements in large populations under normal and/or diseased or stress conditions.

I. ION-EXCHANGE CHROMATOGRAPHY

The major difficulty with most of the commercially available automatic amino acid analysers is that they are designed primarily for analysis of protein hydrolysates but are generally much less efficient with physiological samples. Moreover, although they are programmed to operate at rapid speeds, in most cases relatively high concentrations (0·1–0·5 micromole) of individual amino acids or large volumes (0·5–1·0 ml) of physiological fluids are required. The present discussion will deal with the adaptation of two such systems to high sensitivity micro-techniques and with modifications adapted to allow satisfactory resolution of all the common amino acids found in blood plasma.

TABLE I. Conditions employed with the various systems of ion-exchange chromatography

One-column system[a]		*Neutral and acidic amino acid system*[b]	
Column—	0·9 × 62 cm, 42°/55°C. 60 ml/h, 300 psi	Column—	0·5 × 42 cm, 45°C. 27 ml/h, 450 psi
Resin	20 μm Spherical Bio-Rad Aminex A-4	Resin	15 μm Spherical Type-3 (Technicon)
Sample—	0·01 μM amino acid 0·05 ml plasma	Sample	0·005 μM amino acid 0·025 ml plasma
Buffers—	pH 3·05, 0·2 M Sodium Citrate, 192 min pH 3·65, 0·2 M Sodium Citrate, 233 min pH 5·05, 0·35 M Sodium Citrate, 475 min	Buffers—	pH 2·68, 0·3 M Lithium Citrate, 36 min pH 2·63, 0·3 M Lithium Citrate, 62 min pH 3·28, 0·3 M Lithium Citrate, 30 min pH 4·17, 0·3 M Lithium Citrate, 92 min
Phe, Tyr and basic amino acid system[a]		*Basic amino acid system*[b]	
Column—	0·9 × 35 cm, 55°C. 60 ml/h, 75 psi	Column—	0·4 × 27 cm, 60°C. 27 ml/h, 325 psi
Resin	20 μm Spherical Bio-Rad Aminex A-5	Resin—	15 μm Spherical Type-3 (Technicon)
Sample—	0·01 μM amino acid 0·05 ml plasma	Sample—	0·005 μM amino acid 0·025 ml plasma
Buffers—	pH 5·05, 0·35 M Sodium Citrate, 300 min	Buffers—	pH 3·85, 0·5 M Lithium Citrate, 68 min pH 5·23, 0·5 M Lithium Citrate, 62 min pH 6·00, 0·8 M Lithium Citrate, 50 min

[a] Model K-8200-VG, Phoenix Precision Instrument Co., a subsidiary of Virtis Co., Gardiner, N.Y.

[b] TSM Analyser, Technicon Corp., Tarrytown, N.Y.

A. One-Column System

The complete analysis at the micro-level for the acidic, neutral and basic amino acids in a physiological sample has been accomplished by using a Phoenix Amino Acid Analyser K-8200-VG and modifying the general procedure recommended by the Phoenix Precision Instrument Company, at present a subsidiary of the Virtis Company, Gardiner, N.Y. To allow micro-analysis at high sensitivity a Honeywell recorder equipped

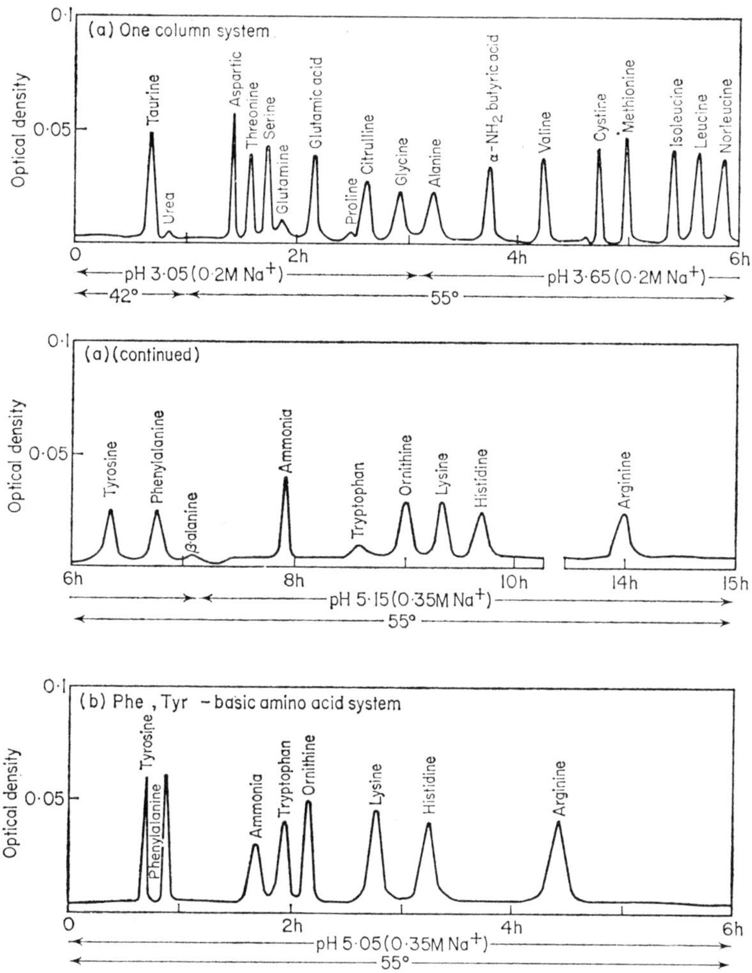

FIG. 1. Elution pattern using a modified procedure of the Phoenix Amino Acid Analyser System. (a) One-column system; (b) Phenylalanine, tyrosine and basic amino acid system

with a 1 millivolt range expander giving a full scale deflection equivalent to 0–0·1 optical density units is used. The major revision of the essential conditions for the analysis relating to the ion-exchange resin, the column size, the buffer sequence, along with other minor changes are outlined in Table I. To maintain the base-line noise at a minimum, highly-purified methylcellosolve, ninhydrin, and thiodiglycol obtained from the Pierce Chemical Company are used as well as a special "demineralizer-deionizer-cartridge" manufactured by the Continental Water Conditioning Company to treat all water used in preparation of buffers and reagents. Prior to use all buffers were washed through a 10 × 18 cm column bed of Dowex AG 50W-X8 (100–200 mesh) resin to remove any ninhydrin-reacting impurities.

With these special precautions and modifications excellent chromatographic analysis at the micro-level (0·01 micromole concentrations equivalent to 0·05 ml of plasma) are obtained as illustrated in Fig. 1a. Although this procedure does require nearly 15 h for a complete run it does provide completely satisfactory separation of all the common amino acids and in particular the three groups which generally pose the greatest problem: (1) aspartic–threonine–serine; (2) valine–cystine, and (3) tryptophan–ammonia–orthinine–lysine. By making the appropriate changes in reaction bath heating time and flow rate of buffer and ninhydrin, the running time can be decreased by 50%. However, such a change will result in less efficient resolution of some amino acids.

B. Phenylalanine, Tyrosine and Basic Amino Acids

This chromatographic system has been devised primarily for the rapid analysis of tyrosine and phenylalanine, and/or the complete analysis of phenylalanine, tyrosine and the basic amino acids in physiological samples. The Phoenix Amino Acid Analyser is employed with a 0·9 × 35 cm column. The special precautions described in the preceding section are followed and the specific conditions for the analysis are given in Table I. Using these special procedures the elution of tyrosine and phenylalanine requires approximately 1 h and the complete analysis including arginine nearly 3 h (Fig. 1b). Recovery of the amino acids from protein hydrolysates or plasma filtrates are within 3% of theoretical values. It has been noted that in carrying out repeated amino acid analysis of plasma or urine samples at the micro-level, some difficulty with base-line noise will eventually develop, apparently from contaminants in the physiological samples which are not completely removed by the normal protein-precipitation procedures. In most cases this difficulty can be overcome by routinely regenerating the column with 0·4 M NaOH instead of the generally recommended 0·2 M base.

C. Neutral and Acidic Amino Acid System

The conditions for this system are outlined in Table I. For this analysis the Technicon TSM Analyser is employed with only minor modifications in column length, buffer time and pH from the general procedure recommended by the Technicon Corporation in their Technical Publication No. TAI-0233-00. In this system a 0·5 × 42·0 cm column is employed with lithium citrate buffers. As shown in Fig. 2a the separation of the

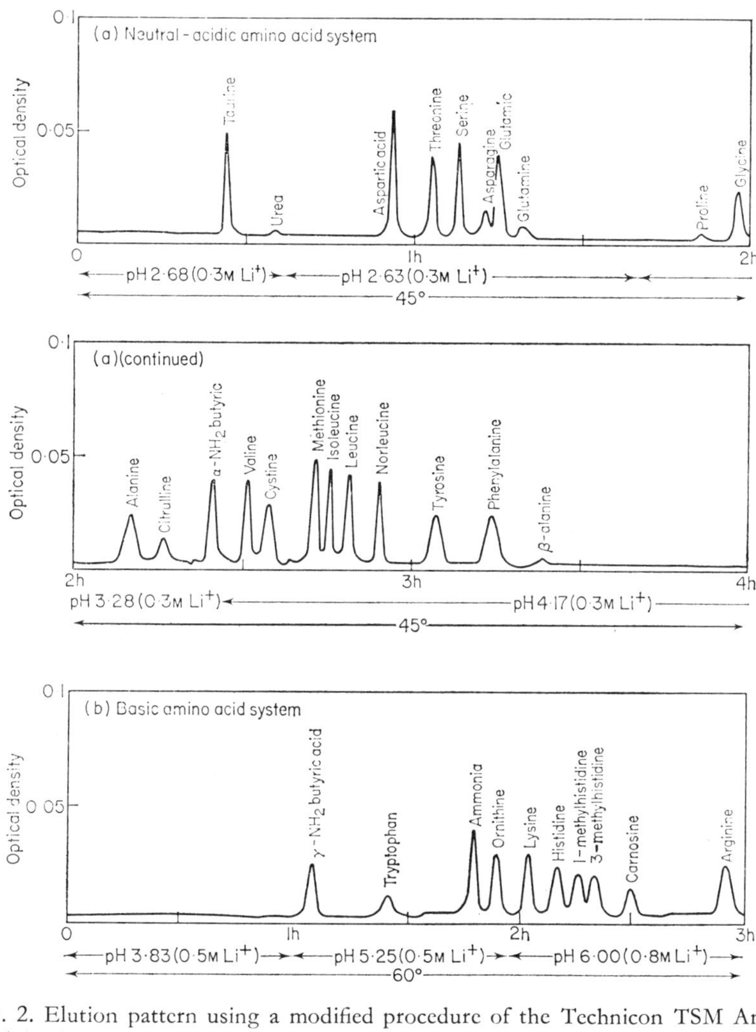

FIG. 2. Elution pattern using a modified procedure of the Technicon TSM Amino Acid Analyser System. (a) Acidic and neutral amino acid system; (b) Basic amino acid system

amino acids, when the conditions outlined in Table I are used, is exceptionally good and allows the complete resolution of the acidic and neutral amino acids in less than 3 h. To minimize base-line noise during high-sensitivity analysis of small samples, the same precautions as described in the previous section are used in the preparation of the buffers and reagents. With these special conditions the range scale expander on the recorder can be employed with a 5–10 × expansion making 1 full scale deflection equivalent to 0·1 optical density units. Two advantages of this system over the previously described Phoenix Analyser are apparent. The Technicon system is somewhat more sensitive, allowing for smaller samples, and permits analysis in approximately one-third the time.

D. Basic Amino Acid System

With the Technicon TSM Analyser the long column for the neutral and acidic amino acid analysis is coupled with a shorter column for analysis of the basic amino acids. In our laboratory a 0·4 × 27 cm column is employed for the basic amino acid system. All the specific conditions for this system are given in Table I and the elution pattern in Fig. 2b. In general the conditions used are similar to those recommended by the Technicon Corporation except for minor changes in column length, buffer time and pH. These changes have been found to provide somewhat better separation of tryptophan, ammonia, orthinine and lysine than generally obtained with the conditions recommended by the Technicon Corporation.

With the Technicon TSM Analyser the neutral and acidic amino acid system can be overlapped with the basic amino acid system and the complete analysis can be effected in approximately $5\frac{1}{2}$–6 h. The greater sensitivity of the TSM Analyser compared with the Phoenix instrument results from a higher electrical expansion of the recorder and also from the greater sensitivity of the ninhydrin reagent employed. However, one disadvantage with this system is that base-line noise can be a problem if extreme care is not taken in preparation of all reagents and buffers, and if careful maintenance of all analyser parts and accessories is not practised routinely.

II. APPLICATION FOR DETERMINING AMINO ACID REQUIREMENTS OF THE RAT

With the availability of micro-methods for amino acid analysis of plasma samples, it has been possible to adapt to the rat our *in vivo* Plasma Amino Acid ratio method which was originally developed to determine amino acid requirements with man or dogs as the test subjects (Thirumurthi and Longenecker, 1966). It has long been known that the levels of the plasma amino acids change markedly after the ingestion of a high protein meal. It has been demonstrated (Denton and Elvehjem, 1954a, b) that the absolute concentration changes of the amino acids of portal blood were generally proportional to the amount of amino acids provided by the dietary protein. However, from our initial studies such a relationship was not apparent when venous blood was analysed (Longenecker and Hause, 1959). This led us to the conclusion that the post-absorptive changes in the blood amino acid levels are due not only to the amino acid composition of the ingested protein but also to the rate at which the amino acids are removed from the blood by the body tissues. Furthermore, it was postulated that the rate of removal of the amino acids from the blood should be proportional to the requirement of the animal for individual amino acids. From experimental results obtained with dogs (Longenecker and Hause, 1959, 1961) Plasma Amino Acid (PAA) ratios that expressed the post-absorptive plasma concentration change for each essential amino acid as a function of its requirement by the test animal were calculated as follows:

$$\text{PAA ratio} = \frac{\text{B} - \text{A}}{\text{R}} \times 100$$

where:

A plasma concentration of essential amino acid after an 18 h fast.
B average post-absorptive concentration of essential amino acid in plasma during 5 h after meal.
R requirement for that individual amino acid.

When the amino acids were listed in a sequence ranging from the lowest to the highest PAA ratio, the order was nearly identical to that in which the amino acids in the dietary protein were limiting. It should be pointed out that it is necessary to have a dietary protein intake of 2–4 g/kg bodyweight with the dog, or 1–2 g/kg with man to obtain significant changes in the amino acid levels in venous blood. In this way conditions can be established whereby amino acids are being absorbed into the blood faster than they are being removed by the body tissues. This PAA ratio method provides a practical approach for direct studies in man to determine not only the sequence in which amino acids become limiting in a particular protein but also the amount of supplement needed to remove a deficiency of the most limiting amino acid, and the time at which to feed an amino acid supplement in relation to the dietary protein to obtain the maximum beneficial effect.

In other studies conducted in our laboratory (Longenecker, 1963), this general procedure was used to obtain results that provided the basis for a proposed ideal dietary amino acid pattern for normal, adult man. This pattern is somewhat different from that generally accepted from the results of nitrogen balance studies. However, it is not yet possible to determine which pattern best defines man's amino acid needs.

A. Adaptation of PAA Ratio Method to Adult Rats

The micro-technique for amino acid analysis has now been used in conjunction with our general PAA ratio procedure (Longenecker, 1963) in making similar studies with rats. For these studies it is necessary to employ a semi-force feeding technique so that the rats consume sufficient protein (3–6 g/kg) in a reasonably short period of time to produce significant changes in the levels of the plasma amino acids in the post-absorptive state. If the animals are allowed to eat a meal voluntarily the time of ingestion is quite variable and this results in large variations in the plasma amino acid changes after feeding. Therefore, in all tests the diet is prepared in a thick slurry and fed to the animal from an eye dropper. In this manner the required amount of food is ingested in approximately 5 min. To obtain the fasting and three post-prandial samples (1, 3 and 5 h after the meal) of blood from a rat several bleeding procedures have been tried but it soon became apparent that the only practicable way to obtain such samples was by an orbital sinus bleeding procedure (Stone, 1954). In this technique a Natelson-type heparinized capillary tube is inserted into the medial corner of the ventral aspect of the orbit. The orbital veins are ruptured and blood rises rapidly into the capillary. Once the technique is mastered the blood sample can be obtained in a few seconds with little stress on the rat and repeated samples can be taken from the same rat during the same day.

The results of PAA ratio studies with three-month-old rats given wheat gluten and wheat gluten supplemented with amino acids are given in Table II. In our theoretical considerations we have postulated that if the dietary amino acid intake meets the amino acid requirements of the test subject the PAA ratios should all be essentially equal. If this is the case it would indicate that the essential amino acids are being absorbed at a rate essentially equal to the rate at which they are utilized by the test animal. In Experiment 1 the two test animals were given the wheat gluten diet alone. The PAA ratios revealed the major deficiency of lysine and the slightly low levels of the sulphur amino acids, threonine and valine, whereas the other essential amino acids appeared to have fairly high ratios, indicating an excess in the dietary protein. In the second experiment, conducted with the same rats, the wheat gluten diet was supplemented with the amino acids which gave low PAA ratios in Experiment 1. With this amino acid supplementation of the wheat gluten, the PAA ratios

TABLE II. PAA ratios for wheat gluten and wheat gluten plus amino acid mixtures[a]

	Lys	*Met+Cys*	*Thr*	*Val*	*Iso*	*Arg*	*Leu*	*Phe+Tyr*	*Try*	*His*
EXPERIMENT 1 (WHEAT GLUTEN)										
Dietary amino acids (g/16 g N)	1·9	3·6	2·9	4·4	4·4	3·2	7·6	9·4	1·9	2·9
PAA Ratios										
Rat No. 1[a]	−10·8	3·2	5·1	8·4	11·6	12·0	8·9	15·1	18·9	19·1
Rat No. 2[a]	−13·1	4·1	5·8	7·1	5·6	11·6	12·5	16·0	17·0	17·2
EXPERIMENT 2 (WHEAT GLUTEN PLUS AMINO ACIDS)										
Dietary amino acids (g/16 g N)	7·5	5·5	4·0	5·0	4·2	3·1	7·4	8·9	1·0	1·9
PAA Ratios										
Rat No. 1[a]	14·6	12·6	10·6	15·4	12·5	9·8	11·6	9·9	7·1	8·1
Rat No. 2[a]	16·1	15·6	12·6	14·6	10·6	10·4	12·6	8·0	8·6	7·0
EXPERIMENT 3 (WHEAT GLUTEN PLUS AMINO ACIDS)										
Dietary amino acids (g/16 g N)[b]	6·6	4·8	4·3	4·8	4·2	3·1	7·1	9·1	1·2	2·2
PAA Ratios										
Rat No. 1[a]	8·5	7·6	8·2	10·1	9·2	7·6	8·5	8·0	8·4	9·6
Rat No. 2[a]	8·8	8·6	8·9	9·4	10·2	8·8	9·8	7·6	11·3	8·1
Ideal amino acid pattern[b]	5·5	4·0	3·6	4·0	3·5	2·6	5·9	7·6	1·0	1·8
Amino acid requirements[c]	8·2	4·6	4·6	5·0	5·0	—	6·4	6·6	1·0	2·3

[a] Three-month-old rats (275 g) semi-force fed 3·0 g of a 40% wheat gluten meal in 5 min after a 15 h fast. Water was not available to the rats during the 5 h post-prandial period and at least 7 days elapsed between experiments

[b] Predicted as the Ideal Dietary Pattern (Tryptophan set to 1·0)

[c] Requirements as given by Rao *et al.* (1964)

revealed that the amino acid balance for this dietary protein had been reversed, that is, the amino acids which were deficient were now in excess, and those which were in excess were now slightly limiting. A third experiment was conducted in which lysine, methionine and cystine, and valine supplements were reduced slightly from the levels employed in Experiment 2. With this change the PAA ratios were all essentially equal with values ranging from 7·6 to 11·3 and indicated that the dietary intake of the essential amino acids was balanced. From our theoretical considerations we should predict that this dietary pattern should be essentially the ideal dietary amino acid pattern of the three-month-old rat.

At the bottom of Table II, by setting tryptophan to 1·0, we have compared the ideal amino acid pattern as determined by the PAA ratio procedure with the amino acid requirement pattern derived from nitrogen balance data (Rao *et al.*, 1964). Although the two patterns are in general agreement, certain differences do exist, particularly for lysine and histidine.

Studies are in progress to use the PAA ratio procedure to determine amino acid requirements for rats of different ages from weanling to adult. After such results have been obtained it will then be possible to carry out long-term feeding and nitrogen balance studies to determine the validity of the requirements determined by the PAA ratio procedure.

B. Possible use of PAA Ratio Method with Newborn Rats

In addition to these studies we have been developing techniques to carry out similar *in vivo* plasma amino acid studies with newborn rats. Since the protein and amino acid needs during the first 2 weeks of life are so extremely critical, it would be valuable to develop the PAA ratio method to assess amino acid needs during this period. Adaptation of the PAA ratio procedure to the newborn rat required the development of a special intubation procedure to feed the pups. The technique developed is a modification of the procedure of Miller and Dymsza (1963) and allows for the direct intubation into the pup's stomach through polyethylene tubing (Intramedic P.E.–50/S by Clay Adams Inc.) which is attached to a 22 gauge needle. The end of the polyethylene tube that enters the oesophagus is cut straight across and the edges are bevelled smoothly with fine emery paper to facilitate easy passage into the stomach. Care must be exercised when inserting the tube, for excessive pressure can puncture the oesophagus and prove fatal to the pup. Using this procedure to feed semi-synthetic diets (containing at least 40% rat milk), we are able to raise young rats during the first 2–3 weeks of life with normal growth and development, so long as the pups are allowed to suckle at least 4–8 h each day with either their mother or a foster mother who is no longer producing milk. In future studies we plan to use the PAA ratio procedure with newborn rats to determine their amino acids requirements during the first few weeks of life.

REFERENCES

DENTON, A. E. and ELVEHJEM, C. A. (1954a). *J. biol. Chem.* **206**, 449–454.

DENTON, A. E. and ELVEHJEM, C. A. (1954b). *J. biol. Chem.* **206**, 455–460.

LONGENECKER, J. B. (1963). *In* "Newer Methods of Nutritional Biochemistry" (A. A. Albanese, ed.) pp. 113–144. Academic Press, New York.

LONGENECKER, J. B. and HAUSE, N. L. (1959). *Archs Biochem. Biophys.* **84**, 46–59.

LONGENECKER, J. B. and HAUSE, N. L. (1961). *Am. J. clin. Nutr.* **9**, 356-362.

LONGENECKER, J. B., REED, P. B., LO, G. S., CHANG, D. Y., NASBY, M. W., WHITE, M. N. and IDE, S. (1970). *Nutr. Rep. int.* **1**, 105–112.

MILLER, S. A. and DYMSZA, H. A. (1963). *Science, N.Y.* **141**, 517–518.

RAMA RAO, P. B., NORTON, H. W. and JOHNSON, B. C. (1964). *J. Nutr.* **82**, 88–92.

STONE, S. H. (1954). *Science, N.Y.* **119**, 100.

THIRUMURTHI, H. R. and LONGENECKER, J. B. (1966). *Ann. N.Y. Acad. Sci.* **134**, 873–884.

CHAPTER 11

Chemical Scores and Availability of Amino Acids

A. E. BENDER

Queen Elizabeth College, London, England

I. INTRODUCTION

The nutritional value of a protein is its usefulness for a defined purpose such as growth in children, maintenance of tissues, restoration of losses caused by damage or disease, lactation, growth of new tissue, or, from the point of view of food supply, production of meat, fish, milk, eggs or offspring. The nutritional value of a protein should be measured for the purpose for which it is intended, yet we generally select a single index, such as biological value, and use this to designate a protein as good or otherwise for all these very different purposes.

Logically, because the protein is to be used for a biological purpose, a biological method of evaluation is preferred but a chemical method might, in practice, provide more information. One major drawback of biological assessment under standardized conditions is that other dietary and environmental factors alter the value of the protein. If, instead, the protein could be chemically defined, it might be possible to calculate its value in any set of circumstances.

Much effort has been devoted to correlating the various biological and chemical measures but even when the intended purpose of the protein is precisely defined there is no criterion: there is no "best" method against which to measure the other indices. For example, Oser's amino acid index takes into account all the essential amino acids but, although there are many reports of good or mediocre correlations between this and biological measures, no correlation should be expected since all biological measures depend only on the limiting amino acid.

Thus there are drawbacks to biological evaluation, and whereas chemical score may offer more information there are also drawbacks to this method. It is suggested below that if c.s. and b.v. are determined under standardized conditions it would be possible to use the results to calculate the biological availability of the amino acids in a protein and so provide information that could be applied to practical feeding conditions.

II. PROBLEMS OF BIOLOGICAL EVALUATION

The biological methods suffer from various disadvantages.

(a) Results obtained from all methods, growth and N balance, depend on the limiting amino acid and provide no information about other amino acids; these may be present in relative surplus or at as low a level as the limiting amino acid. Therefore these results do not allow any predictions of the effects of mixing protein foods. For example, when milk, limited by the sulphur amino acids, suffers mild heat-damage, there is a reduction in available lysine, but until this becomes the limiting amino acid the biological assay result remains unchanged. If, however, the damaged milk is tested together with cereal, and lysine is the limiting amino acid in the mixture, then the damage is revealed.

(b) The biological results vary with the experimental conditions, including the presence of other dietary factors and the level and amount of protein given. Indeed, there still appears to be controversy on the effect of protein level (Hegsted and Neff, 1970). Calloway and Spector (1954) concluded from available evidence that on a fixed adequate protein intake, the energy level is the deciding factor in N balance; on fixed adequate energy intake, protein level is the determinant. Animal assays of protein value may therefore have little relevance to conditions in developing countries.

(c) Although there is considerable evidence that the various biological measures correlate well with one another (Campbell and McLaughlan, 1970) and, indeed, with chemical composition, it is possible to obtain misleading results if conditions influence the amount of food eaten by experimental animals. For example, Shyamala and Kennedy (1962) reported that cooking of wheat increased its nutritive value but Milner and Carpenter (1969) showed that this was simply due to improved palatability. White *et al.* (1958) indicated that quinua protein was as good as milk protein but Bender (1956) gave evidence to suggest that this was due to an artificially low value for milk resulting from a low food intake. Not only has it been established that some measures, such as protein efficiency ratios, are influenced by food intake but that food intake (of the rat) is influenced by nutritive value (Bender 1956).

(d) Since the rat is the most commonly used test animal and the results are often applied to man, there is a need for evidence to permit this extrapolation. Although there are differences between different experimental animals—Eggum (1971) showed that the b.v. wheat was 0·59 by rat test and 0·71 by pig test; the corresponding figures for soya-bean were 0·62 and 0·71—there does appear to be agreement between results obtained with the weanling rat and the young baby. Table I shows results

TABLE 1. Biological values of protein foods measured with rats and with children[a]

Protein	*Children*	*Young rats*
Dried skim milk	0·84	0·80
Peanut flour	0·61	0·48
Cottonseed flour	0·62	0·65
Sesame flour	0·62	0·58

[a] After Bender (1969)

obtained with the same samples of protein and measured with rats by carcass analysis and with babies by the Thomas-Mitchell procedure. Similarly Bernhard (1970) showed that apart from the sulphur amino acids the requirements of amino acids calculated per gram weight gain were similar in weanling rat and human infant; the ratios of the requirements of rat : infant were between 0·8 and 1·2.

Cremer *et al.* (1951) found that the b.v. of wheat bread alone was 0·42 in man, and 0·62 when fortified with lysine. Bender (1958) obtained results of 0·46 and 0·57 respectively for these foods in rats.

On the other hand Barness *et al.* (1961) and Bressani *et al.* (1963) both showed that wheat fortified with lysine was retained by children as well as was milk. As far as adults are concerned the b.v. of many cereals appears to be higher than for the rat; recorded rat values include 0·76 (Klein, 1926), 0·68, 0·67 (Boas-Fixsen, 1935), 0·64 (Morgan, 1931), 0·40 (FAO, 1970); and those for man shredded whole wheat, 0·90 (Murlin *et al.*, 1938) and puffed and flaked wheat, 0·80. Other results are: wheat germ, rat, 0·75, man, 0·89; oats, rat, 0·66, man, 0·89; wheat gluten, 0·40 for both.

Campbell and McLaughlan (1970) reviewed evidence to show that although in adult man all the dietary protein is used for maintenance whereas in the growing rat it is mainly used for growth, nevertheless the amino acid requirements of young and adult for both species are similar. (Table II; estimates of sulphur amino acids and methionine are excluded because they may be inaccurate for man.) The same workers found good

TABLE II. Relative essential amino acid requirements of man and rat, expressed as per cent of total for the six amino acids[a]

	Man		*Rat*		
	Boys	*Adult*	*Growing*	*Adult*	*n.p.u. Target*[b]
Tryptophan	4	6	4	5	4
Lysine	26	19	27	7	19
Threonine	16	12	15	22	15
Leucine	24	24	21	13	28
Isoleucine	16	17	17	33	16
Valine	14	22	17	20	18

[a] From Campbell and McLaughlan (1970)
[b] Target values from Table III

agreement between the values obtained for 9 proteins assayed for PER with rats or b.v. with children. They concluded that assays carried out with the growing rat at 8–10% dietary level can be used to predict the value for man.

(e) Amino acid imbalance, can, at least under experimental conditions where the amino acid is added in excessive quantities, reduce the nutritive value of a protein food.

III. CHEMICAL SCORE

A. Procedure

Chemical score is based on the assumption that the nutritive value of a protein is that of its constitutent amino acids. Two measurements are required, the chemical composition of the protein and that of a standard for comparison. In the original definition of Block and Mitchell (1946–7) egg protein was used as the standard of reference; in the subsequent definition, Protein score, an amino acid mixture was used.

Block and Mitchell (1946–7) introduced the concept by comparing the analyses and b.v.'s of a series of 37 proteins published from various laboratories. The relation between c.s. and b.v. was a straight line, not from zero to 1·0 but from b.v. 0·40, c.s. 0 to 1·0 (Fig. 1). Bender (1954)

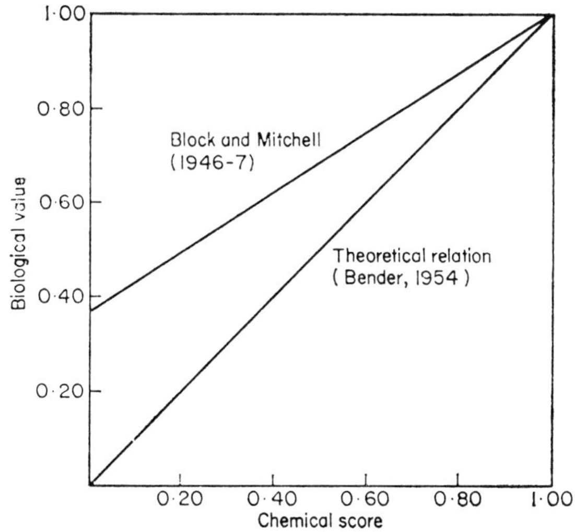

FIG. 1. Chemical score and biological value

and Fisher (1954) postulated a theoretical relationship between c.s. and b.v. as a straight line running from zero to 1·0.

More precise comparisons were made by Bender (1960, 1961, 1965) by measuring the b.v. of egg protein diluted to various levels and of amino acid mixtures. The "target" mixture (Table III) had a b.v. (duplicate esti-

TABLE III. Target amino acid mixture compared with levels used by Block and Mitchell (1946–7)

Amino acid	*Target mixture*	*Expressed as per cent of levels used by Block and Mitchell*
Histidine	1·8	86
Lysine	5·2	72
Tryptophan	1·0	67
Phenylalanine	4·9	
Methionine	2·7 }	73
Cystine	2·0 }	
Threonine	4·1	84
Leucine	7·8	85
Isoleucine	4·3	54
Valine	5·0	69

mations) of 0·92 and 0·99. It differed from the various mixtures that have been formulated for maximum growth, as would be expected. Growth depends to a large extent on the amount of food eaten as well as on its quality, and maximum growth rate will require a different mixture of amino acids from lower rates since the needs for maintenance are proportionately less. Maximum b.v. can be achieved at any growth rate.

The relation between c.s. and b.v. is shown in Fig. 2. There is a 1 : 1 relation for values of b.v. between 0·50 and 1·0; at lower values the b.v. depends on the limiting amino acid. In the absence of lysine, the b.v. is about 0·40; Block and Mitchell's original data show a b.v. of 0·37 when c.s. was zero. In the absence of valine and the sulphur amino acids the

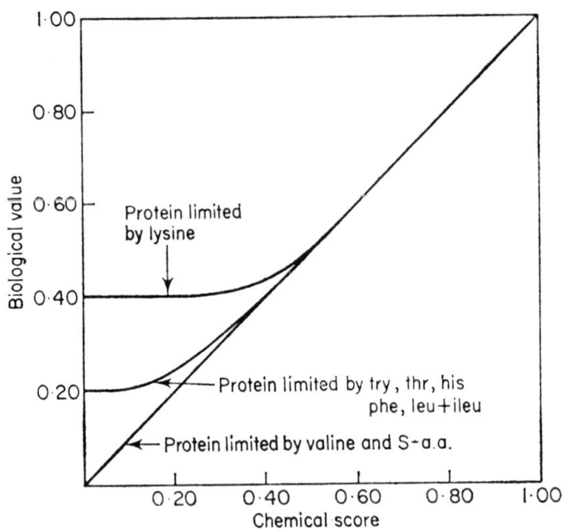

FIG. 2. Measured relationship between chemical score and biological value

b.v. is zero; in the absence of the other essential amino acids the b.v. is about 0·20. Leucine and isoleucine, as has been shown by others (Harper *et al.*, 1955; Lojkin, 1970) provide a special case of interaction; an amino acid mixture containing 50% of the target value of isoleucine had a b.v. of 0·35, when the leucine level was simultaneously reduced to 50% the b.v. increased. The ability to synthesize at least a limited amount of tissue protein in the absence of dietary lysine may be due to endogenous synthesis of these small quantities, reduced catabolism of the lysine from degraded protein tissues, or, partly at least, to the consumption of faeces (Bender, 1961).

Evidence to support the relationship between c.s. and b.v. is shown in Table IV with nine proteins and five mixtures.

TABLE IV. Comparison of chemical score with biological value

Protein	*Limiting amino acid*	*c.s.*	*b.v.*
Dried milk	S-a.a.	0·72	0·80
Dried fish	S-a.a.	0·69	0·67
Coconut protein 1	S-a.a.	0·56	0·66
Coconut protein 2	S-a.a.	0·54	0·54
Cottonseed flour 1	S-a.a.	0·68	0·65
Cottonseed flour 2	S-a.a.	0·62	0·63
Maize meal	Lysine	0·50	0·35
Yellow pea flour	S-a.a.	0·43	0·43
Mixture, maize and pea	S-a.a.	0·72	0·70
Bread	Lysine	0·38	0·50
+lysine	Threonine	0·66	0·61
+lys+thr	S-a.a.	0·87	0·80
+lys+thr+met	Valine	0·82	0·85
+lys+thr+met+val			0·93

B. Criticisms of Chemical Score as an Index of Nutritional Value

(a) Chemical analysis carried out after acid hydrolysis yields total, not available, amino acid content. In practice most of the reports of unavailable amino acids refer to animal feedingstuffs such as fish and meat meals and oilseed residues which have been badly processed, but there are a few reports of low availability in processed foods intended for human consumption.

Losses of lysine from bread on baking have been estimated at 32% (Rosenberg and Rohdenburg, 1951) and 25% (Gates and Kennedy, 1964), but Bender and Doell (unpublished results) found that the lysine in bread was 100% available, measured chemically and biologically. The accurate forecast of the b.v. of bread with supplements of lysine, threonine, methionine and valine (Table IV) indicates that the availability of all these four amino acids is 100%.

Corned beef, its n.p.u. reduced by processing from 0·75 to 0·55, has all the lysine available. Similarly the lysine of cheese is fully available (Table V).

(b) Said and Hegsted (1969) stated that if mixtures with a c.s. of zero can have a b.v. of 0·40 then the method is valueless. They stated that "these results are quite incongruous, since, in theory at least, a protein with an n.p.u. of 0·40 can meet the needs of an animal when fed in amounts 2·5 times the minimal protein need. Similarly if 5 times the minimal protein need is supplied by protein with an n.p.u. of 0·20 the protein requirements should be met. . . . There must be something wrong with either the theory or the method."

The reason why the relation changes below b.v. 0·40 is, as Said and Hegsted point out, because of the differing needs for maintenance and growth. An n.p.u. of 0·40 approximately equals a PER of zero, i.e. maintenance but not growth. Campbell and McLaughlan (1970) showed the quantitative differences between the requirements for growth and maintenance and verified the difference experimentally. Protein amino acid mixtures made to suit maintenance had an n.p.u. of 0·80 when fed at maintenance level, 2·5% protein, but this was inadequate for growth since the n.p.u. fell to 0·41 when the mixture was fed at 10%. Lactalbumin,

TABLE V. Net protein utilization and lysine availability[a]

Protein source	*Total lysine* (g/16 g N)	*Available lysine* *Biological* (%)	*Chemical* (%)	*n.p.u.*
Meat meal (animal feed)	6·2	80	78	0·41
Corned beef	8·3	99	105	
Skim milk	7·1	90	81	0·74
Cheese	7·4	101	107	
Bread	2·0	103	99	0·46
crust				0·48
crumb				0·48

[a] Bender and Doell (unpublished results)

with an amino acid composition close to the mixture needed for growth, had an n.p.u. of 0·93 when fed at 3·2% and this value remained as high as 0·79 when fed at 10%.

Biological assays at low values of n.p.u. show considerable variability, and, since the c.s./b.v. curves become almost horizontal, b.v. provides little information about the amino acid composition of the protein (conversely, c.s. is misleading). However, this does not invalidate c.s. at values above 0·40, and values below 0·40 are not a matter of any practical importance since nearly all proteins (and in all probability, every diet) have n.p.u. values greater than 0·40. According to the data collected by FAO, out of 133 values listed for different foods only 9 fall below n.p.u. 0·40 (FAO, 1970).

The textbook value of n.p.u. 0·25 for gelatin (c.s. zero) has been adduced as evidence in this discussion (Said and Hegsted, 1969), but the value is incorrect and is, in fact, zero (Bender *et al.*, 1953). The values for gelatin that had previously been reported were, in one instance, measured on pork crackling and, in the other, on a mixture of gelatin with one-tenth part of the dietary N supplied by yeast used as a source of the B vitamins.

(c) It has been shown that amino acids are released from proteins during digestion at different rates. A similar difficulty arises from the finding of Eggum (1971b) that the different amino acids in some proteins differed in digestibility. For example the digestibility of lysine in wheat was 0·79, that of histidine 0·96; that of lysine in rye was 0·65, of histidine 0·84; and that of lysine in soya-bean 0·92. Similar values were obtained with both rats and pigs. However, there is no evidence that for these reasons two proteins of the same amino acid composition differ in nutritional value.

(d) Amino acid mixtures do not always simulate proteins of the same apparent composition. Rose *et al.* (1954) found that to maintain N balance with amino acid mixtures required more dietary energy than with whole protein of the same composition. This may possibly be explained by the rate of supply of energy, an explanation that has been offered for the reduced N retention that follows when dietary starch is replaced by sucrose. It is suggested that the more rapid absorption of the sucrose leaves the absorbed protein with insufficient energy for full anabolism, compared with starch which is absorbed more slowly. It is possible that in Rose's experiments the amino acid mixture was absorbed more rapidly than the energy supply (in contrast with whole protein) and so the amino acid mixture required more energy than did the whole protein.

C. Chemical Score and Biological Analysis

The procedure for using c.s. to forecast b.v. is based on a chemical analysis of the protein or, if possible, a measure of the available limiting amino acid, with the drawbacks already discussed. It is possible, however, to use the predetermined c.s./b.v. relation as a biological measure of the available limiting amino acids in the protein. The relation shown in Fig. 2 was determined under standardized conditions: mixtures and proteins of known composition were assayed biologically. If the protein in question is assayed biologically under the same conditions, the c.s. can be read from Fig. 2 (subject to the limitations of low values). Repeated assays with supplements of amino acids would provide information of the content of available amino acids, and so permit calculations of the usefulness of the protein for any required purpose in any set of circumstances where the effects on protein utilization are known.

IV. GENERAL CONCLUSIONS

Apart from the difficulties of putting a value on a protein which may be used for a variety of different purposes, this value can vary.

(a) Human beings appear to vary in their ability to use protein. Calloway and Margen (1971) showed that the minimum daily amount of egg protein required to maintain N balance in men varied from 3·9 g to 6·8 g; the b.v. of egg protein varied from 0·45 to 0·85. Rice *et al.* (1970) reported such considerable individual variation that the results from groups of subjects had to be pooled.

(b) Nutritional value depends to some extent on the level of protein in the diet. Kies and Fox (1970) found that the second limiting amino acid in maize was trytophan when 4 g were given and methionine when 13 g were given, at the same intake of essential amino acids.

(c) Animals (in the instance of protein measurement) and man (in the instance of utilization of the protein) adapt to dietary change and alter the utilization of the protein. Pitot and Peraino (1963) showed that dietary glucose had an inhibitory effect on the inducible formation of threonine dehydratase and ornithine transaminase, whereas olive oil was not effective. Nakano and Ashida (1970) showed that starch and fat exert their protein-sparing action by retarding the inducible formation of amino acid degrading enzymes. Further, these enzymes were affected by the previous diet and the levels were lower when the previous diet had been high in fat compared with diets high in starch.

Stephen and Waterlow (1968) showed that babies adapt to changes in protein intake by similar enzyme changes, and Khan (1971) showed that adult rats adapt to energy and protein restriction after 10 days. There is abundant evidence to show that N retention is reduced when dietary starch is replaced by sucrose.

Finally, the true nutritional value of a protein, if it were known, is a matter of limited importance when that protein is used to supplement a practical diet. Firstly, the maximum range of n.p.u. of proteins likely to be used is from 0·75 for the highly-prized animal foods to about 0·50–0·60 for the despised vegetable proteins such as wheat, rice and barley. Secondly, since the best diets of the western world have an n.p.u. of 0·70 and the poor diets of the developing countries have n.p.u.'s of 0·50–0·60, supplementary foods, whether high or low in nutritional value (i.e. whether they have n.p.u.'s of 0·75 or 0·50) can have only a small effect on the protein quality of the total diet.

REFERENCES

Barness, L. A., Kaye, R. and Valyasevi, A. (1961). *Am. J. clin. Nutr.* **9**, 331–334.

Bender, A. E. (1954). *J. Sci. Fd Agric.* **5**, 305–318.

Bender, A. E. (1956). *Br. J. Nutr.* **10**, 135–143.

Bender, A. E. (1958). *Science, N.Y.* **127**, 874–875.

Bender, A. E. (1960). *Clinica chim. Acta* **5**, 1–5.

Bender, A. E. (1961). *In* "Progress in Meeting Protein Needs of Infants and Preschool Children": proc. symp. 1960 (L. Voris, ed.) pp. 407–424. *Publs natn. Res. Coun., Wash.* no. 843.

Bender, A. E. (1965). *Proc. Nutr. Soc.* **24**, 190–202.

Bender, A. E. (1969). *Chemy Ind.* pp. 904–909.

Bender, A. E., Miller, D. S. and Tunnah, E. J. (1953). *Chemy Ind.* p. 799.

Bernhart, F. W. (1970). *J. Nutr.* **100**, 461–466.

Block, R. J. and Mitchell, H. H. (1946–7). *Nutr. Abstr. Rev.* **16**, 249–278.

Boas-Fixsen, M. A. (1935). *Nutr. Abstr. Rev.* **4**, 447–459.

Boas-Fixsen, M. A., Hutchinson, J. C. D. and Jackson, H. M. (1934). *Biochem. J.* **28**, 591–601.

Bressani, R., Wilson, D., Béhar, M., Chung, M. and Scrimshaw, N. S. (1963). *J. Nutr.* **79**, 333–339.

Calloway, D. H. and Margen, S. (1971). *J. Nutr.* **101**, 205–216.

Calloway, D. H. and Spector, H. (1954). *Am. J. clin. Nutr.* **2**, 405–412.

Campbell, J. A. and McLaughlan, J. M. (1970). Symposium on Biological Evaluation of the Nutritive Value of Foods. *Int. Congr. Fd Sci. Technol. 3*, pp. 336–343. Washington, D.C.

Cremer, H. D., Lang, K., Hubbe, I. and Kulik, U. (1951). *Biochem. Z.* **322**, 58–67.

Eggum, B. O. (1971a). International symposium: "Amino Acids in Animal Husbandry": Private Communication.

Eggum, B. O. (1971b). Research Co-ordination Meeting on the Use of Nuclear Techniques for Improvement of Seed. New Delhi, India.

FAO (1970). "Amino Acid Content of Foods and Biological Data on Proteins." *F.A.O. nutr. Stud.* no. 24.

Fisher, R. B. (1954). "Protein Metabolism." Methuen, London.

Gates, J. C. and Kennedy, B. M. (1964). *J. Am diet. Ass.* **44**, 374–377.

Harper, A. E., Benton, D. A. and Elvehjem, C. A. (1955). *Archs Biochem. Biophys.* **57**, 1–12.

Hegsted, D. M. and Neff, R. (1970). *J. Nutr.* **100**, 1173–1179.

Kahn, M. A. (1971). Ph.D. Thesis, University of London.

Kies, C. and Fox, H. M. (1970). *J. Nutr.* **100**, 1275–1285.

Klein, M. (1926). *Am. J. Physiol.* **76**, 237.

Lojkin, M. E. (1970). *J. Nutr.* **100**, 51–58.

Milner, C. K. and Carpenter, K. J. (1969). *Cereal Chem.* **46**, 425–434.

Morgan, A. F. (1931). *J. biol. Chem.* **90**, 771–792.

MURLIN, J. R., NASSET, E. S. and MARCH, M. E. (1938). *J. Nutr.* **16**, 249–269.
NAKANO, K. and ASHIDA, K. (1970). *J. Nutr.* **100**, 208–216.
PITOT, H. C. and PERAINO, C. (1963). *J. biol. Chem.* **238**, 1910–1912.
RICE, H. L., SHUMAN, A. C., MATTHIAS, R. H. and FLODIN, N. W. (1970). *J. Nutr.* **100**, 847–854.
ROSE, W. C., COON, M. J. and LAMBERT, G. F. (1954). *J. biol. Chem.* **210**, 331–342.
ROSENBERG, H. R. and ROHDENBURG, E. L. (1951). *J. Nutr.* **45**, 593–598.
SAID, A. K. and HEGSTED, D. M. (1969). *J. Nutr.* **99**, 474–480.
SHYAMALA, G. and KENNEDY, B. M. (1962). *J. Am. diet. Ass.* **41**, 115–118.
STEPHEN, J. M. L. and WATERLOW, J. C. (1968). *Lancet* **i**, 118–119.
WHITE, P. L., ALVISTUR, E., DÍAS, C., VIÑAS, E., WHITE, H. S. and COLLAZOS, C. (1958). *J. agric. Fd Chem.* **3**, 531–534.

CHAPTER 12

Evaluation of Protein Quality by Dye-binding Procedures

A. L. LAKIN

Department of Food Science, University of Reading, England

I. INTRODUCTION

Three classes of dyestuffs have either been used for the evaluation of protein quality or may have potential application for this purpose. They are:

Phthalein dyes: for example, phenolphthalein and cresol red.

Reactive dyes: for example, C.I. Reactive Blue 19* or Remazol Brilliant Blue R (Hoechst).

Acid azo dyes: for example, C.I. Acid Orange 10 or Orange G, C.I. Acid Orange 12 or Acilane Orange G (Bayer) and C.I. Acid Black 1 or Amido Black 10B.

The published literature contains only a few reports on the use of phthalein dyes and reactive dyes and these will therefore be considered separately.

II. PHTHALEIN DYES AND REACTIVE DYES

A. Phthalein Dyes

1. Experimental Procedure

Phthalein dyes were introduced by Frölich (1954a,b) as a means of assessing the heat treatment given to soya-bean meal and the method was

* In order to avoid the confusion brought about by the indiscriminate use of trade names for dyestuffs, nomenclature will be based on the "Colour Index" (2nd ed.), Society of Dyers and Colourists (1956), Bradford, England.

subsequently modified by Olomucki and Bornstein (1960). In principle, the procedure involves mixing the sample with a solution of the dye dissolved in 0·1M hydrochloric acid, allowing about 1 h for equilibration, separating the supernatant by filtration and measuring its absorbance after the addition of alkali to convert the indicator to the baso-form.

It was found that the amount of dye bound by the sample progressively increased as it was subjected to more drastic heat treatment. Frölich (1954a) first reported the effect with respect to the binding of phenolphthalein by heated soya-bean meal and in a second paper (Frölich, 1954b) stated that all phthalein dyes behaved in a similar manner. He investigated particularly the use of cresol red and found that it could be used to detect the heat treatment of soya-bean meal, rapeseed meal, linseed meal and dried milk. In later work by Olomucki and Bornstein (1960) and by Ascarelli and Gestetner (1962) the growth of chicks was correlated with the binding of cresol red by heated soya-bean meals, and this work has shown that the procedure readily differentiates between unheated, properly heated and over-heated samples.

2. *Mechanism*

The nature of the association between phthalein dyes and food materials at low pH is not known. Indeed it may be that proteins are not involved in the mechanism because Frölich (1954b) has suggested that products of non-enzymic browning are responsible for the binding. One thing is certain, namely that phthalein dyes form internal salts at low pH (Tomiček, 1951) so that they are not present as anions (Fig. 1). This means that they cannot behave as acid azo dyes even though the experimental conditions employed with both groups of dyes appear to be similar.

B. Reactive Dyes

1. *Experimental Procedure*

The method described by Ney and Wirotama (1970) is much more complicated than other dye-binding techniques. After activating the dye, the pH is lowered and then the sample is added and the reaction allowed to proceed. The unreacted dye is then separated from the sample by gel-filtration and its concentration determined spectrophotometrically. This value was found to increase with time when milk was maintained at 95°C; that is, the milk proteins bound less dye because their content of available lysine fell.

2. *Mechanisms*

Reactive dyes have been employed in the dyeing industry for many years and of the several types available there are some which form covalent

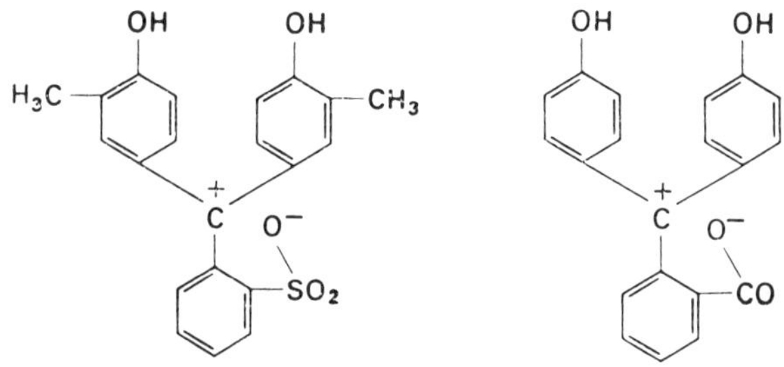

FIG. 1. Structure of phthalein dyes at pH 1·0

bonds with the free amino groups of proteins. It should be understood, however, that other groupings may also associate with these dyes, the degree of specificity depending on the structure of the dye molecule and the reaction conditions (Shore, 1968a,b,c; Beech, 1970). Even so, Ney and Wirotama (1970) have published an account of the use of Reactive Blue 19 for the determination of available lysine in milk and cheese. It may be, therefore, that these dyes are potentially useful reagents for the evaluation of protein quality.

The mechanisms responsible for the dye–protein interaction vary according to the structure of the dye molecule. Reactive Blue 19 is a vinyl sulphone dye and is believed to react as follows (Ney and Wirotama, 1970):

(a) Dye activation (maintain at 35°C for 1 h at pH 10·8)

$$\text{DYE–SO}_2.\text{CH}_2.\text{CH}_2.\text{O.SO}_3.\text{Na} + \text{NaOH} \rightarrow \text{DYE–SO}_2.\text{CH=CH}_2 + \text{Na}_2\text{SO}_4 + \text{H}_2\text{O}$$

(b) Dye–protein reaction (maintain at 60°C for $2\frac{1}{2}$ h at pH 8·0)

$$\text{DYE–SO}_2.\text{CH=CH}_2 + \text{H}_2\text{N–PROTEIN} \rightarrow \text{DYE–SO}_2.\text{CH}_2.\text{CH}_2.\text{NH–PROTEIN}$$

III. ACID AZO DYES

A. Experimental Procedure

1. Basic Technique and Applications

Nearly all the dye-binding procedures that have been used for the evaluation of protein quality employ acid azo dyes and originate from a method devised by Fraenkel-Conrat and Cooper (1944) for the determination of basic groups in proteins. Although there have been many modifications of almost every aspect of this procedure, the basic technique is always the same and it may be summarized as follows:

(a) The sample is intimately mixed with a solution of the dye which is buffered at about pH 2.
(b) During an equilibration period, which may take a few minutes or many hours, the dye and the proteins of the sample react to form insoluble complexes.
(c) A clear supernatant is obtained by filtration or centrifugation.
(d) The absorbance of the supernatant, which must contain a large excess of dye, is then measured either after dilution or in a cuvette with a very short path-length (e.g. 0·5 mm).

Although the mechanism for the dye–protein interaction will be considered later, it may be stated at this stage that the dominant factor is an electrovalent attraction between the dye anion and the proteins which are positively charged at the ambient pH value. The positive charges originate from terminal amino groups and from residues of histidine, arginine and lysine and it would therefore seem reasonable to expect a direct stoichiometric equivalence between the amount of dye bound and the number of basic groups of the proteins in the sample. It is very doubtful if this is being achieved by most of the methods in current use but there are good reasons to believe that they yield results which bear a very close relationship to the total content of basic amino acids.

It should also be noted that if the amino acid composition of the proteins of a food material remains constant, then the amounts of dye bound by samples will be a function of their total protein content. This has been found to occur with many products and this quantitative relationship has found wide application for the determination of the total protein content of many materials (Cole, 1969). These dye-binding procedures have proved to be most successful in providing rapid, inexpensive analytical methods that are highly reproducible and that are officially recognized for the analysis of certain materials (AOAC, 1970; AACC, 1962). Furthermore, their versatility has been greatly enhanced by the introduction of automatic and semi-automatic equipment which has greatly increased the throughput of samples (Udy, 1971; O'Connell, 1970).

It is because of the theoretical potential of dye-binding procedures and their practical advantages, that work has been initiated in this Department and at other centres with the object of developing these techniques as rapid, routine methods for the evaluation of protein quality, and in particular for the assessment of the content and availability of lysine.

2. *Experimental Considerations*

Although dye-binding procedures are usually simple to use, it must be emphasized that their chemistry is somewhat complex and is not fully understood. It follows, therefore, that these methods are invariably used on an empirical basis and it is essential that the experimental conditions are standardized in every respect. In particular, it is important to ensure thorough mixing of the sample and the dye so that a state of equilibrium is either attained or approached. If this condition is not fulfilled, the result will not be reproducible and a quantitative measure of total basic amino acids will not be obtained.

Soluble protein systems, such as milk, attain equilibrium within minutes (Dolby, 1961) whereas insoluble protein systems may take many hours. For example, Fraenkel-Conrat and Cooper (1944) stated that wool took more than 24 h to attain equilibrium, and Veis and Cohen (1954) found that hide collagen needed at least 36 h. However, equilibrium can be accelerated by reducing the particle size of the sample (Bunyan, 1959) and by increasing the rate of agitation of the system (Mossberg, 1969). It should be mentioned that equilibrium is rarely attained with the commercial equipment which has been developed for the determination of total protein in food commodities. This means that rigid standardization of procedure would be essential when using this type of apparatus for the evaluation of protein quality. It is also reasonable to postulate that lipid material may hinder dye penetration and that solvent extraction should be considered as a pre-treatment. Indeed Moran *et al.* (1963) found that this was necessary before comparing the dye-binding of a series of fish meals of differing fat contents.

There have been occasional reports of acid azo dyes being bound by food components other than proteins but in most cases the errors caused are negligible. Carbohydrates are known to bind small amounts of dye, and Udy (1956a, 1971) suggested that large variations in the starch content of a material might constitute a source of error. However, Ashworth (1971) stated that starch did not interfere with the use of Acid Orange 12 and this accords with our recent findings in experiments in which starch granules and gelatinized starch were added to solutions of diluted milk (Jones, G. P. and Lakin, A. L., unpublished results). We used Acid Orange 10, Acid Orange 12 and Acid Black 1 and found that, although small amounts of the dyes were bound by starch, the values were insignificant when compared with the amounts bound by milk proteins.

Udy (1956a) also suggested that the bran of cereals could be another source of interference since it bound significant amounts of Acid Orange 10, and Schou (1972) has reported a similar effect with Acid Orange 12.

Unfortunately, it is not yet resolved whether or not the amount of dye bound by bran is in excess of that bound by the proteins present in the bran. Since these proteins are known to be rich in basic amino acids (Kasarda *et al.*, 1971) it is possible that this "interference" is a true reflection of the protein content of bran. Even so, it is essential, when working with whole cereal products, to ensure that the bran is uniformly distributed throughout the samples and allowed to attain equilibrium with the dye.

Fortification of animal feeds with calcium compounds and contamination of feeds with soil may also give rise to sources of error, but such interference seems to be overcome by the addition of oxalic acid to the buffer systems (Udy, 1971; A/S N. Foss Electric, 1972a).

B. Practical Significance of Dye-binding Data

1. Variations in Protein Composition

When dye-binding procedures are used to determine the total protein of food materials, they are used on the assumption that the relative amounts of the proteins in a series of samples will either remain constant or have similar dye-binding properties. Indeed these methods are only satisfactory when this condition is fulfilled (Dolby, 1961; Mossberg, 1969). When individual proteins are investigated, however, it is usually found that their dye-binding properties vary considerably and that these differences are determined by their total content of basic amino acids. This effect was demonstrated by Fraenkel-Conrat and Cooper (1944) who examined several proteins and found excellent agreement between the numbers of basic sites and the amounts of bound Acid Orange 10; by Veis and Cohen (1954) using the same dye with different types of hide collagen, and by Alais *et al.* (1961) using Acid Black 1 and casein.

In addition to these stoichiometric relationships, the hypothesis that the binding of acid azo dyes is primarily due to association with basic amino acids is well substantiated by other work. For example, Udy (1954) found that the "soluble" proteins of wheat bound more Acid Orange 10 than the "insoluble" proteins and similar, more detailed, observations, were reported by Mossberg (1965). Subsequently, Lawrence *et al.* (1970) separated a series of wheat protein fractions by gel electrophoresis and showed that their ability to bind Acid Black 1 increased with their content of basic amino acids. Mossberg (1969) has examined several varieties of different types of cereals and has obtained good correlations between the binding of Acid Orange 12 and the total content of basic amino acids ($r = 0{\cdot}940$) and the total content of lysine (r = 0·819). Similarly, Schou (1972) has used this dye and has found good agreement between the amounts bound and the total contents of basic amino acids in lysozyme, egg albumin, insulin, protamine and barley albumin. Good correlations have also been obtained between the available lysine contents of fish meals and the binding of Acid Orange 10 (Boyne *et al.*, 1961; Baba *et al.*, 1964) and of Acid Orange 12 (A/S N. Foss Electric, 1972a).

2. *Effect of Heat on Proteins and Protein Foods*

Mild heat treatment of proteins for short periods would not be expected to cause losses of basic amino acids and so dye-binding properties should not be affected. This has been found to be so in practice. For example, the binding of Acid Orange 10 by albumin is not affected by mild heat treatment (Fraenkel-Conrat and Cooper, 1944) and neither is the binding of Acid Black 1 by milk (Vanderzant and Tennison, 1961).

On the other hand, severe heat treatment is known to affect all basic amino acids, and in particular lysine, when carbohydrates are present (Bjarnason and Carpenter, 1970). In these circumstances, therefore, dye-binding properties should be reduced and there are many reports to this effect. For example:

(a) The binding of Acid Orange 10 by "soluble" wheat proteins (Udy, 1954), by dried skim milk, whale meat meal and fish meal (NIRD, 1961), by meat and bone meal (Choppe and Kratzer, 1963), by soya-bean meal (Moran *et al.*, 1963; Pomeranz, 1965), by wheat flour (Mossberg, 1965) and by barley (Mossberg, 1966).
(b) The binding of Acid Orange 12 by soya-bean meal (Hymowitz *et al.*, 1969; Udy, 1971), and by soya-beans, wheat flour and rye meal bread (Udy, 1971).
(c) The binding of Acid Black 1 by milk (Alais *et al.*, 1961).

The only anomalous report concerning the effect of severe treatment was that the binding of Acid Orange 10 by milk proteins was not affected during the production of commercial sterilized evaporated milk (Ashworth, 1966). This appears to be surprising in that this process is known to effect a decrease in available lysine (NIRD, 1966), but it is possible that the loss was offset by the production of free amino groups from the thermal decomposition of milk proteins (Grimbleby, 1954). Ashworth (1971) has also stated that the heat treatments used to process foods have little effect on the ability of the foods to bind Acid Orange 12. It is possible, however, that the losses of available lysine were so small under the conditions studied that they were not detected by the method employed.

3. *Relevance to Evaluation of Protein quantity*

It will be evident from the foregoing discussion that, when the biological value of a food protein is limited by its content of a basic amino acid, its dye-binding properties should correlate with the results of biological tests of protein quantity. Again, there are several examples to support this inference: the binding of Acid Orange 10 has been found to be correlated with the nutritive value of fish meals (Thurston, 1957; Boyne *et al.*, 1961; Moran *et al.*, 1963; Bunyan and Woodham, 1964), whale meat meals and meat meals (Bunyan and Price, 1960; Boyne *et al.*, 1961) meat and bone meal (Choppe and Kratzer, 1963), soya-bean meal (Moran *et al.*, 1963), heat-damaged barley samples (Mossberg, 1966) and a range of miscellaneous materials (Bunyan and Price, 1960).

There have been relatively few experiments reported in which dye-binding results have not been in agreement with those of biological tests and when such disagreement has occurred it is likely that the diets were not limiting in their content of basic amino acids. For example, Moran *et al.* (1963) reported that when fish meal samples were low in sulphur-containing amino acids, dye-binding results did not agree with those of chick growth tests.

C. Theoretical Significance of Dye-binding Results

1. *Association of Acid Azo Dyes with Protein*

Although the primary mechanism in the dye–protein interaction is an electrovalent association between the dye anions and positive sites on the proteins, it is well known that secondary mechanisms may also be involved. Unfortunately, exact information is not available about the conditions employed in some dye-binding procedures but excellent reviews are available on the interactions of dyes and proteins at near-to-neutral pH values (Rosenberg and Klotz, 1960) and on the dyeing of wool (Vickerstaff, 1954). It must be stressed, however, that care should be exercised in extrapolating concepts from one set of conditions to another. For example, milk proteins bind much more Acid Orange 10 at pH 2 than they do at pH 6 (Seals and Rippie, 1966) and milk proteins do not bind acid azo dyes in the presence of 30% w/v urea (Jones, G. P. and Lakin, A. L., unpublished results), whereas wool may be dyed under these conditions (Asquith and Booth, 1971).

In addition to the electrovalent association, several possible secondary mechanisms can be postulated:

(a) Hydrogen bonding between dye molecules and proteins: all the dyes used in these methods contain groupings (—N=N—, —OH,

—NH_2, etc.) which are capable of forming hydrogen bonds with proteins.

(b) Hydrophobic bonding between dye molecules and proteins: acid azo dyes are hydrophobic structures which are made water-soluble by the substitution of polar groups, consequently they tend to associate with hydrophobic sites on proteins so as to reduce the free energy content of the system.

(c) Association, perhaps by hydrogen and/or hydrophobic bonding between free dye molecules and other dye molecules already bound to protein.

These secondary mechanisms are largely responsible for what is termed the substantivity of a dye. Dyes with poor substantivity are mainly dependent upon the electrovalent mechanism for their association with proteins, whereas this is supplemented by secondary mechanisms in dyes with good substantivity. This property is determined by the structure of the dye molecule; it is decreased by the incorporation of more sulphonic acid groups and it is raised by increasing the complexity of the molecule, particularly with respect to its aromatic and aliphatic character.

It would seem that these considerations have been used on an empirical

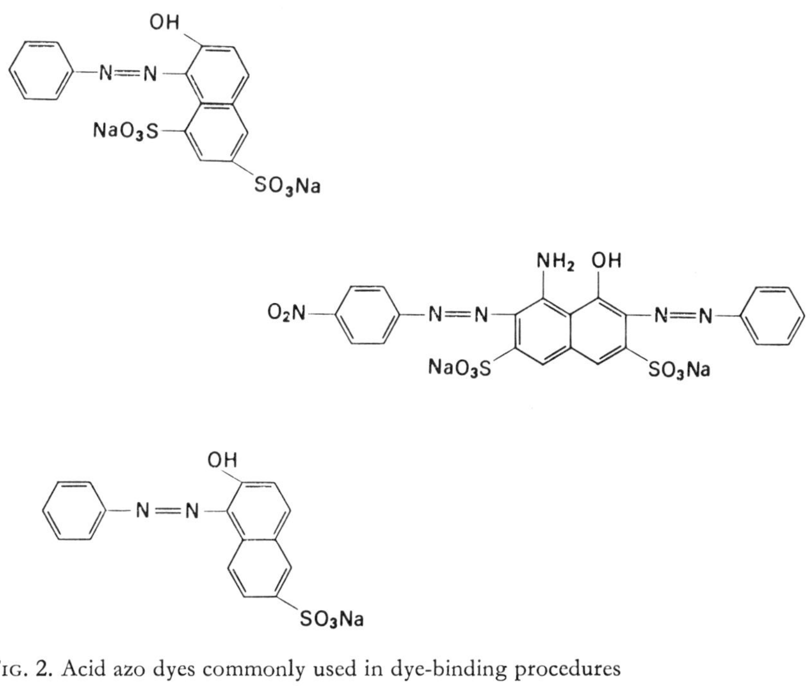

FIG. 2. Acid azo dyes commonly used in dye-binding procedures

basis during the evolution of dye-binding procedures (Fig. 2). Whether by accident or by design, Fraenkel-Conrat and Cooper (1944) selected Acid Orange 10, a dye with poor substantivity, to determine the basic groups of proteins and they obtained stoichiometric equivalence. However, this dye reacts slowly and so it has been superseded by more substantive dyes which react more quickly. Böhle and Fischer (1953) replaced it with Acid Black 1 in a method for the determination of blood proteins, and Udy (1956b) replaced it with Acid Orange 12 in methods for the determination of milk and cereal proteins. There is no doubt that these changes have been advantageous for the routine determination of total protein, but it can no longer be assumed that stoichiometric relationships still apply when these more substantive dyes are used.

We are currently investigating the effect of substantivity and have found that both milk and wheat proteins bind these dyes (milliequivalents/g protein) in the order: Acid Orange 10 < Acid Orange 12 < Acid Black 1 (i.e. in order of their substantivities). These findings suggest that secondary forces play a major role in the binding of the faster-reacting dyes and so it is likely that routine procedures based on their use could not be employed to determine basic groups without some modification.

2. *Effect of Experimental Conditions*

Of the several buffer systems which have been employed in dye-binding procedures, the most widely used are those based on citrate, citrate-phosphate and phosphate. In addition to these, complex buffer systems containing 1·0 M acetic acid have been introduced by the manufacturers of equipment for dye-binding procedures (Udy, 1971; A/S N. Foss Electric, 1972b). For example, Udy's 0·05 M phosphate buffer (AOAC, 1970) contains propionate (0·01 M), oxalate (0·02 M), phosphate (0·05 M) and acetate (1·05 M). These relatively large concentrations of acetate have been found to improve the reproducibility of routine procedures for total protein and the other components have also enhanced the versatility of the procedure (Udy, 1971).

It should be appreciated, however, that the anions associated with a buffer system compete with the dye anions for the positive sites on the protein and so the amount of dye bound will be the resultant of these two effects. The experimental evidence indicates that these equilibria are largely displaced in favour of the dye anion once it exceeds a certain concentration. Even so, dye-binding results are not absolute because the amounts of dye bound are affected by the composition of the buffer system. For example, proteins bind less Acid Orange 10 in the presence of a citrate buffer than they do in the presence of a phosphate buffer (Ashworth, 1964) and the incorporation of 1·0 M acetic acid into a phosphate buffer causes proteins to bind less Acid Orange 12 (Udy, 1971). The reasons for these effects have not yet been resolved and so for the present it would seem advisable to employ simple, well-defined buffer systems when using dye-binding procedures to evaluate protein quality.

Similar considerations apply to the selection of dyes to be used. Commercial dyestuffs are invariably contaminated with inert impurities such as sodium chloride and with interfering impurities such as other acid azo dyes (Vickerstaff, 1954). Inert impurities create difficulties in measuring the amount of dye bound by a protein (Lakin, to be published), whereas subsidiary dyes may compete with the principal component for the same sites on a protein (Dolby, 1961). These are important considerations in fundamental studies, but for empirical work dye purity is of less importance, though it can create problems in standardization. It is fortunate that the two dyes which have been most commonly used for the evaluation of protein quality can be easily purified by recrystallization; Acid Orange 10 from 90% ethanol, and Acid Orange 12 from 50% ethanol.

3. *Interpretation of Dye-binding Results*

Most of the dye-binding results reported in the literature have been obtained either with dyestuffs of unspecified purity or with complex buffer systems, or with both. Such empirical findings are very useful when associated with a particular experiment or set of conditions, and so long as the regressions are re-determined when the experimental conditions are changed or a new batch of dye is employed. However, no theoretical significance can be attached to information obtained in this way and attention must be drawn to the indiscriminate use of the term "dye-binding capacity" or "DBC". This is an almost pseudo-scientific term which implies that a given amount of protein has an affinity for a given amount of dye and values for dye-binding capacities have been widely quoted. It has been shown, however, that this value must depend upon the experimental conditions, the structure of the dye molecule, the composition of the buffer system and the purity of the dye. The temperature of the system and its pH are also important factors. It follows, therefore, that unless these parameters are specified a statement of dye-binding capacity has no real meaning and may even prove to be misleading (Lakin, unpublished results).

The results from work with pure dyes under clearly defined conditions are likely to have some fundamental significance. Such studies should provide a better understanding of dye-binding phenomena and could lead to methods for the routine determination of the total content of basic amino acids in proteins. There are good reasons to believe that this can be achieved with Acid Orange 10, a dye with poor substantivity

(Fraenkel-Conrat and Cooper, 1944; Veis and Cohen, 1954), but when reaction times are reduced by the use of more substantive dyes, it may be necessary to introduce a correction to compensate for secondary binding mechanisms.

D. Potential Application of Dye-binding Procedures

Dye-binding procedures are rapid, inexpensive methods which have been successfully adapted to automatic and semi-automatic systems of analysis. They give an empirical measurement of the total content of the basic amino acids in the proteins of a sample and this is a function of two factors: (i) the total protein content of the sample; and (ii) the amino acid composition of those proteins. Thus if the protein composition of samples remains constant, then total protein content can be determined and, conversely, if the protein contents of samples are known, then variations in basic amino acid composition can be measured. Furthermore, this second measurement will also provide an index of biological value when basic amino acids are limiting.

1. Selection of Strains for Plant Breeding

In plant breeding work there is often a need for rapid chemical methods to determine the protein and lysine contents of cereals and other seeds. If a genotype has a high dye-binding capacity it is identified as being worthy of further examination by more expensive techniques such as the determination of nitrogen content and, possibly, amino acid analysis. For example, Munck *et al.* (1969) used a dye-binding procedure to search the world barley collection for types with a high lysine content and were able to select several promising varieties. Similar work has been undertaken in India by Kaul *et al.* (1970) who are using the method to screen thousands of strains of cereals, pulses and millets. These workers have also devised a micro-method whereby the determinations are made on the endosperms of single grains so that the embryos can be saved and grown. In this way superior genotypes can be selected within two crop seasons.

2. Harvesting and Storage of Cereals

Mossberg (1970) has suggested that dye-binding procedures offer a convenient means of evaluating the various factors associated with the harvesting and storage of grain, and hence ensuring that maximum yields of protein or lysine are obtained.

In our own work with cereals we have found that the heterogeneity of grain is such that great care must be taken to avoid sampling errors. Manufacturers of equipment for dye-binding procedures suggest that grain samples may be as small as 15 g (A/S N. Foss Electric, 1971a) and the AACC (1962) stipulate that a minimum of 25 g be milled prior to the dye-binding determination. We have found that these small samples are not representative of bulk material. In order to obtain values accurate to within 1% of the mean we recommend that at least four 100 g samples of grain be taken for milling and that from each of these at least four samples be taken for the dye-binding procedure (Jones and Lakin, unpublished results).

3. *Quality Control of Foods and Animal Feeds*

There is ample evidence to suggest that dye-binding procedures can be used to monitor losses of lysine and possibly other amino acids during the processing of food proteins. When the protein content of the material is relatively constant, a simple dye-binding procedure suffices for this purpose, but with samples of variable protein content it is necessary to measure the amount of dye bound per unit weight of total nitrogen or of protein nitrogen. It is somewhat surprising that applications of this kind have been mainly confined to animal feed supplements such as fish meal and soya-bean meal and there seems to be no reason why a similar approach could not be usefully applied to the quality control of dehydrated foods such as milk, egg, meat, and other protein concentrates.

A further, logical extension of this work would be to use these methods to investigate the behaviour of food proteins during processing. It was for this reason that studies on dye–protein interactions were initiated in this University and it is hoped that our work will lead to a better understanding of the properties of food proteins.

ACKNOWLEDGEMENTS

The author wishes to thank the Agricultural Research Council and the Sainsbury Centenary Fund for grants enabling work to be carried out on the theory and application of dye-binding procedures.

REFERENCES

Alais, C., Ribadeau-Dumas, B. and Saint-Lebe, L. (1961). *Lait* **41**, 241–273.

American Association of Cereal Chemists (1962). "Cereal Laboratory Methods", 7th ed. AACC Method 46-14, AACC, St Paul, Minn.

Ascarelli, I. and Gestetner, B. (1962). *J. Sci. Fd Agric.* **13**, 401–410.

Ashworth, U. S. (1964). *J. Dairy Sci.* **47**, 672–673.

Ashworth, U. S. (1966). *J. Dairy Sci.* **49**, 133–137.

Ashworth, U. S. (1971). *J. Dairy Sci.* **54**, 752.

Asquith, R. S. and Booth, A. K. (1971). *J. Soc. Dyers Colour.* **87**, 334–337.

Association of Official Analytical Chemists (1970). "Official Methods of Analysis", 11th ed., p. 248. AOAC, Washington, D.C.

Baba, H., Matuno, N. and Niizeki, S. (1964). *Rep. natn. Inst. Nutr. Tokyo.* 6–7.

Beech, W. F. (1970). "Fibre-Reactive Dyes." Logos, London.
Bjarnason, J. and Carpenter, K. J. (1970). *Br. J. Nutr.* **24**, 313–329.
Böhle, E. and Fischer, H. (1953). *Klin. Wschr.* **31**, 798–802.
Boyne, A. W., Carpenter, K. J. and Woodham, A. A. (1961). *J. Sci. Fd Agric.* **12**, 832–848.
Bunyan, J. (1959). *J. Sci. Fd Agric.* **10**, 425–430.
Bunyan, J. and Price, S. A. (1960). *J. Sci. Fd Agric.* **11**, 25–37.
Bunyan, J. and Woodham, A. A. (1964). *Br. J. Nutr.* **18**, 537–544.
Choppe, W. and Kratzer, F. H. (1963). *Poult. Sci.* **42**, 642–646.
Cole, E. R. (1969). *Rev. pure appl. Chem.* **19**, 109–130.
Dolby, R. M. (1961). *J. Dairy Res.* **28**, 43–55.
A/S N. Foss Electric (1971a). "Operating Instructions for Pro-Meter Mk. II." Hillerød, Denmark.
A/S N Foss Electric (1971b). "Introduction of New Working Liquid for Pro-Meter Mk. II; Service Note no. 44." Hillerød, Denmark.
A/S N Foss Electric (1972a). "Measuring of Lysine and Protein in Fishmeal with Pro-Meter Mk. II; Application Note no. 4." Hillerød, Denmark.
A/S N Foss Electric (1972b). "Measuring of Protein in Alfalfa (Lucerne and Grasspills) with Pro-Meter Mk. II; Application Note no. 7." Hillerød, Denmark.
Fraenkel-Conrat, H. and Cooper, M. (1944). *J. biol. Chem.* **154**, 239–246.
Frölich, A. (1954a). *Nature, Lond.* **173**, 132–133.
Frölich, A. (1954b). *Nature, Lond.* **174**, 879.
Grimbleby, F. H. (1954). *J. Dairy Res.* **21**, 207–211.
Hymowitz, T., Collins, F. I. and Gibbons, S. J. (1969). *Agron. J.* **61**, 601–603.
Kasarda, D. D., Nimmo, C. C. and Kohler, G. O. (1971). *In* "Wheat Chemistry and Technology", 2nd ed. (Y. Pomeranz, ed.), pp. 227–299. American Association of Cereal Chemists, St Paul, Minn.
Kaul, A. K., Dhar, R. D. and Raghaviah, P. (1970). *J. Fd Sci. Technol.* **7**, 11–16.
Lawrence, J. M., Liu, S. C. and Grant, D. R. (1970). *Cereal Chem.* **47**, 110–117.
Moran, E. T., Jensen, L. S. and McGinnis, J. (1963). *J. Nutr.* **79**, 239–244.
Mossberg, R. (1965). *Agri Hort. Genet.* **23**, 206–218.
Mossberg, R. (1966). *Agri Hort. Genet.* **24**, 193–203.
Mossberg, R. (1969). *In* "New Approaches to Breeding for Improved Plant Protein", pp. 151–160. International Atomic Energy Agency, Vienna.
Mossberg, R. (1970). *Proc. Nutr. Soc.* **29**, 39–48.
Munck, L., Karlsson, K.-E. and Hagberg, A. (1969). *In* "Second International Barley Genetics Symposium", pp. 544–558. Washington State University, Pullman, Washington.
National Institute for Research in Dairying (1961). *Rep. natn. Inst. Res. Dairy.* 1960, p. 102.
National Institute for Research in Dairying (1966). *Rep. natn. Inst. Res. Dairy.* 1965, p. 144.
Ney, K. H. and Wirotama, I. P. G. (1970). *Z. Lebensmittelunters. u. -Forsch.* **144**, 92–95.

O'Connell, J. A. (1970). *Lab. Pract.* **19**, 1119–1120.
Olomucki, E. and Bornstein, S. (1960). *J. Ass. off. agric. Chem.* **43**, 440–442.
Pomeranz, Y. (1965). *J. Fd Sci.* **30**, 307–311.
Rosenberg, R. M. and Klotz, I. M. (1960). *In* "A Laboratory Manual of Analytical Methods of Protein Chemistry (Including Polypeptides). Vol. 2. The Composition, Structure and Reactivity of Proteins" (P. Alexander and R. J. Block, eds.) pp. 131–168. Pergamon, Oxford.
Schou, J. (1972). Private Communications. A/S N. Foss Electric, Hillerød, Denmark.
Seals, R. G. and Rippie, E. (1966). *J. Dairy Sci.* **49**, 617–620.
Shore, J. (1968a). *J. Soc. Dyers Colour.* **84**, 408–412.
Shore, J. (1968b). *J. Soc. Dyers Colour.* **84**, 413–422.
Shore, J. (1968c). *J. Soc. Dyers Colour.* **84**, 545–555.
Thurston, C. (1957). *Comml Fish. Rev.* **19** (5a), 7–9.
Tomiček, O. (1951). "Chemical Indicators", pp. 37–62. Butterworths, London.
Udy, D. C. (1954). *Cereal Chem.* **31**, 389–395.
Udy, D. C. (1956a). *Cereal Chem.* **33**, 190–197.
Udy, D. C. (1956b). Addendum to Udy, D. C. (1956a) *Nature, Lond.* **178**, 314–315.
Udy, D. C. (1971). *J. Am. Oil Chem. Soc.* **48**, 29A–33A.
Vanderzant, C. and Tennison, W. R. (1961). *Fd Technol., Champaign* **15**, 63–66.
Veis, A. and Cohen, J. (1954). *J. Am. chem. Soc.* **76**, 2476–2478.
Vickerstaff, T. (1954). "The Physical Chemistry of Dyeing", 2nd ed. Oliver and Boyd, London.

CHAPTER 13

Some Observations on the Use of Microbiological Techniques for the Determination of Protein Quality

H. HAENEL

Central Institute of Nutrition, Potsdam-Rehbrücke, GDR

and

S. G. KHARATYAN

Institute of Organo-Element Compounds, Moscow, USSR

I. INTRODUCTION

Our aim in this chapter is to discuss generally the role of microbiological assays in protein research. We should like to begin by drawing a parallel with their role in the development of vitamin research, where microbiological assays have an important role in the determination of vitamins in food, feed, clinical material and in metabolic studies. Historically, the following stages can be distinguished: (1) The recognition of a practical problem manifest as a deficiency disease, e.g. beri-beri; (2) The production and cure of the deficiency in experimental animals; the isolation and characterization of the vitamin; the study of its distribution in nature, and its metabolic role and its metabolism; (3) The development of biological assays with experimental animals of various species; (4) The development of quicker and simpler laboratory methods of vitamin assay, leading to the elaboration of a number of microbiological methods, the results from which were compared with those of biological assays; (5) The adoption of the most satisfactory laboratory methods for routine use.

Protein quality research has proceeded through similar stages but has proved more complicated and we are now at the intermediary stage of evaluating several promising chemical and microbiological assays to find simple and quick methods of estimating protein quality. A particular problem is to decide on the reference standard against which to judge them, since we are primarily interested in the application of the laboratory methods to problems of human and animal nutrition.

It is well established that the quality of a protein is dependent on its amino acid composition, its digestibility, and the amounts of its constituent amino acids that are absorbed and retained. Unfortunately, the quality of a protein is also dependent on the species, strain or method used for its evaluation, and different results may be obtained for the same protein by different laboratories using the same method. Protein quality may also be affected by a number of other factors including: amount and composition of the diet, stage of growth, lactation, infection, physiological and/or micro-ecological status of the gastro-intestinal tract, hormonal factors, environmental temperature, and stress. It is most necessary, therefore, to establish the relevance of the laboratory test to the particular problem of animal nutrition that is under investigation.

II. GENERAL ASPECTS OF MICROBIOLOGICAL ASSAYS

What are the advantages and limitations of microbiological assays in the evaluation of protein quality? In general, such tests are rapid, comparatively cheap and provide a means of testing large numbers of samples in a short time. They are widely used for three main purposes: the determination of amino acids in acid hydrolysates; determination of protein quality, expressed as relative nutritive value (RNV), as assessed by the growth of the test organism relative to that with a standard protein, usually casein or whole egg; and the determination of amino acid availability.

Micro-organisms have no gastro-intestinal tract and are therefore without the processes of chewing, crushing and mixing of the food protein in the gut; utilization of the protein may therefore be less efficient and particle size may be important. The pattern of enzymes in the gastro-intestinal tract of animals usually achieves more efficient digestion than that in most micro-organisms, and predigestion of the test proteins may be necessary for satisfactory results from microbiological assays. In our experience with *Tetrahymena pyriformis* W such predigestion was especially necessary in the evaluation of cereal proteins. In two of the micro-organisms that have been much investigated as indicators of protein quality, the pattern of requirement for exogenous amino acids is broadly similar to that in higher animals, but there are important differences which may influence the results of the tests. Thus *Streptococcus zymogenes* does not require lysine, and *Tetrahymena pyriformis* requires serine which is not an indispensable amino acid for higher animals. Differences may also exist in the utilization of small peptides.

Microbiological assay procedures require particular attention to experimental detail. Small and accidental changes in, for instance, the composition of the nutrient medium, in aeration, in temperature of incubation or in the age of the inoculum can markedly affect the results. Even the change of an assistant in the laboratory can lead to surprises.

It is necessary in the microbiological tests to sterilize the test proteins by autoclaving, and this may lead to changes in their properties. With *Tetrahymena pyriformis*, the size of individual cells can be markedly influenced by the energy source used in the medium (Reynolds, 1970). A further consideration in the *Tetrahymena pyriformis* test is that the organism often grows poorly in media containing free amino acids. We found that a solution of amino acids simulating the composition of egg protein gave an RNV of 50–60, as against 100 for the intact protein. We have occasionally found a similar effect with acid hydrolysates of proteins, and it may be due to inhibition of growth by single amino acids or to amino acid imbalances (Dewey and Kidder, 1958). Except with lysine, increasing the concentration of individual essential amino acids always leads to inhibition.

III. APPLICATIONS

There is an extensive literature covering the use, application and results of microbiological methods for evaluating protein quality (Baum and

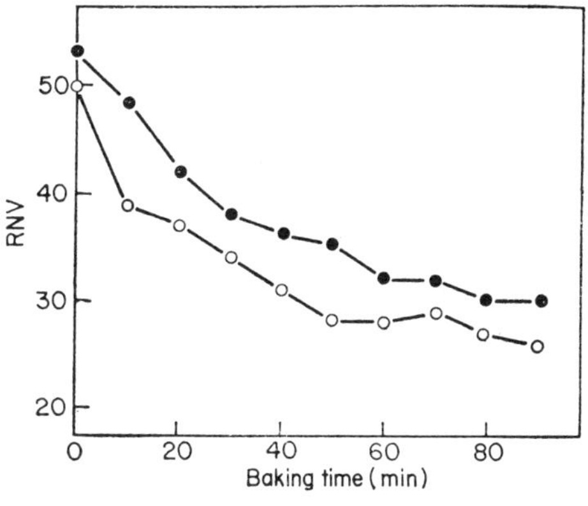

FIG. 1. Relative Nutritive Values (whole egg protein = 100) determined with *Tetrahymena pyriformis* for two rye/wheat breads (•——•, 85% rye; 15% wheat. o——o, 60% rye; 40% wheat) baked at 245° for different times (Baum, 1968)

Haenel, 1965; Fernell and Rosen, 1956; Ford, 1960, 1964; Helms and Rølle, 1970; Pilcher and Williams, 1954; Rosen and Fernell, 1956; Stott *et al.*, 1963). Whereas some methods gave results agreeing with those of animal assays, others did not, though there is general agreement that all the methods are satisfactory for differentiating good from poor proteins.

A. Relative Nutritive Value (RNV)

As shown in Fig. 1 the RNV measured with *Tetrahymena pyriformis* of two rye/wheat breads containing different proportions of the cereals decreased with increase in the length of time for which they were baked. Whereas the dietary lysine content of the samples was reduced by 28–33%, the RNV of the crust fell by 72–75% and of the whole bread by 43–48% (Baum, 1968). In another study the effect of storage on the RNV of cereal flours was determined. The results in Table I (Baum, 1966b)

TABLE I. Relative nutritive value (*Tetrahymena pyriformis*) of cereal flours before and after storage at 20°C
(Whole egg = 100)

Flour	*Storage time* (months)	*RNV*
Rye	0	58
	6·5	42
Wheat	0	36
	6·5	25
Rice	0	19
	6	14
Maize	0	43
	7	32
Oat	0	61
	5·5	59

indicated that, except for oats, the values fell by 26–30% during six months' storage. However, since all the values were low the investigation was repeated and the samples were predigested with pepsin. Table II shows that the effect of this predigestion was to give markedly higher and probably more accurate results. We have also found *Tetrahymena pyriformis* useful for grading different batches of the same cereal (Baum, 1966a), and for assessing the protein quality of other micro-organisms (*Candida*, *Hansenula*, *Mycococcus*, *Pseudomonas*). The results of RNV determinations

TABLE II. Relative nutritive values (*Tetrahymena pyriformis*) of some foods (expressed as PER) (Baum, 1970)

	PER Block and Mitchell (1946–7)	*RNV Tetrahymena calculated as PER*	
		Without predigestion	*Digestion with papain*
Casein	2·0	2·0	2·0
Soya-bean	2·3	2·4	2·5
Oat	2·2	2·4	2·6
Rice	1·7	0·8	1·5
Wheat	1·5	1·2	1·5
Maize	1·2	0·7	1·2

of protein quality in Table III illustrate values obtained with *Tetrahymena pyriformis* by different workers. Further comparisons were made by Boyne *et al.* (1961) and, as shown in Table IV, RNV as determined with *Tetrahymena pyriformis* correlated well with gross protein values for three of the four groups of materials tested; with only one of these three groups was there a significant correlation with n.p.u. Net protein utilization and GPV were correlated only in two of the three groups.

Kofrányi (1967) and Kofrányi *et al.* (1970) found that a mixture of egg protein and potato protein had a higher biological value (b.v. *ca* 1·3) than egg protein alone, when given to human subjects at nitrogen balance. We have made similar findings with *Tetrahymena pyriformis* (Fig. 2) and have shown that a combination of 70% egg protein and 30% potato

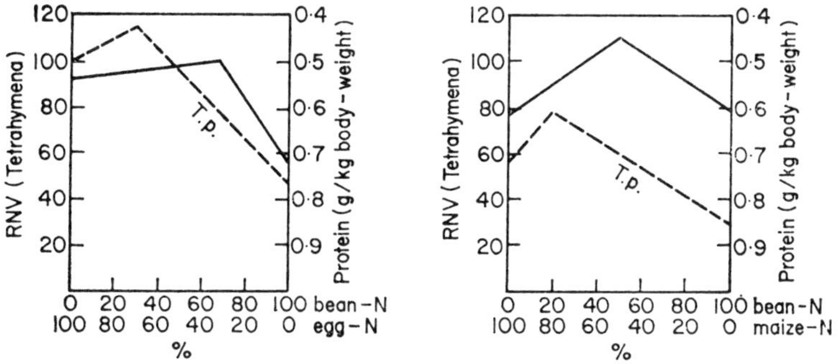

FIG. 2. Relative Nutritive Values determined with *Tetrahymena pyriformis* for protein mixtures (----) compared with the minimum daily protein requirements per kg body-weight for N balance (——) (Kofrányi, 1967)

TABLE III. Comparison for selected proteins of Relative Nutritive Values determined with *Tetrahymena pyriformis* W and rat assay values. All values are expressed relative to casein = 100

Protein source	*Tetrahymena pyriformis* W				
	Fernell and Rosen (1956)	*Helms and Rølle* (1970)	*Baum and Haenel* (1965)	*Calculated from Block and Mitchell* (1946–7)	*Calculated from Miller and Bender* (1955)
Dried whole egg	137	115	124	1·37	1·52
Egg white	121			1·22	1·37
Dried skim milk		97	108	1·22	1·16
Wheat germ	115			1·05	1·15
Soya-bean meal	80	87	107	1·06	0·93
Cottonseed meal	78			0·78	0·98
Sesame meal	52			0·96	
Groundnut meal	50		68	0·84	0·83

protein gave an RNV 16% higher than that of egg protein alone. The reason for these effects is not known.

TABLE IV. Correlation coefficients for determinations of Relative Nutritive Value, Gross Protein Value and Net Protein Utilization (Boyne *et al.*, 1961)

Protein source	*GPV/RNV*	(100 × *n.p.u.*)/*RNV*	*GPV*/(100 × *n.p.u.*)
Whale meat meals	0·89[a] (15)	0·82[a] (14)	0·90[a] (14)
Meat meals	0·63[b] (13)	0·30 (13)	0·42 (13)
Fish meals	0·07 (18)	0·10 (6)	0·92[a] (6)
Cottonseed meals	0·66[a] (17)	—	—

[a] Significant correlation at 1% level
[b] Significant correlation at 5% level
( ) number of pairs of samples

B. Total and Available Amino Acids

It is well known that the determination of amino acids in acid hydrolysates of closely related proteins may reveal only small differences in amino acid content, whereas biological tests with the unhydrolysed proteins may show large differences in apparent or available amino acid content. Microbiological tests can be used to determine available amino acids, after enzymic hydrolysis, and total amino acids, after acid hydrolysis (Bender, 1969; Boyne *et al.*, 1967; Ford, 1962, 1965; Guggenheim, 1970;

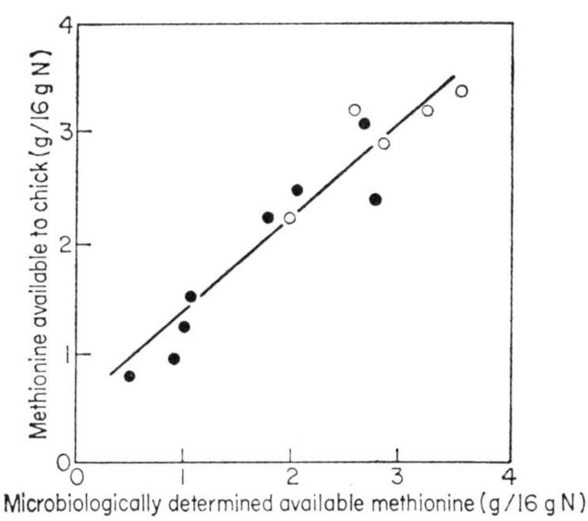

FIG. 3. Comparison of values for available methionine in protein concentrates determined biologically by chick assay and microbiologically with *Streptococcus zymogenes* (Miller *et al.*, 1965a)

Reynolds, 1964; Stott and Smith, 1966; Waterworth, 1964; Szklarska-Cygańska and Kakowska-Lipińska, 1970).

A good example of the correlation found between assays for available methionine with animals (chicks) and with micro-organisms (*Streptococcus zymogenes*; predigestion with papain) is shown in Fig. 3 (Miller *et al.*,

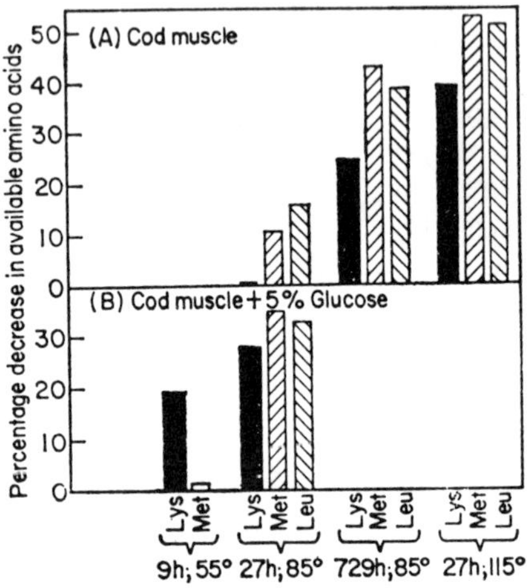

FIG. 4. Percentage decreases in available methionine and leucine (*Strep. zymogenes*) and in FDNB available lysine caused by heat treatment (Miller, *et al.*, 1965c)

TABLE V. The chemically determined tryptophan content of foods and its percentage availability as determined in rat and microbiological assays[a]

Assay method	*Chemical* (mg/g N)	*Rat growth*	*Streptococcus zymogenes*[b]	*Lactobacillus arabinosus*[b]
Casein	87		94	91
Egg white	90	100	103	86
Dried skim milk	93	88	94	75
Fish meal	78	35	99	82
Soya-bean flour, toasted	82	87	96	60
Sesame flour	87	92	99	83
Wheat flour	64		88	58
Rice flour	81		96	67
Chick-peas, autoclaved	70	27	81	67
Zein	27		93	37

[a] Taken from Pongpaew and Guggenheim (1968)

[b] After digestion with pepsin, trypsin and erepsin

TABLE VI. Microbiological determination of essential amino acid content (g/16 g N) of native albumin using *Streptococcus faecalis* (F), *Streptococcus zymogenes* (Z) and *Lactobacillus arabinosus* (A) after hydrolysis with HCl or with papain, leucine aminopeptidase and prolidase[a]

	Isoleucine			*Leucine*			*Lysine*	*Phenyl-alanine*	*Methionine*			*Threo-nine*	*Tryptophan*			*Valine*		
	F	Z	A	F	Z	A	F	A	F	F	A	F	F	Z	A	F	Z	A
After acid hydrolysis	2·61	2·25	2·48	11·85	11·85	12·00	12·73	6·38	0·89	0·83	0·85	5·68				5·50	5·50	5·78
After enzymic hydrolysis	2·39	2·61	2·35	11·74	11·79	11·89	12·79	6·68	0·89	0·80	0·77	5·49	0·58	0·53	0·61	5·85	5·54	5·76

[a] Taken from Dvořák (1968)

1965a). Miller *et al.* (1965c) also found correlations between available methionine and leucine determined microbiologically and available lysine determined chemically (Carpenter, 1960) in samples of unheated and heated cod muscle (Fig. 4).

Less satisfactory correlations between different methods for the measurement of the available tryptophan content of various foods were found by Pongpaew and Guggenheim (1968) (Table V). They considered that *Strep. zymogenes* overestimated and *Lactobacillus arabinosus* underestimated tryptophan availability and that neither assay was suitable for prediction of availability for animals. Similar conclusions were reached by Szmelcman and Guggenheim (1967) who pointed out that the distinction between

TABLE VII. Available leucine (g/16 g N) in the proteins of beef muscle after hydrolysis by pepsin, leucine aminopeptidase and prolidase

	Leucine after:					
	Initial 24 h hydrolysis by pepsin	*Further 24 h hydrolysis by leucine amino-peptidase* (0·6 ml)	*Further 24 h hydrolysis by leucine aminopeptidase (0·6 ml) + prolidase* 0·1 ml	0·2 ml	0·3 ml	*Percentage of total leucine*
Streptococcus zymogenes	6·68	7·34	8·00	8·00	8·00	100
Streptococcus faecalis	4·37	7·16	8·05	8·05	8·05	100·5
Lactobacillus arabinosus	4·67	6·66	7·98	—	7·98	99·8

available and unavailable amino acids is arbitrary and relates to the particular conditions of the assay. However, the procedure using digestion with papain, leucine aminopeptidase and prolidase (Hill and Schmidt, 1962) has led to reproducible results and was used by Dvořák (1968a) with bovine serum albumin (Table VI). Dvořák (1968b) obtained excellent agreement between the results of enzymic and acid hydrolysis using as test organism *Streptococcus faecalis*, *Strep. zymogenes* and *L. arabinosus*. The decrease found in digestibility of cod protein after heating with glucose agreed closely with the decrease in its content of available amino acids (Miller *et al.*, 1965b). The different effects of the three enzymes, used singly or in combination, are shown in Table VII. However, it remains to be established whether the results that can be achieved with such predigestion agree with the findings of other assessments of protein quality.

IV. CONCLUSIONS

Microbiological assays of protein quality, expressed as RNV, have proved a valuable tool for the control of technological processes in the food and feed industries, and for screening groups of materials such as seeds and micro-organisms to select samples of desired quality. Measurements of RNV are suitable for differentiating between good and poor proteins but the results are not an absolute measure of protein quality and should not be applied in human or animal nutrition without further confirmation.

Microbiological assays can be used to determine the available and total amino acid content of proteins. For the determination of available amino acids predigestion with appropriate enzymes is generally necessary, and conditions should be chosen such that results of microbiological tests agree with those of biological assays.

REFERENCES

Baum, F. (1966a). *Nahrung* **10**, 453–459.

Baum, F. (1966b). *Nahrung* **10**, 571–580.

Baum, F. (1968). *Nahrung* **12**, 61–67.

Baum, F. (1970). *Wiss. Z. Ernst Moritz Arndt-Univ. Greifswald* **19**, 13.

Baum, F. and Haenel, H. (1965). *Nahrung* **9**, 517–525.

Bender, A. E. (1969). *Chemy Ind.* p. 904–909.

Block, R. J. and Mitchell, H. H. (1946–7). *Nutr. Abstr. Rev.* **16**, 249–278.

Boyne, A. W., Carpenter, K. J. and Woodham, A. A. (1961). *J. Sci. Fd Agric.* **12**, 832–848.

Boyne, A. W., Price, S. A., Rosen, G. D. and Stott, J. A. (1967). *Br. J. Nutr.* **21**, 181–206.

Carpenter, K. J. (1960). *Biochem. J.* **77**, 604–610.

Dewey, V. C. and Kidder, G. W. (1958). *Archs Biochem. Biophys.* **73**, 29–37.

Dvořák, Z. (1968a). *J. Sci. Fd Agric.* **19**, 71–76.

Dvořák, Z. (1968b). *J. Sci. Fd Agric.* **19**, 77–82.

Fernell, W. R. and Rosen, G. D. (1956). *Br. J. Nutr.* **10**, 143–156.

Ford, J. E. (1960). *Br. J. Nutr.* **14**, 485–497.

Ford, J. E. (1962). *Br. J. Nutr.* **16**, 409–425.

Ford, J. E. (1964). *Br. J. Nutr.* **18**, 449–460.

Ford, J. E. (1965). *Br. J. Nutr.* **19**, 277–293.

Guggenheim, K. (1970). *In* "Evaluation of Novel Protein Products": proc. symp. 1968 (A. E. Bender *et al.*, eds), pp. 235–246. Pergamon Press, Oxford.

Helms, P. and Rølle, G. (1970). *In* "Evaluation of Novel Protein Products": proc. symp. 1968 (A. E. Bender *et al.*, eds), pp. 259–264. Pergamon Press, Oxford.

Hill, R. L. and Schmidt, W. R. (1962). *J. biol. Chem.* **237**, 389–396.

Kofrányi, E. (1967). *Nahrung* **11**, 863–873.

KOFRÁNYI, E., JEKAT, F. and MÜLLER-WECKER, H. (1970). *Hoppe-Seyler's Z. physiol. Chem.* **351**, 1485–1493.
MILLER, D. S. and BENDER, A. E. (1955). *Br. J. Nutr.* **9**, 382–388.
MILLER, E. L., CARPENTER, K. J. and MILNER, C. K. (1965c). *Br. J. Nutr.* **19**, 547–564.
MILLER, E. L., CARPENTER, K. J., MORGAN, C. B. and BOYNE, A. W. (1965a). *Br. J. Nutr.* **19**, 249–267.
MILLER, E. L., HARTLEY, A. W. and THOMAS, D. C. (1965b). *Br. J. Nutr.* **19**, 565–573.
PILCHER, H. L. and WILLIAMS, H. H. (1954). *J. Nutr.* **53**, 589–599.
PONGPAEW, P. and GUGGENHEIM, K. (1968). *Nutritio Dieta* **10**, 297–308.
REYNOLDS, H. (1964). *J. Wash. Acad. Sci.* **53**, 99–108.
REYNOLDS, H. (1970). *J. Bact.* **104**, 719–725.
ROSEN, G. D. and FERNELL, W. R. (1956). *Br. J. Nutr.*, **10**, 156–169.
STOTT, J. A. and SMITH, H. (1966). *Br. J. Nutr.* **20**, 663-673.
STOTT, J. A., SMITH, H. and ROSEN, G. D. (1963). *Br. J. Nutr.* **17**, 227–233.
SZKLARSKA-CYGAŃSKA, R. and KAKOWSKA-LIPIŃSKA, I. (1970). *Roczn. państ. Zakl. Hig.* **21**, 379–388.
SZMELCMAN, S. and GUGGENHEIM, K. (1967). *J. Sci. Fd Agric.* **18**, 347–350.
WATERWORTH, D. G. (1964). *Br. J. Nutr.* **18**, 503–517.

CHAPTER 14

An Improved Procedure for the Determination of Available Lysine and Methionine with Tetrahymena

C. SHORROCK* AND J. E. FORD

National Institute for Research in Dairying, Shinfield, Reading, England

I. INTRODUCTION

The amino acid composition of a food protein is of fundamental importance in determining its nutritional quality, but other characteristics may also be important, especially in proteins that have been heated during manufacture. In such proteins the amino acid composition represents only the potential nutritive quality, and the biological availability of the amino acids must also be taken into account. This concept of "biological availability" has been much studied in recent years, and a number of biological, chemical, microbiological and enzymic methods for determining amino acid availability have been proposed.

One such method has been described by Stott and Smith (1966). It is a microbiological procedure using *Tetrahymena pyriformis* W as the test organism, and is based on the method of Fernell and Rosen (1956) who used *Tetrahymena* to predict the nutritive value of a variety of proteins. *Tetrahymena* is a ciliated protozoan which can be grown in pure culture on a chemically defined medium. The observed nutritional requirements (Kidder and Dewey, 1951) proved to be remarkably similar to those of the rat. *Tetrahymena* requires the same amino acids as are essential for normal growth of the rat. In addition, serine, not essential for the rat, is

* Present address: Colborn Group Limited, Barton Mills, Canterbury, Kent.

synthesized too slowly by most strains of *Tetrahymena* to permit normal growth without an exogenous supply. Efforts to apply *Tetrahymena* to the evaluation of proteins stem from the observations of Lawrie (1937) that the organism is strongly proteolytic, and of Rockland and Dunn (1946) that it readily utilizes intact protein as its sole source of amino acids.

Stott and Smith (1966) developed a procedure with *Tetrahymena* for measuring the availability of lysine, methionine, arginine and histidine in intact protein sources, but the technique they employed is complex and unfamiliar to most microbiological assayists. The technique was adopted as the basis of the present investigation and further developed empirically. The results obtained were evaluated by comparison with those from rat growth tests, from microbiological tests with *Streptococcus zymogenes* and with available lysine values determined by reaction with 1-fluoro-2,4-dinitrobenzene (FDNB) by the method of Carpenter (1960).

II. EXPERIMENTAL

Most of the samples used in the investigation have been the subject of a collaborative study on biological, chemical and microbiological methods of assessing protein quality, conducted under the aegis of the Protein Evaluation Group of the Agricultural Research Council. The samples were chosen to represent a wide variety of protein sources, and to include a wide range of protein quality. The code letters and numbers are those given to the samples by the Protein Evaluation Group.

In the assay procedure described by Stott and Smith (1966) the growth responses of the organism to graded supplements of the test protein are compared with the responses to graded doses of the amino acid under test. The test samples are prepared simply by suspending the material in water to give concentrations of 2, 3, 4 and 5 mg N/assay tube. Growth is assessed, after 4 days' incubation, by counting the numbers of organisms/ml of culture fluid, using a Fuchs–Rosenthal counting chamber. Organisms in eight 1 mm squares are counted and the mean number/1 mm square gives the final population of the test culture in units of 10^4 organisms/ml. This procedure was modified, in that a camera attachment was fitted to the eyepiece of the microscope and each haemocytometer slide was photographed. The numbers of organisms on each photograph were counted with the aid of a digital counter with a marking pen attachment which provided a simple method of marking the cells on each photograph and counting the total numbers marked (Shorrock, 1972).

III. RESULTS AND DISCUSSION

A. Results Obtained by the Modified Stott and Smith Procedure

The available lysine values for fifteen proteins as measured with *Tetrahymena* are shown in Table I, together with the corresponding rat assay and FDNB values. The rat assay values were determined by the growth method first described by Carpenter (1957) and later used by Bjarnason and Carpenter (1969) to determine the biological availability of lysine in heat-damaged proteins. The test protein was added to a low-lysine diet based on zein and sesame-seed meal. Growth with the diet supplemented with the test protein was compared with that with the basal diet supplemented with graded doses of L-lysine. The FDNB values were determined by the method of Carpenter (1960), except that the hydrolysis was carried out using 8·1 M hydrochloric acid as recommended by Booth (1971), who

TABLE I. Available lysine values (g/16 g N) for a variety of food proteins as determined microbiologically with *Tetrahymena* (Method of Stott and Smith, 1966), chemically by reaction with FDNB and in growth tests with rats

	Tetrahymena[a]	*FDNB*	*Rat growth tests*
Fish meal, FM 101	4·8	6·1	6·9[b]
Meat meal, MM 101	1·1	4·1	4·3[b]
Whalemeat meal, WM 1	1·2	4·1	4·2
WM 3	2·7	6·1	6·7
WM 7	0·8	3·0	1·8
Hydrocarbon yeast, HY 101	1·9	5·7	7·0
HY 104	2·6	5·8	7·1
Groundnut meal, GN 101	2·4	2·6	3·5[b]
Groundnut meal, GN	2·1	3·0	3·2
Groundnut meal, heated, HGN	0·6	1·3	1·0
Soya-bean meal, SB	4·2	5·4	5·0
Soya-bean meal, heated, HSB	1·0	2·4	1·3
Cod muscle, unheated, CM	6·4	8·5	10·9[c]
Cod muscle, heated, HCM	1·0	5·6	4·3[c]
Casein	8·1	8·4	8·6

[a] Samples were not predigested before assay
[b] Unpublished values determined by the Biological Panel of the Agricultural Research Council's Protein Quality Group
[c] Values from Ford and Salter (1966)

found that DNP-proteins were not completely hydrolysed using 5·5 M acid as recommended by Carpenter (1960).

The *Tetrahymena* values ranged from 8·1 g/16 g N for casein to 0·6 g/16 g N for heated groundnut meal. The heat-damaged samples all showed a loss in lysine availability. For the heated cod muscle, heated soya-bean meal and heated groundnut meal the losses were 85%, 75% and 72% respectively.

All the available lysine values as determined by all the different methods were lower than the corresponding total lysine values, indicating that some portion of the lysine in all the test proteins was unavailable. An exception was the rat assay value for available lysine in the freeze-dried cod muscle which, at 10·9 g/16 g N, was higher than the total value. Similar values for the available lysine content of cod muscle were found in chick growth tests by Carpenter *et al.* (1963) and also by Miller *et al.* (1965a). Miller *et al.* (1965a) suggested that a value representing 120% availability for lysine was meaningless, and that the values from such chick assays could only be regarded as indicative of the relative values of protein supplements.

Comparison of the *Tetrahymena* with the rat and FDNB available lysine values shows that, except for casein, the microbiological values were lower. *Tetrahymena* underestimated the rat assay values by from 8% for GN 101 up to 77% for the heated cod muscle and similarly underestimated the corresponding FDNB values by from 21% to 82%. Despite this, however, there was a fair correlation between the *Tetrahymena* and the rat assay values ($r = 0{\cdot}775$) and between the *Tetrahymena* and FDNB values ($r = 0{\cdot}703$).

Stott and Smith (1966) similarly found that their *Tetrahymena* values for available lysine in fish meals, meat meals and whalemeat meals were generally lower than the FDNB values. Haenel (see Chapter 13) reported that unless samples of cereals were predigested with enzymes before assay they were poorly utilized by *Tetrahymena*. Similarly, in the assay of the relative nutritive value (RNV) and available amino acid content of proteins with *Strep. zymogenes*, predigestion of the test sample with papain speeded growth and improved the linearity and reproducibility of the dose-response curves. Ford (1960, 1964) and Miller *et al.* (1965b) showed that, in the *Strep. zymogenes* assay of available methionine content of cod muscle preparations, the degree of enzymic hydrolysis to which the test protein was subjected was critically important in determining the test results.

Clearly, under the conditions of the test described above, *Tetrahymena* gave improbably low values for the available lysine content of some proteins, and did not accurately predict either the rat assay or the FDNB assay values. The low values determined with *Tetrahymena* were probably due to the incomplete digestion of the proteins by the organism's own proteolytic enzymes, resulting in incomplete utilization. It seemed possible that enzymic predigestion of the test proteins might increase the amount of lysine available to *Tetrahymena* and give values in better agreement with the biological assay results.

B. Effect of Enzymic Predigestion on the Available Lysine Value of Proteins for Tetrahymena

The effect of introducing an enzymic predigestion stage into the assay of available lysine with *Tetrahymena* was determined using the same fifteen test samples. The samples were predigested with papain, as described by Boyne *et al.* (1967) for the assay of available methionine with *Strep. zymogenes*. The digests were then diluted to contain 5 mg N/3 ml and assayed as described previously. Lysine contributed by the enzyme itself

TABLE II. Influence of predigestion of the test samples with papain on the available lysine content (g/16 g N) as measured with *Tetrahymena*

	No predigestion	*Predigestion*
Fish meal, FM 101	4·8	7·0
Meat meal, MM 101	1·1	3·1
Whalemeat meal, WM 1	1·2	3·6
WM 3	2·7	4·2
WM 7	0·8	2·3
Hydrocarbon yeast, HY 101	1·9	5·9
HY 104	2·6	7·1
Groundnut meal, GN 101	2·4	3·5
Groundnut meal, GN	2·1	3·0
Groundnut meal, heated, HGN	0·6	1·7
Soya-bean meal, SB	4·2	4·4
Soya-bean meal, heated, HSB	1·0	2·4
Cod muscle, unheated, CM	6·4	8·6
Cod muscle, heated, HCM	1·0	5·0

was determined from an enzyme blank set up at twice the concentration present in the test protein digests, and a suitable blank correction was made in the calculation of the results. Table II shows the results of the assays together with the corresponding values for the undigested samples.

Introduction of this enzymic predigestion stage into the assay gave higher results for all the test proteins, especially for the heat-damaged samples. The value for the heat-damaged cod muscle was increased fivefold, from 1·0 to 5·0 g/16 g N; the value for heated soya-bean meal increased from 1·0 to 2·4 g/16 g N and that for heated groundnut meal from 0·6 to 1·7 g/16 g N. These values determined with the predigested samples correlated closely with the rat assay (r = 0·928) and FDNB values (r = 0·923).

These results showed clearly that it was essential to predigest the samples before assay with *Tetrahymena* in order to obtain results that were in sensible agreement with rat assay and FDNB available lysine values.

C. Measurement of Growth Response in Tetrahymena assays

A major practical disadvantage of the *Tetrahymena* procedure is the need for laborious microscopic counting of the cells in the test cultures. Microscopic cell counting is tedious and time-consuming and subject to error as it is often difficult to distinguish between cells and particles of food in the cultures. Difficulties in filling the haemocytometer often occur with cultures containing particles of undigested protein and before counting it is essential to ensure that there is uniform distribution of *Tetrahymena* cells over the whole of the haemocytometer grating.

One result of introducing an enzymic predigestion stage into the *Tetrahymena* assay was that the test extracts were relatively clear and free from material in suspension. With these clearer extracts it seemed that it might often be possible to assess growth simply by reading the optical densities of the test cultures rather than by counting the cells. To facilitate the measurement of optical density the test cultures were grown in 19 × 150 mm optically matched Pyrex test-tubes. The enzyme digests were diluted to contain 0·3 mg N/ml, which gave nitrogen concentrations of 0, 0·15, 0·30, 0·45, 0·60, 0·75 and 0·9 mg N/assay tube. The standard was set up in duplicate tubes from 0 to 540 μg L-lysine HCl, in 90 μg increments. To ensure sufficient aeration during growth the baskets of inoculated tubes were incubated at 25°, with continuous shaking. After 4 days' incubation a 1 ml sample of each culture was taken for determination of cell counts. The remaining 9 ml of culture was steamed. This had the effect of disrupting the cells, so that each cell made a much greater contribution to the optical density of the culture. Thus, non-specific interference from undigested food residues was further reduced. The tubes were cooled to room temperature, shaken and allowed to stand for 2–3 min to allow air bubbles to rise and food particles to settle. Optical densities were then read at 580 nm in a Lumetron Model 401A colorimeter.

Table III shows the available lysine content of five proteins, assessed both from measurement of the optical density of the cultures and by counting the numbers of organisms. Soya-bean and groundnut were included because they are comparatively rich in carbohydrate, and might be expected to leave a large quantity of non-protein material in suspension in the digests, which might interfere with optical density readings. In the event, only the groundnut meal showed a marked difference between the results calculated by the different methods—optical density measurements gave a result of 5·4 g/16 g N, as against only 3·6 from cell counts. The value of 5·4 g/16 g N was higher than the total lysine content and was clearly incorrect. With casein, cod muscle and fish meal FM 101, optical densities and cell counts gave essentially the same answers. Thus, the use of optical density measurements for assessing the growth of *Tetrahymena* is simple and time saving, but it is only possible with materials of high protein content that leave very little material in suspension after enzymic predigestion.

TABLE III. Comparison of results obtained from direct microscopical counts and from measurements of optical density

	Available lysine (g/16 g N)	
	Optical density (580 nm)	*Cell counts*
Casein	7·8	8·1
Cod muscle	8·1	8·6
Fish meal, FM 101	5·6	5·3
Groundnut meal	5·4	3·6
Soya-bean meal	5·5	5·3

D. Period of Incubation

The introduction of an enzymic predigestion stage into the assay procedure increased the rate of growth of *Tetrahymena*, and it seemed possible that this increase would shorten the 4-day incubation period needed for the test. To examine this possibility the available lysine content of a number of proteins was determined, using four different periods of incubation. Five meals—FM 101, FM 102, FM 113, HY 101 and casein—were chosen so that growth could be measured optically. The growth response to the L-lysine standard at 48, 72, 90 and 96 h, and the corresponding available lysine values for the meals are shown in Fig. 1.

Increasing the period of incubation increased the growth response to the L-lysine standard up to 90 h, after which there was no further increase. Lengthening the period of incubation increased the measured available lysine values for all the samples examined, and especially for the poorer quality protein FM 102. The measured available lysine value of FM 102 increased from 2·9 g/16 g N at 48 h to 4·3 g/16 g N at 90 h. It was evident that during the early hours of growth *Tetrahymena* utilizes free amino acids

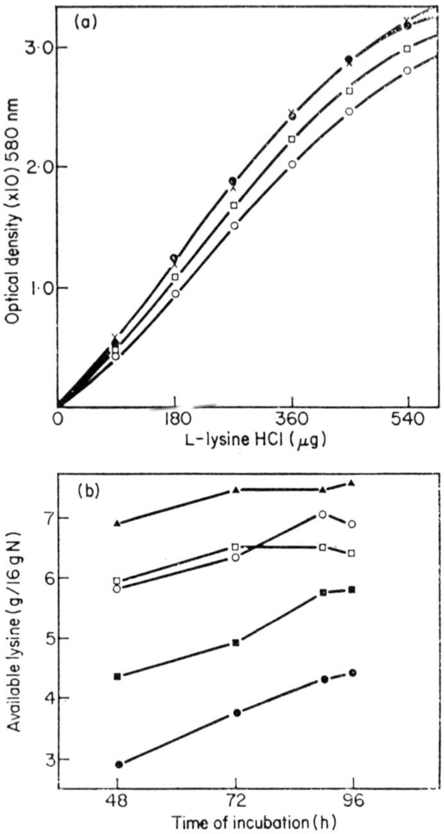

FIG. 1 (a) Growth response of *Tetrahymena* at graded concentrations of L-lysine HCl after incubation for 48, 72, 90 and 96 h

○——○, 48 h
□——□, 72 h
●——●, 90 h
×——×, 96 h

(b) Available lysine determined for five proteins at different incubation periods

●——●, Fish meal, FM 102
■——■, Fish meal, FM 101
□——□, Fish meal, FM 113
○——○, Hydrocarbon yeast, HY 101
▲——▲, casein

more rapidly than protein-bound amino acids, but that ultimately the protein-bound lysine was digested and utilized. It is possible that if the incubation had been carried out for an even longer period there might have been a still further increase in the measured available lysine value. However, the maximum value that can be obtained is not necessarily the correct value, since the aim in the microbiological test is to predict the results of the biological tests. There was little increase in the available lysine values between 90 and 96 h incubation, and since the 96 h values agreed with the rat assay and FDNB values, this period was adopted as standard.

E. Aseptic Addition of Medium Ingredients

A disadvantage of the *Tetrahymena* assay procedure proposed by Stott and Smith (1966) is the need for separate sterilization of the medium ingredients. The authors sterilized the test protein and solution E (nucleic acids) separately from solution A (vitamins), solution F (amino acids) and glucose, to prevent possible sugar–amino acid and sugar–vitamin interactions. Although they recommended separate sterilization they did not in fact report on whether this had any effect on the assay. To test this point, two proteins—casein and whalemeat meal WM 7—were assayed for available lysine using separate sterilization and "all in" sterilization of the medium ingredients. Figure 2 shows the results with casein.

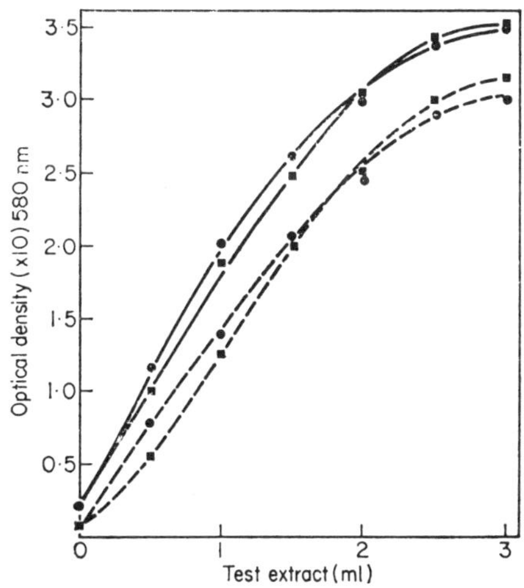

FIG. 2. Effect of separate sterilization of medium ingredients on growth of *Tetrahymena*

■——■, casein, separate sterilization
■- - - ■, casein, "all in" sterilization
●——●, standard, separate sterilization
●- - - ●, standard, "all in" sterilization

Separate sterilization gave slightly better growth with the lysine standard and with casein, the difference at the top level of the standard being 0·05 optical density units, equivalent to about 15% extra growth. However, the method of sterilization had no significant effect on the assay results. Calculation of the available lysine values for casein showed 7·4 g/16 g N after "all in" sterilization and 7·6 g/16 g N after separate sterilization. Similarly with WM 7, "all in" sterilization gave a value of 2·2 g/16 g N and separate sterilization a value of 2·3 g/16 g N. The heating conditions—110° for 10 min—during the "all in" sterilization were less drastic than those—121° for 10 min—employed by Stott and Smith (1966). No contamination was found in assays sterilized under these milder conditions, which were adopted to minimize amino acid–sugar interaction. In all subsequent assays the test samples and medium ingredients were sterilized together at 110° for 10 min. This simplified the test procedure and, by avoiding aseptic addition, reduced the possibility of bacterial contamination of the assay.

F. Conditions of Enzymic Predigestion

In the assay for available methionine with *Strep. zymogenes*, the conditions of enzymic predigestion are important, and influence the extent of the agreement with biological assay values (cf. Ford, 1964; Miller *et al.* 1965b). Similarly, with *Tetrahymena* it is clear that the enzymic pretreatment of the samples is equally important. The conditions of predigestion initially chosen gave results that were in fair agreement with rat assay and FDNB values. If a different proteolytic enzyme or different conditions of papain pretreatment had been used quite different results might have been obtained. To test this possibility six different proteins were assayed for available lysine after predigestion with papain or pepsin.

The papain predigestion was carried out using 2 ml of a 4% suspension of crude papain per 100 mg protein N, and incubated for 3 h or 5 h at 56° in an end-over-end shaker. Pepsin digestion was carried out by suspending a sample of test protein containing 100 mg N in 20 ml of 0·05 M hydrochloric acid in a 1 oz screw-capped bottle and adjusting the pH to 1·8. One ml of a 1% w/v solution of three times crystallized pepsin in 0·05 M hydrochloric acid was then added and the sample was incubated for 3 h at 56° in the end-over-end shaker. The pH was adjusted to 7·1 and the digest diluted to contain 300 μg N/ml.

The influence of pepsin and papain predigestion on the growth response of *Tetrahymena* to FM 101 is shown in Fig. 3. The measured available lysine values for the six protein samples are given in Table IV. With all the samples, except casein, the effect of predigestion before assay was to increase the available lysine value. Digestion with pepsin and papain gave

TABLE IV. Measurement of available lysine (g/16 g N) with *Tetrahymena*. Influence of conditions of pretreatment of the test proteins

		Predigested with			
	Undigested	*Pepsin*	*Papain* 3 h	*Papain* 5 h	6 M HCl
Fish meal, FM 101	2·0	5·3	5·1	4·8	6·7
Whalemeat WM 1	1·2	2·8	3·1	3·3	7·1
WM 3	2·7	3·8	3·9	4·2	8·8
WM 7	0·8	1·5	1·7	2·0	7·2
WM 9	1·6	7·1	7·3	6·8	9·0
Casein	7·7	7·5	7·6	7·5	8·1

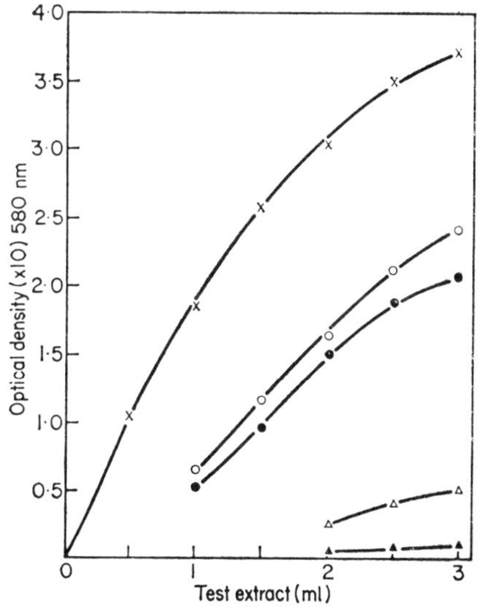

FIG. 3. Influence of pepsin and papain predigestion on the growth response of *Tetrahymena* to fish meal FM 101

×——×, L-lysine standard, 180 μg/ml
○——○, FM 101; papain digest
●——●, FM 101; pepsin digest
△——△, papain blank
▲——▲, pepsin blank

similar values, and increasing the period of incubation with papain from 3 to 5 h gave no consistent increase in the available lysine values. It is apparent in Fig. 3 that there was more growth when FM 101 was digested with papain than with pepsin, but this was due entirely to the greater concentration of lysine present in the papain. For casein the available lysine value was close to the total value, as would be expected since casein is known to be highly digestible and its amino acids are completely available for higher animals.

It seems from the results with this limited range of samples that the conditions of enzymic predigestion are not highly critical. However, before we can conclude that the papain pretreatment, arbitrarily chosen as it was, is generally suitable, experience will be needed from comparative biological and microbiological testing of a wider range of protein foods.

G. Determination of Available Lysine in Sixteen High-protein Materials

From all the foregoing, a modified test procedure was provisionally selected. The assay medium consisted of two stock solutions—the basal medium and the amino acid supplement. The composition of the basal medium was the same as in the Stott and Smith (1966) procedure except that the ingredients of solutions A, B, C, D and E and glucose were all dissolved into one solution which was made up at ten times final strength.

The amino acid supplement was the same as that used by Stott and Smith (1966) but was also made up at ten times final strength. The test proteins were predigested for 3 h with papain, as previously described. The assay was carried out in optically matched tubes. The test samples were assayed at dose levels of 0, 0·15, 0·30, 0·45, 0·60, 0·75 and 0·90 mg N/assay tube, and the L-lysine HCl standard at dose levels of 0, 90, 180, 270, 360, 450 and 540 μg/assay tube. After incubation for 96 h at 25° in a shaker incubator, the baskets of tubes were steamed and growth was measured turbidimetrically.

This procedure was applied to the determination of the available lysine content of sixteen high-protein feedstuffs. The results of the assays and the corresponding FDNB values are given in Table V. There was a good correlation between the results obtained by the two methods ($r = 0·931$) and the results were quantitatively closely similar. The main discrepancies occurred with the heat-damaged cod muscle and the poorer-quality whale-meat meals WM 1 and WM 7. The FDNB values for these three samples were on average 25% higher than the corresponding *Tetrahymena* values, reflecting the inability of the chemical test to take digestibility into account.

Ten of these high-protein materials were assayed repeatedly for their available lysine content in a number of independent assays to determine the reproducibility of the assay results. The results of these assays are shown in Table VI. The between-assay reproducibility was judged from the magnitude of the coefficient of variation of the available lysine values. The coefficients of variation for the ten samples ranged from 6·9% for FM 113 to 14·4% for FM 102. The largest coefficient of variation was

TABLE V. Available lysine values (g/16 g N) for sixteen proteins determined with *Tetrahymena* and by reaction with FDNB

	Tetrahymena	*FDNB*
Fish meal, FM 101	5·9	6·1
FM 102	4·0	4·0
FM 108	5·8	6·3
FM 113	6·4	7·0
FM 122	6·0	6·7
FM 123	6·5	6·6
Meat meal, MM 101	3·8	4·1
Whalemeat meal, WM 1	2·9	4·1
WM 3	4·5	6·1
WM 7	2·1	3·0
WM 9	6·6	6·6
Hydrocarbon yeast, HY 101	6·0	5·7
HY 104	6·6	5·8
Cod muscle, unheated, CM	8·2	8·5
Cod muscle, heated, HCM	4·4	5·6
Casein	7·9	8·4

found for an atypical fish meal of low lysine availability, and reflected the difficulty of obtaining a representative sample of the material.

Although the coefficient of variation for available lysine as measured with *Tetrahymena* was larger than that reported by Booth (1971) for the FDNB procedure (3·8%), the microbiological test has the advantage that it takes digestibility into account and does not overestimate the lysine availability in heat-damaged proteins. Thus the results, though less precise, may be more accurate.

H. Use of Tetrahymena for the Determination of Available Methionine

In further experiments *Tetrahymena* was used for measuring the available methionine content of the sixteen feedstuffs described above. The assay procedure was similar to that described for the determination of available lysine, except that lysine was included in the amino acid supplement and methionine omitted. The L-methionine standard was set up at dose levels of 0, 40, 80, 120, 160, 200 and 240 μg/tube. The results were evaluated by comparison with those obtained in parallel tests on the same samples using the *Strep. zymogenes* procedure (Ford, 1962, 1964; Ford and Salter, 1966). The *Strep. zymogenes* assay for available methionine is now well established and has been shown, for certain categories of protein foods, to give good agreement with biological assay values with chicks and rats (cf. Miller *et al.*, 1965b; Carpenter *et al.*, 1972).

The results obtained using the two different organisms are shown in

TABLE VI. Reproducibility of available lysine values as determined with *Tetrahymena*

Test protein	*No. of assays*	*Mean* (g/16 g N)	*Standard deviation*	*Coefficient of variation* (%)
Fish meal, FM 101	16	5·44	0·49	9·0
FM 102	8	3·94	0·57	14·4
FM 113	6	6·48	0·45	6·9
Whalemeat meal, WM 1	5	2·95	0·23	7·9
WM 3	5	4·47	0·47	10·5
WM 7	8	2·10	0·23	11·2
WM 9	5	7·15	0·82	11·5
Hydrocarbon yeast, HY 101	9	5·97	0·56	9·3
HY 104	9	7·13	0·51	7·2
Casein	14	7·40	0·64	8·7

Table VII. The available methionine values, measured with *Tetrahymena*, ranged from 3·1 g/16 g N for freeze-dried cod muscle to 0·4 g/16 g N for whalemeat meal WM 7. As with lysine, there was some variation between samples of the same type; for example the available methionine values for whalemeat meals ranged from 0·4 to 2·2 g/16 g N. The available methionine values obtained by the two microbiological methods were closely correlated (r = 0·963) and quantitatively similar. Both methods graded the whalemeat meals in the same order, and both identified the poor-quality fish meal FM 102. Although the remaining fish meals were broadly similar in quality, both methods indicated that FM 113 was marginally superior.

The *Tetrahymena* assay takes 96 h, as against the 48 h required for the

Strep. zymogenes test. Besides being quicker, the *Strep. zymogenes* test is more easily applied to samples rich in carbohydrate, as growth can be assessed not only from optical density measurements but also from measurement of the acid produced during growth of the test cultures. However, *Tetrahymena* offers the compensating advantage that it can be employed to measure both lysine and methionine in the same test extract.

TABLE VII. *Tetrahymena* and *Strep. zymogenes* values for available methionine (g/16 g N) in a variety of food proteins

	Tetrahymena	*Strep. zymogenes*
Fish meal, FM 101	2·5	2·3
FM 102	1·6	1·7
FM 108	2·4	2·4
FM 113	2·9	2·6
FM 122	2·4	2·5
FM 123	2·7	2·5
Meat meal, MM 101	1·1	0·9
Whalemeat meal, WM 1	1·0	1·1
WM 3	1·0	1·5
WM 7	0·4	0·5
WM 9	2·2	2·1
Hydrocarbon yeast, HY 101	1·5	1·6
HY 104	1·6	1·5
Cod muscle, unheated, CM	3·1	3·0
Cod muscle, heated, HCM	1·6	1·6
Casein	2·7	3·1

IV. CONCLUSIONS

The *in vitro* methods for protein evaluation must ultimately be checked in comparative tests with the animal species for which the proteins are intended. However, animal feeding trials are expensive and laborious, and they are quite unsuitable for routine use. For such applications as quality control in food manufacture, for monitoring the commercial development of new protein foods, and for rapid screening of novel protein sources, the *in vitro* procedures have much to offer, and they will clearly increase in importance in the future. They must be used with discrimination, but properly used they are becoming an indispensable adjunct to animal assays.

The *Tetrahymena* assay for available lysine has not yet been widely adopted, partly for the reason that the use of protozoa in analysis is unfamiliar to most analysts, and partly because the published procedure is complex and laborious. Nevertheless, in the course of the present study it has become apparent that *Tetrahymena* is of great potential value as a test animal in protein nutrition research. Compared with the chemical test, any shortcomings it may have in precision are amply offset by its biological specificity, and by the fact that it is applicable to a much wider range of foods. The advantage of biological specificity was nicely illustrated in the wide discrepancy between *Tetrahymena* and FDNB values for heat-damaged cod muscle. The *Tetrahymena* values were much lower, and agreed closely with the results of rat growth tests.

In general, the present findings illustrate that the *Tetrahymena* assay can predict accurately the results of growth tests with rats but it would be premature to recommend the present assay procedure for general use. Further development is still needed and, in particular, the problem of finding a quicker alternative to cell counting remains to be solved. Another unsatisfactory feature in the present procedure is the non-specific stimulation at high levels of the test extracts. Errors from this cause have been avoided by restricting the upper dose limit in the test, and this points to the need for more fundamental information on the nutritional requirements of the organism.

REFERENCES

Bjarnason, J. and Carpenter, K. J. (1969). *Br. J. Nutr.* **23**, 859–868.

Booth, V. H. (1971). *J. Sci. Fd Agric.* **22**, 658–665.

Boyne, A. W., Price, S. A., Rosen, G. D. and Stott, J. A. (1967). *Br. J. Nutr.* **21**, 181–206.

Carpenter, K. J. (1957). *Int. Congr. Nutr. 4, Paris, Abstr. Pap.* pp. 154–155.

Carpenter, K. J. (1960). *Biochem. J.* **77**, 604–610.

Carpenter, K. J., McDonald, I. and Miller, W. S. (1972). *Br. J. Nutr.* **27**, 7–17.

Carpenter, K. J., March, B. E., Milner, C. K. and Campbell, R. C. (1963). *Br. J. Nutr.* **17**, 309–323.

Fernell, W. R. and Rosen, G. D. (1956). *Br. J. Nutr.* **10**, 143–156.

Ford, J. E. (1960). *Br. J. Nutr.* **14**, 485–497.

Ford, J. E. (1962). *Br. J. Nutr.* **16**, 409–425.

Ford, J. E. (1964). *Br. J. Nutr.* **18**, 449–460.

Ford, J. E. and Salter, D. N. (1966). *Br. J. Nutr.* **20**, 843–860.

Kidder, G. W. and Dewey, V. C. (1951). *In* "Biochemistry and Physiology of Protozoa" (A. Lwoff, ed.), pp. 323–400. Academic Press, New York.

Lawrie, N. R. (1937). *Biochem. J.* **31**, 789–798.

Miller, E. L., Carpenter, K. J. and Milner, C. K. (1965a). *Br. J. Nutr.* **19**, 547–564.

MILLER, E. L., CARPENTER, K. J., MORGAN, C. B. and BOYNE, A. W. (1965b). *Br. J. Nutr.* **19**, 249-267.
ROCKLAND, L. B. and DUNN, M. S. (1946). *Archs Biochem. Biophys.* **11**, 541–543.
SHORROCK, C. (1972). Ph.D. Thesis. University of Reading, England.
STOTT, J. A. and SMITH, H. (1966). *Br. J. Nutr.* **20**, 663-673.

CHAPTER 15

Methods of Protein Evaluation with Rats, I

P. L. PELLETT

University of Massachusetts, Amherst, Massachusetts, USA

The methodology of protein quality evaluation in foods has been discussed frequently (Allison, 1959; Pellett, 1963; Campbell, 1963), the most recent review being that of McLaughlan and Campbell (1969) who cite over 150 references to the literature. Biological methods with rats are usually subdivided into those based on weight gain and those based on nitrogen retention in the whole body either by direct carcass analysis or by N balance techniques. In addition there are several miscellaneous procedures involving either liver protein, enzymes, blood amino acids or repletion of the deprived animal; these are all discussed by McLaughlan and Campbell (1969).

This chapter will be concerned mainly with the carcass analysis method for determination of net protein utilization, however some consideration will be given to the relative nutritive value procedure of Hegsted and his associates (Hegsted and Chang 1965a,b; Hegsted *et al.*, 1968; Hegsted and Neff, 1970), together with their criticisms of the net protein utilization procedure as used at present.

I. NET PROTEIN UTILIZATION

Net protein utilization derives from the Thomas-Mitchell procedure (Mitchell, 1923–4) for the determination of biological value (b.v.). As originally described it was called net protein value (Bender and Miller,

1953a) and was a measure of the proportion of food N that was retained by the rat, it was thus indicative of the relative protein values of various protein sources. Definitions of biological value, digestibility, net protein utilization (n.p.u.), as it was renamed by Miller and Bender (1955), and apparent n.p.u. have been given elsewhere (Pellett, 1963; FAO/WHO, 1965) but are repeated here for convenience:

BALANCE — CARCASS

$$\text{b.v.} = \frac{R}{A} = \frac{I - (F - F_k) - (U - U_k)}{I - (F - F_k)} \quad \text{or} \quad \frac{B - B_k}{I - (F - F_k)}$$

$$\text{Digestibility} = \frac{A}{I} = \frac{I - (F - F_k)}{I}$$

$$\text{n.p.u. (True)} = \frac{R}{I} = \frac{I - (F - F_k) - (U - U_k)}{I} \quad \text{or} \quad \frac{B - B_k}{I}$$

$$\text{n.p.u. (Apparent)} = \frac{I - F - U}{I} \quad \text{or} \quad \frac{B - B_0}{I}$$

where A = absorbed N
R = retained N
B = body N at end of test period
B_k = body N at end of test period for animals fed a non-protein diet
B_0 = body N at zero time
F = faecal N
F_k = endogenous faecal N
I = nitrogen intake
U = urinary N
U_k = endogenous urinary N

Note: For complete accuracy the N intake on the non-protein diet should be included in the equations, see Miller and Bender (1955) and Bender and Miller (1957a).

Thus, n.p.u. can, by definition, be derived either by estimating carcass gain from faecal and urinary excretion (Rippon, 1959; Henry and Toothill, 1962) or directly from carcass analysis (Bender and Miller, 1953a). A full description of the methodology has been given by Miller (1963) and our own slightly modified procedure is appended.

A. Nitrogen/Water Ratio

The brief procedure (Bender and Miller, 1953a) using carcass analysis gave a considerable saving in time over the original balance-sheet method but could be shortened further if one assumed that the nitrogen to water ratio was constant for a strain of rats at any specific age. That such an assumption was justified originates from the work of Moulton (1923) who showed that body constituents including N and water were a constant proportion of the body when measured on a fat-free basis. Bender and Miller (1953b) thus showed that n.p.u. could be calculated from body water provided that one knew the N/H_2O ratio for the rats being used; they later (Miller and Bender, 1955) showed that the ratio changed with age in a predictable manner for their own colony of black and white rats (Table I). Good correlations between body water and body N and the

TABLE I. Some published values for regression equations relating age and N/H_2O ratio

Investigators	*Age range (days)*	*No. of rats*	*Strain*	*Regression equation*[a]
Dreyer (1957)	32–49	300	Wistar	$Y = 0{\cdot}015X + 3{\cdot}39$ (male)
Bender and Miller (1953b)	33–57	147	Black and white hooded	$Y = 0{\cdot}024X + 2{\cdot}92$ (both sexes)
Miller and Bender (1955)	0–503	107	Black and white hooded	$Y = 4{\cdot}83\text{-antilog}_{10}(0{\cdot}4304\text{–}0{\cdot}0115X)$
Henry and Toothill (1962)	36–42	—	Hooded Norwegian	$Y = 0{\cdot}034X + 2{\cdot}63$ (male)
				$Y = 0{\cdot}034X + 2{\cdot}71$ (female)
Pellett (1967)	30–40	766	Sprague-Dawley	$Y = 0{\cdot}027X + 2{\cdot}86$ (male)

[a] X = age in days, $Y = (100 \times N\%)/(H_2O\%)$

usefulness of the N/H_2O ratio for n.p.u. calculation were demonstrated by Henry and Toothill (1962), Donoso and Yáñez (1962) and Rafalski and Nogal (1966). Moreover, Hegsted *et al.* (1968) showed that body water determinations were highly correlated with N gain in the determination of relative nutritive value (RNV) of proteins. There have, however, been criticisms of the short cut N/H_2O ratio procedure by Stucki and Harper (1962), Scrimshaw (1962) and Henry (1965) who have questioned the assumption that the N/H_2O ratio is constant at any given age regardless of the previous dietary treatment.

That the N/H_2O ratio was not constant, at least for the Sprague-

Dawley rat, was demonstrated by Pellett (1967). It was shown that for 33 and 40-day-old animals there were significant differences in body composition including N/H_2O ratio between animals given a protein-free diet and those given protein at the 10% dietary level. This could lead to errors in the calculation of n.p.u. of about 0·05–0·06. The results obtained are shown in Table II. An additional finding confirmed the observation of Donoso and Yáñez (1962) that body N could be calculated with equal accuracy from either water content or from total weight, as has also been observed by Hegsted, *et al.* (1968). This indicated that under the experimental conditions the proportion of fat did not change significantly. The correlation coefficients obtained are also shown in Table II; in all cases the correlation between determined body N and that calculated was slightly higher when using body weight for calculation rather than body water. Campbell (1963) and Henry (1965) have pointed out that if body weight is used to calculate n.p.u. then it becomes the same as Net Protein Ratio (NPR), i.e. protein retention efficiency (PRE) as described by Bender and Doell (1957b), since both are calculated from the differences in weight between rats given a non-protein diet and those given test diets.

For Sprague–Dawley rats it was thus recommended that body N determinations be used routinely for the determination of n.p.u. rather than be calculated from body water. It was, however, shown by Kaba (1971), working in the author's laboratory, that if the two N/H_2O ratios be used (Pellett, 1967), one for animals given test diets and the other for those given the protein-free diet, then there was an extremely high correlation between determined N and predicted N ($r = 0{\cdot}99$; $P < 0{\cdot}001$) and that the regression equation was $Y = 0{\cdot}977X + 0{\cdot}205$ where Y is the determined N and X is that calculated from N/H_2O ratios. Thus even with the Sprague-Dawley rat N/H_2O ratios can be used for accurate prediction of n.p.u.

B. Carcass Amino Acid Composition

An underlying assumption of the n.p.u. carcass analytical procedure is that the amino acid composition of the carcass is unaffected by diet; that this assumption was justified has recently been demonstrated by Pellett and Kaba (1972) who determined carcass amino acids in rats under the experimental conditions of net protein utilization determination. Diets based on gluten, chick-pea, casein and egg were fed at different concentrations such that the levels of utilizable protein (n.d.–p : e) were similar. At the end of the 10-day experimental period the amino acid compositions of the rat carcasses were determined together with those of rats receiving the protein-free diet and of the zero-day control groups (Table III). Except for increases in glycine and proline concentrations between the zero-day

TABLE II. The relationship of body composition of Sprague-Dawley rats with diet and age and correlation coefficients between determined body N and N calculated from body weight or body water[a]

Diet	*Age* (days)	*No. of rats*	N % *Dry body-weight*	*Water* (%)	N (%)	N : H_2O *ratio*	*Correlation Coefficients* *Calculated from body weight*	*Calculated from body water*
Protein-free	30	18	10·73	72·64	2·71	3·66	0·23	−0·24
10% protein	30	52	9·41	74·42	2·58	3·59	0·86	0·77
Combined	30	70	—	—	—	3·61	0·90	0·82
Protein-free	33	102	10·20	71·14	2·94	4·16	0·55	0·28
10% protein	33	400	8·88	70·47	2·60	3·70	0·95	0·93
Combined	33	502	—	—	—	3·79	0·96	0·95
Protein-free	37	17	10·54	72·14	2·93	4·08	0·83	0·66
10% protein	37	57	9·38	69·79	2·83	4·06	0·93	0·90
Combined	37	74	—	—	—	4·07	0·96	0·94
Protein-free	40	33	9·94	71·14	2·86	4·04	0·95	0·92
10% protein	40	87	8·53	68·55	2·67	3·90	0·96	0·94
Combined	40	120	—	—	—	3·94	0·97	0·96

[a] Adapted from Pellett (1967)

control group and the test groups, all other amino acid compositional differences were small and were only of the same order as the differences produced between replicate analyses of the same sample. These results contradicted in some degree the experiments of Bunce and King (1969a,b) who had claimed that when rats were given diets which resulted in a growth reduction of more than 50% "the resultant animal showed a

TABLE III. Amino acid composition (mg/g N) of rat carcasses after 10 days' growth on various diets at similar levels of utilizable protein. Pooled sample, four animals per group; mean of four analyses[a]

	DIET					
Amino acid	*Zero day control*	*Protein-free*	*Gluten* (4·13% N)	*Chick-pea* (1·84% N)	*Casein* (2·08% N)	*Egg* (1·44% N)
Ileu	230	227	213	221	229	223
Leu	476	476	456	478	472	474
Lys	451	446	441	438	455	454
Met	126	130	129	130	138	130
Cys	121	120	115	110	110	115
Total S.A.A.	247	250	244	240	248	245
Phe	249	252	241	249	251	248
Try	226	229	213	212	218	220
Total Aromatic	475	480	454	462	469	468
Thr	285	292	286	278	286	286
Try	74	73	72	72	74	74
Val	293	278	279	289	282	268
Arg	446	435	427	417	430	438
His	185	193	197	199	210	191
Ala	390	415	414	402	410	404
Asp	542	563	551	547	545	566
Glu	860	896	875	885	877	894
Gly	532	621	607	582	589	600
Pro	360	415	410	403	403	406
Ser	293	320	303	294	292	310
Total E.A.A. (g)	2·48	2·51	2·43	2·46	2·49	2·46

[a] Adapted from Pellett and Kaba (1972) who give standard deviations for all values

severe disruption of his usual carcass amino acid pattern and that the long term consequences could be profound". Certainly the growth reduction on the protein-free diet was more than 50% but no significant changes in amino acid composition occurred. The reason for the discrepancy is discussed by Pellett and Kaba (1972) but probably lies in the calculation method used by Bunce and King (1969a,b) in that the inherent variability in amino acid analysis could amplify small differences in composition when growth and hence amino acid gain were low but which did not occur to the same degree when growth was normal or high.

From the carcass amino acid results and the amino acid composition of diets given it was possible to calculate values that were analogous to the net protein utilization both true and apparent for each individual amino acid, the results obtained are shown in Table IV. Assuming amino acids were used for tissue building purposes only, there should be 100% incorporation of the limiting amino acid. In practice the highest value (excluding synthesis) will be that for the limiting amino acid but the efficiency of utilization will vary depending on the degree of use of the amino acid for purposes other than protein synthesis. In this way total sulphur amino acids were limiting for chick-pea and casein whereas lysine was limiting for gluten and egg. There was no evidence of any methionine synthesis under the conditions of this experiment, in contrast to the claims of Bunce and King (1969a,b) when lactalbumin was given at low levels.

It may well be that there are changes in the proportions of the various proteins present in the carcass after the animal has consumed different diets, as was observed for blood proteins by Tagle *et al.* (1970), however any such changes were not accompanied by any demonstrable alterations in the proportions of amino acids in the carcasses, even of those rats receiving the protein-free diet. Any changes in amino acid composition that did occur were more a reflection of age differences than of effect of diet.

C. Net Protein Utilization, Operative and Standardized

Since the percentage of protein retained falls with increasing concentration of protein in the diet (Barnes *et al.*, 1946) and thus in contrast to the protein quality score, n.p.u. value is not constant for any specific protein, it has been proposed (Platt and Miller, 1959; Miller and Payne, 1961a) that two terms be used: net protein utilization (standardized) and net protein utilization (operative) (n.p.u.$_{st}$ and n.p.u.$_{op}$). These are, respectively, a value obtained at or about maintenance levels of protein intake and a value obtained at any other (stated) protein level. Thus n.p.u.$_{st}$ is a measure of quality and, unless amino acid availability or toxic factors impinge, should be a function of amino acid composition and score,

TABLE IV. Percentage amino acid retention on various diets expressed for growth and maintenance and for growth alone

	Try	*Thr*	*Ile*	*Leu*	*Lys*	*Met*	*Cys*	*Total SAA*	*Phe*	*Tyr*	*Total arom.*	*Val*	*Arg*	*His*
Growth + maintenance, compared to protein-free group														
Gluten	24	32	17	20	**86**[a]	27	18	22	14	19	16	25	40	29
Chick-pea	59	61	42	56	54	83	60	**72**	29	52	36	53	42	**72**
Casein	43	62	40	45	53	55	288	**82**	44	34	39	29	102	75
Egg	64	74	53	71	**92**	50	61	54	59	55	57	51	93	80
Growth alone, compared to zero-day control group														
Gluten	13	20	8	11	**51**	18	10	13	8	10	9	12	21	20
Chick-pea	39	43	27	39	37	62	36	**49**	20	34	25	34	26	57
Casein	32	48	29	33	40	45	198	**63**	34	25	30	25	73	63
Egg	44	55	36	50	**68**	38	41	39	43	39	41	30	66	62

[a] Probable limiting amino acids are in bold type. From Pellett and Kaba (1972)

whereas $n.p.u._{op}$ is a measure of the overall protein value of the diet at a particular level of protein, i.e. a combined measure involving both amino acid composition and the lower utilization with increasing protein concentration. Thus $n.p.u._{op}$ is only meaningful for a specific diet at a specific level of protein. The prediction of the rate of fall of n.p.u. with increasing concentration of protein has engaged the attention of several workers; Miller and Payne (1961a) concluded that n.p.u. decreased in a linear fashion with the slope varying with protein quality, whereas Morrison *et al.* (1963) and Tagle and Donoso (1967) have proposed logarithmetric equations thus giving curvilinear responses, and Payne (1968), in the light of the failure of the original equation at high levels of intake (Carpenter

TABLE V. Prediction equations relating $n.p.u._{op}$ with protein concentration

$n.p.u._{op} = \dfrac{100s\,(1-1{\cdot}9p)}{100-7{\cdot}6/s}$	Miller and Payne (1961a)
$n.p.u._{op} = \dfrac{(100s-4)\log(1/p)}{100\log(25s)} + 0{\cdot}04$	Morrison *et al.* (1963)
$n.p.u._{op} = 0{\cdot}09 + \dfrac{(9-100s)\log p}{100\,(\log s + 1{\cdot}4)}$	Tagle and Donoso (1967)
$n.p.u._{op} = \dfrac{1{\cdot}25s}{1 + 6{\cdot}4\,ps}$	Payne (1968)

The equations of Miller and Payne (1961a) and of Morrison *et al.* (1963) are in the form as derived by Carpenter and Anantharaman (1968), and all are expressed according to the current convention.
s = protein quality score, as a decimal fraction of unity.
p = energy from protein as a fraction of total metabolizable energy.

and Anantharaman, 1968), proposed a modified equation which also predicted a curvilinear response. These equations are shown in Table V. The fall of utilization with increasing concentration is thus well established; however the biochemical reasons behind the fact are not clear. Miller and Payne (1963) have suggested that protein synthesis is controlled by energy availability, whereas Tagle and Donoso (1967) believe that the free amino acids that enter the liver pool may have a smaller chance of being channelled into the urea cycle when protein concentration in the diet is low than when it is high, since Schimke (1962) had demonstrated that the enzymes of the urea cycle became increasingly active as the protein concentration increased. Very recently Brookes *et al.* (1972) using radioactive techniques have shown that when lysine is limiting or deficient in the diet the major proportion is utilized for protein synthesis and little accumulated in the plasma, however when it was present at higher concentrations, plasma levels increased and more of the amino acid was oxidized and that after an initial threshold the quantity of lysine oxidized increased in a linear manner.

In contrast to these findings Hegsted and Chang (1965a,b) have claimed that they were unable to confirm the conclusions of Miller and Payne (1961a,b) and that n.p.u. was constant for four different proteins—

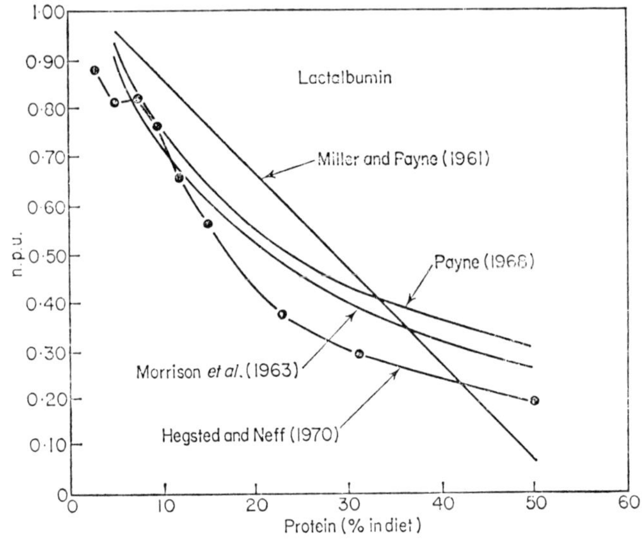

(A)

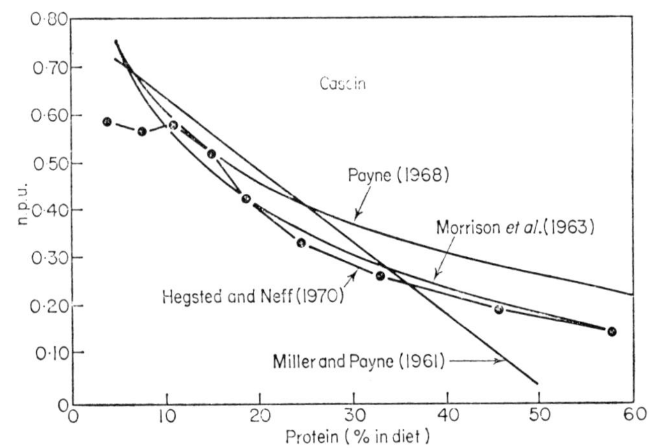

(B)

lactalbumin, casein, soya-bean protein and wheat gluten, given at seven different dietary levels during three-week growth periods. Certainly the linear relationship originally proposed by Miller and Payne (1961a,b) does not meet the facts, especially at higher levels of protein, and can be justly criticized (Hegsted and Chang, 1965b; Carpenter and Anantharaman, 1968). However the results of Hegsted and Neff (1970) can be presented in an alternative manner which shows continuously falling values for percentage N retention as the N concentration increases. The curves shown in Fig. 1 were obtained directly from the results presented by Hegsted and Neff (1970) for animals given both test and protein-free diets. Body N was calculated from body water by the use of a constant factor for the N/H_2O ratio, an assumption whose validity is confirmed by the original authors. The ratio used was 3·84 (Pellett, 1967), the choice of another ratio would not alter the relative values obtained. Thus from body water and the ratio, values for B and B_k could be calculated. The values for N intake (I) were calculated from protein consumption by the use of the 6·25 factor, other factors for each protein would change the absolute values but not the relative values as the concentration increased. For casein the n.p.u. appeared to be almost constant in the range 4–11% protein although from then onwards the percentage utilization fell predictably though not in a linear fashion. For lactalbumin and soya-bean protein utilization fell with increasing concentration not only at high levels but also in the region below 20% protein that is important with diets for man. Also shown in Fig. 1 are the predictions of n.p.u.$_{op}$ by several authors for the same proteins using generally accepted n.p.u. values (FAO, 1970). The equation

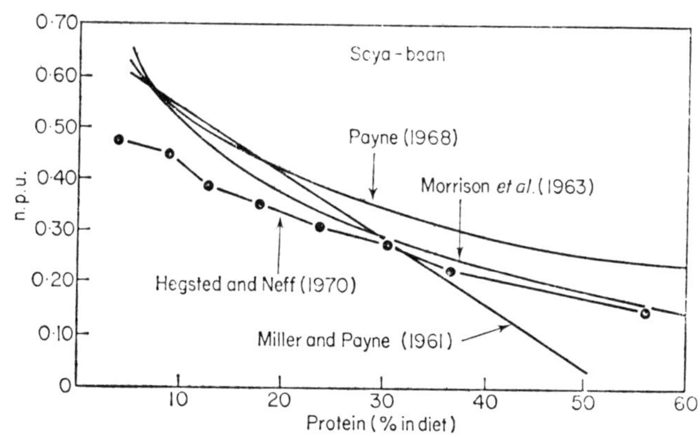

(C)

FIG. 1. The changes in net protein utilization with protein concentration for lactalbumin (A), casein (B) and soya-bean (C). Calculated from the data of Hegsted and Neff (1970) and the prediction equations of various authors

of Morrison *et al.* (1963) shows the closest fit to the data of Hegsted and Neff (1970); however only the slopes, not the numerical relations, should be compared because of the assumptions made in the calculation of the n.p.u. values from the results of Hegsted and Neff. For clarity the results as calculated by the equations of Tagle and Donoso (1967) have not been included, these were also curves which paralleled and fell between those of Payne (1968) and Morrison *et al.* (1963).

However, the fact that the results of Hegsted and Neff (1970) can be shown to fall predictably with concentration of protein does not affect the position of Hegsted and his associates, who relate protein consumption (not concentration) with response (N gain, water gain or weight gain) and claim that this response is linear over the range used for measurement of the relative nutritive value. This implies that utilization is not affected by the protein level, and that they believe that the concept of n.p.u.$_{op}$ and thence n.d.–p : e is invalid for the measurement of protein value of human dietaries. However, Hegsted and Neff (1970) admit that above about 10–13% protein the intake–gain relationship becomes curvilinear and Payne (1968) has also modified his position from the original claim of a straight line relationship between protein concentration and percentage utilization, both in fact have become "curvilinear". The differences between Hegsted and Payne thus seem somewhat reconciled and more a question of interpretation. In practice protein concentration would be highly correlated with protein intake over the limited range used for dietary protein measurement, and since protein concentration is an analytical value and is a property of the diet alone, this rather than intake should be the value of choice for the prediction of utilization. The question thus becomes how should this value be measured, are rat methods and protein-scoring methods valid for providing the answers we need to be able to predict N retentions in human beings eating their customary diet? These questions have been discussed recently (Hegsted, 1969; Campbell and McLaughlan, 1970; Bernhard, 1970) and are also considered elsewhere in this volume.

II. RELATIVE NUTRITIVE VALUE

The criticisms made by Hegsted and his associates of the n.p.u. procedure have been discussed above but the actual method proposed for determining relative nutritive value has not yet been considered. A series of papers (Hegsted and Chang 1965a,b; Hegsted *et al.*, 1968; Said and Hegsted, 1969; Hegsted and Neff, 1970; Hegsted, 1971) describe the method for determining what was first called "relative growth index" and which bears some relation to the nitrogen growth index of Allison (1959). A group of rats receiving a protein-free diet was included and at least three levels of each test protein were used, a modified slope-ratio analysis was used to calculate the slope of the response which was then compared to the slope obtained with lactalbumin as a standard (RNV = 100) to give the relative nutritive value (RNV). Full details of the procedure are given by Hegsted *et al.* (1968).

Hegsted and Chang (1965a) developed their method because of certain inconsistencies in the n.p.u. procedure: some proteins, especially those limited by lysine, were overestimated in quality by the n.p.u. procedure, for example wheat gluten is recorded as 0·40 whereas it appears to have a relative growth index of only 0·20. Bender (1961) showed that a lysine-free amino acid mixture had a n.p.u. of about 0·40, rather than the theoretical value of zero from its chemical score. The different needs of lysine for growth and for maintenance have been discussed by Campbell and McLaughlan (1970) and by Said and Hegsted (1969). McLaughlan and Noel (1970) have also shown that there is no fixed relationship between protein quality determined at maintenance levels and at levels supporting growth, thus indicating that n.p.u.$_{st}$ and biological value measurements can give erroneously high values for lysine-limited proteins. Rakowska *et al.* (1970) confirmed this observation for lysine-limited diets but concluded that the method of choice for the evaluation of dietary value should be the measurement of n.p.u.$_{st}$ at or about maintenance. Said and Hegsted (1969) indicated that for lysine-low proteins their slope-ratio method shared the inadequacies of the other methods because of mechanisms which permitted a relative conservation of body proteins when proteins low in lysine were given at levels below maintenance. These or similar conservation mechanisms are shared by children, at least when malnourished, as is evident from the N^{15} studies of Read *et al.* (1971). Rafalski and Nogal (1966) have further shown that at very low levels of protein intake (1% of the diet) n.p.u. values are about 0·20 and are not correlated with nutritive values at higher levels. These relationships, although important theoretically, are not relevant to the practical problems of measuring protein utilization from diets which usually have n.d.-p : e of 0·10–0·20.

III. MISCELLANEOUS METHODS

Various miscellaneous methods have been introduced over the years based on gain or repletion of certain body tissues rather than the whole animal; these have also been reviewed recently by McLaughlan and Campbell (1969) together with consideration of methods based on changes in the blood amino acids. A newer method based on changes in liver protein has been proposed by Mokady *et al.* (1969). These workers showed a high correlation between protein utilization using total carcass N and that using liver N. They claimed that more uniform homogenates could be obtained from the liver than from the whole carcass and that the whole procedure was more convenient. However anomalous results were obtained when lysine was added to wheat or maize gluten, for with these proteins lysine addition significantly increased protein utilization as measured by carcass N but not as measured by liver N.

IV. RELATIONSHIP BETWEEN SCORE AND BIOLOGICAL PROTEIN VALUE

Protein scoring systems are discussed elsewhere but how they relate to biological methods such as n.p.u. is important. Several studies have demonstrated that protein quality can be predicted with moderate accuracy by chemical score (Miller and Payne, 1961b; Rama Rao *et al.*, 1964; Morrison and Narayana Rao, 1966; Payne, 1968; Pellett and Srouji, 1970). The relationship between the score obtained and the true limiting amino acid in a diet requires three separate steps: (a) amino acid analysis of the diet; (b) supplementation with appropriate amino acids, and (c) biological determination of protein value before and after supplementation, followed by comparison of the scores with the n.p.u. values obtained. Such an experiment was performed by Kaba and Pellett (1971) using diets based on (i) wheat and milk and (ii) rice with lentil, both at 13–15% protein level. These diets were then supplemented with the potential limiting amino acids both singly and in combination. The amino acid composition and the n.p.u. values were obtained for 45 such amino acid-supplemented diets. The true limiting amino acid as determined was compared with that predicted using various scoring procedures. In the light of these results a modified scoring system was proposed and is shown in Table VI while Table VII shows the correctness of the prediction of the limiting amino acid by this and various other scoring systems. It is of interest that the pattern proposed by Kaba and Pellett (1971) was similar to the proposed FAO (1973) scoring pattern which was based on the requirements for preschool children but modified by the experience gained in using the

TABLE VI. Reference pattern (mg/g N) modified from FAO (1957) to fit rat n.p.u. data[a]

Ile	210	Met	144	Phe	180	Thr	270
Leu	306	Cys	126	Tyr	180	Try	70
Lys	360	Total SAA	270	Total arom.	360	Val	270

[a] From Kaba and Pellett (1971)

TABLE VII. The correctness of the prediction (+) of the limiting amino acid using various scoring systems[a]

Diets	*Actual limiting amino acid*	*Whole egg* (*FAO* '68)	*Human milk* (*FAO* '65)	*Human milk* ((*FAO* '68)	*FAO* '57 *pattern*	*Whole rat carcass*[b]	*FAO* '57 *pattern modified*[c]	*FAO* '57 *pattern modified*[d]	*FAO* '72 *pattern*
BM	Lys	+	+	+		+	+	+	+
BM + 0·10× Lys	Lys	+	+	+		+	+	+	+
BM + 0·15× Lys	Thr, Try			+				+	+
BM + 0·35× Lys	Thr, Try			+		+		+	+
BM + 0·35% Lys + 0·2% Thr	Try			+					
BM + 0·35% Lys + 0·2% Try	Thr			+		+		+	+
BM + 0·5% Lys + 0·2% Thr + 0·2% Try	Met	+			+	+	+	+	+
RL	Met	+				+	+	+	+
RL + 0·05% Met	Met	+				+	+	+	+
RL + 0·10% Met	Met	+					+	+	+
RL + 0·15% Met	Thr								
RL + 0·3% Met + 0·2% Thr	Try	+	+	+	+	+		+	+

DIETS: BM = Burghol-Milk (Protein–energy ratio 0·152) RL = Rice-Lentil (Protein–energy ratio 0·131)

[a] From Kaba and Pellets (1971)
[b] Pellett and Kaba (1972)
[c] Payne, P. R., Personal Communication
[d] As in Table VI

FAO (1957) reference pattern. Both these patterns were clearly superior to previous ones in predicting the true limiting amino acid for the rat as determined under n.p.u. conditions.

Said and Hegsted (1969) have, however, questioned the validity of attempting to relate chemical score to protein utilization. For very low levels of protein intake their criticisms are justified, but for the levels present in most actual diets the relationship between score and biological response (when allowance is made for protein concentration) can predict utilization with sufficient accuracy for most purposes, especially if it be accepted that in areas where protein–energy malnutrition (p.e.m.) occurs the cause may be more related to total energy intake than to either the total protein present or to its quality (Gopalan, 1969; Narasinga Rao *et al.*, 1969; Pellett and McGregor, 1971). Much still needs to be known, especially about the protein requirements and actual food consumption of children who later succumb to p.e.m.; the interrelationships between protein and energy are also only beginning to be understood, and especially their relationship to bodily activity. Further, the immediate cause of p.e.m. in an individual child is still unclear in all its complex socio-economic and hygienic aspects. However what does seem clear is that over the years, because it is scientifically interesting, we have over-emphasized the importance of protein quality to the partial exclusion of the protein–energy relationships which increasingly seem to be the most immediate dietary cause of protein–energy malnutrition.

ACKNOWLEDGEMENT

The author wishes to express his grateful thanks to all members of the Department of Food Technology and Nutrition, American University of Beirut, Beirut, Lebanon, for the facilities and technical assistance which made the work reported in this paper possible.

V. APPENDIX

Procedure for determination of n.p.u. Using Rats Body N Technique

Fifty 21-day-old weanling rats of one strain but of mixed sexes are obtained from a reputable animal supplier, introduced to the experimental room at 27°C* and fed on stock diet for one week. The animals are weighed, those of high and low weight are rejected and groups are selected so that the weight range is not greater than 10 g between the heaviest and the lightest and the group weights do not differ by more than 5 g. As many groups are used as can be obtained using these criteria;

* See Payne, P. R. and Jacob, M. (1965).

usually this is not more than 9 or 10; the remaining rats are rejected. Each group of four rats is placed in a single cage with a mesh bottom, under which should be paper on top of a layer of sawdust. One group is given the protein-free diet, the remaining groups are given the test diets; water and food are given *ad libitum* and the dry powdered diets previously equilibriated in the experimental room are dispensed in weighed quantities in pots designed to minimize spillage. The daily group weights are recorded together with the weights of food presented.

At the end of 10 days the animals are killed with chloroform or ether and the head, abdomen and thorax are opened with scalpel and scissors to aid drying. Small trays are made from aluminium foil and the groups of four carcasses are placed in them and weighed. These are then dried in a forced-draught air oven at 105°C for 48 h and reweighed, body water and dry weight are thus calculated.* The dry carcasses are passed through an electric grinder and then twice through a Wiley Mill. The powder is stored in a desiccator until N analysis. The spilt food is separated from faeces and is dried together with the residue in the pot and weighed. Moisture is also determined on a sample of the food as presented to the rats and dry food consumption is thus calculated.

The N contents of the diet and of the carcasses are determined by either macro or semi-micro Kjeldahl procedures, depending on their homogenity. Net protein utilization is thus calculated:

$$\text{n.p.u.} = \frac{B - B_k + I_k}{I}$$

where B is body N of test group; B_k, body N of protein-free control group; I, N intake and I_k, N intake of protein-free control group.

All test diets should be assayed in duplicate with different sets of rats at different times, if duplicates are not within 0·04 a third replicate should be performed.† Results should be rejected if the group weight curves are not smooth.

Protein-free diet‡—The percentages by weight were: maize oil, 15; glucose, 15; mineral mixture (USP XIV, supplied by General Biochemicals, Laboratory Park, Chagrin Falls, Ohio), 5; vitaminized carbohydrate (prepared by mixing 5 g of vitamin fortification mixture supplied by Nutritional Biochemicals Corporation, Cleveland, Ohio [see J. Nutr. **101**: 787 (1971) for composition] with 95 g of maize starch, 5; maize starch, 60. The complete protein-free diet should contain less than 0·1% N.

* Body N can be calculated from body water by use of appropriate factors, see Table I.

† As described by Miller (1963) the standard deviation of the method is 0·037 n.p.u. units; thus two-thirds of the results should fall within ± 0·040.

‡ Variation of this formula within moderate limits is acceptable.

REFERENCES

Allison, J. B. (1959). *In* "Protein and Amino Acid Nutrition" (A. A. Albanese, ed.) pp. 97–116. Academic Press, New York.

Barnes, R. H., Bates, M. J. and Maack, J. E. (1946). *J. Nutr.* **32**, 535–548.

Bender, A. E. (1961). *In* "Progress in Meeting Protein Needs of Infants and Preschool Children": proc. symp. 1960 (L. Voris, ed.) pp. 407–424. *Publs natn. Res. Coun., Wash.* no. 843.

Bender, A. E. and Doell, B. H. (1957a). *Br. J. Nutr.* **11**, 138–139.

Bender, A. E. and Doell, B. H. (1957b). *Br. J. Nutr.* **11**, 140–148.

Bender, A. E. and Miller, D. S. (1953a). *Biochem. J.* **53**, vii.

Bender, A. E. and Miller, D. S. (1953b). *Biochem. J.* **53**, vii–viii.

Bernhart, F. W. (1970). *J. Nutr.* **100**, 461–466.

Brookes, I. M., Owens, F. N. and Garrigus, U. S. (1972). *J. Nutr.* **102**, 27–35.

Bunce, G. E. and King, K. W. (1969a). *J, Nutr.* **98**, 159–167.

Bunce, G. E. and King, K. W. (1969b). *J. Nutr.* **98**, 168–176.

Campbell, J. A. (1963). Publ. 21, American University of Beirut. Beirut, Lebanon.

Campbell, J. A. and McLaughlan, J. M. (1970). *Int Congr. Fd Sci. Technol. 3*, Washington. 336–343.

Carpenter, K. J. and Anantharaman, K. *Br. J. Nutr.* **22**, 183–197.

Donoso, G. and Yáñez, E. (1962). *Nutr. Bromatol. Toxicol.* **1**, 37–42.

Dreyer, J. J. (1957). *Br. J. Nutr.* **11**, 22–27.

FAO (1957). "Protein Requirements." *F.A.O. nutr. Stud.* no. 16.

FAO (1970). "Amino Acid Content of Foods and Biological Data on Proteins." *F.A.O. nutr. Stud.* no. 24.

FAO/WHO (1973). "Energy and Protein Requirements", *F.A.O. Nutr. Mtg Rep. Ser.* no. 52.

FAO/WHO (1965). "Protein Requirements." *F.A.O. Nutr. Mtg Rep. Ser.* no. 37.

Gopalan, C. (1969). *In* "Protein-Calorie Malnutrition" (A. von Muralt, ed.) pp. 77–85. Springer-Verlag, Berlin.

Hegsted, D. M. (1969). *In* "Protein-enriched cereal foods for world needs" (M. Milner, ed.) pp. 38–48. American Association of Cereal Chemists, St. Paul, Minn.

Hegsted, D. M. (1971). *In* "Amino Acid Fortification of Protein Foods" (N. S. Scrimshaw and A. M. Altschul, eds), pp. 157–178. M.I.T., Cambridge, Mass.

Hegsted, D. M. and Chang, Y. (1965a). *J. Nutr.* **85**, 159–168.

Hegsted, D. M. and Chang, Y. (1965b). *J. Nutr.* **87**, 19–25.

Hegsted, D. M. and Neff, R. (1970). *J. Nutr.* **100**, 1173–1179.

Hegsted, D. M., Neff, R. and Worcester, J. (1968). *J. agric. Fd Chem.* **16**, 190–195.

Henry, K. M. (1965). *Br. J. Nutr.* **19**, 125–135.

Henry, K. M. and Toothill, J. (1962). *Br. J. Nutr.* **16**, 125–133.

Kaba, H. (1971). M.S. Thesis, American University of Beirut. Beirut, Lebanon.
Kaba, H. and Pellett, P. L. (1971). Proc. 6th Symposium on Nutrition and Health in the Near East. American University of Beirut. Beirut, Lebanon. (In press.)
McLaughlan, J. M. and Campbell, J. A. (1969). *In* "Mammalian Protein Metabolism" (H. N. Munro, ed.), Vol. 3, pp. 391–422. Academic Press, New York.
McLaughlan, J. M. and Noel, F. J. (1970). *Nutr. Rep. int.* **2**, 281–288.
Miller, D. S. (1963). *In* "Evaluation of Protein Quality" (P. L. Pellett, ed.) *Publs natn. Res. Coun., Wash.* no. 1100, p. 34.
Miller, D. S. and Bender, A. E. (1955). *Br. J. Nutr.* **9**, 382–388.
Miller, D. S. and Payne, P. R. (1961a). *Br. J. Nutr.* **15**, 11–19.
Miller, D. S. and Payne, P. R. (1961b). *J. Nutr.* **74**, 413–419.
Miller, D. S. and Payne, P. R. (1963). *J. theoret. Biol.* **5**, 398–411.
Mitchell, H. H. (1923–4). *J. biol. Chem.* **58**, 873–903.
Mokady, S., Viola, S. and Zimmermann, G. (1969). *Br. J. Nutr.* **23**, 491–495.
Morrison, A. B. and Narayana Rao, M. (1966). *In* "World Protein Resources". *Adv. Chem. Ser.* **57**, 159–177.
Morrison, A. B., Sabry, Z. I., Gridgeman, N. T. and Campbell, J. A. (1963). *Can. J. Biochem. Physiol.* **41**, 275–281.
Moulton, C. R. (1923). *J. biol. Chem.* **57**, 79–97.
Narasinga Rao, B. S., Visweswara Rao, K. and Nadamuni Naidu, A. (1969). *Indian J. Nutr. Diet.* **6**, 238–244.
Payne, P. R. (1968). Equation cited by Carpenter, K. J. and Anantharaman, K. (1968). *Br. J. Nutr.* **22**, 183–197.
Payne, P. R. and Jacob, M. (1965). *J. Nutr.* **87**, 211–227.
Pellett, P. L. (ed.) (1963). "Evaluation of Protein Quality." *Publs natn. Res. Coun., Wash.* no. 1100.
Pellett, P. L. (1967). *Br. J. Nutr.* **21**, 609–616.
Pellett, P. L. and Kaba, H. (1972). *J. Nutr.* **102**, 61–68.
Pellett, P. L. and McGregor, L. (1971). Proc. 6th Symposium on Nutrition and Health in the Near East. American University of Beirut. Beirut, Lebanon. (In press.)
Pellett, P. L. and Srouji, A. (1970). *In* "Nutrition" (J. Mašek *et al.*, eds) *Int. Congr. Nutr. 8*, Prague, 1969. pp. 582–586. Excerpta Medica, Amsterdam.
Platt, B. S. and Miller, D. S. (1959). *Proc. Nutr. Soc.* **18**, vii–viii.
Rafalski, H. and Nogal, E. (1966). *Int. Congr. Nutr. 7*, Hamburg. Abstr. p. 167.
Rakowska, M., Kunachowicz, H. and Szkilladziowa, W. (1970). *Nutr. Metab.* **12**, 160–170.
Rama Rao, P. B., Norton, H. W. and Johnson, B. C. (1964). *J. Nutr.* **82**, 88–92.
Read, W. W. C., McLaren, D. S. and Tchalian, M. (1971). *Clin. Sci.* **40**, 375–380.
Rippon, W. P. (1959). *Br. J. Nutr.* **13**, 243–260.
Said, A. K. and Hegsted, D. M. (1969). *J. Nutr.* **99**, 474–480.
Schimke, R. T. (1962). *J. biol. Chem.* **237**, 459–468.
Scrimshaw, N. S. (1962). *Fd Technol., Champaign* **16** (5), 26–31.

STUCKI, W. P. and HARPER, A. E. (1962). *J. Nutr.* **78**, 278–286.
TAGLE, M. A., COLOMBARA, E., PAK, N., ARAYA, J. and DONOSO, G. (1970). *Nutr. Metab.* **12**, 96–110.
TAGLE, M. A. and DONOSO, G. (1967). *Archos lat.-am. Nutr.* **17**, 295–310.

CHAPTER 16

Methods of Protein Evaluation with Rats, II

J. J. DREYER

National Food Research Institute, Pretoria, RSA

I. INTRODUCTION

Whatever the animal or the method used in the biological assessment of protein quality, the result will always depend on at least two quantities, the extent to which the protein can be digested (d.) and the extent to which the digestible fraction can be assimilated (b.v.). From the many publications of Mitchell and his co-workers (Nevens, 1921; Mitchell and Villegas, 1923; Mitchell, 1923–4, 1943, 1944, 1948, 1962, 1964; Mitchell and Carman, 1926) on this subject have emerged the following equations for d. and b.v.

$$\text{d.} = \frac{N_{\text{consumed}} - N_{\text{faecal}} + N_{\text{metabolic}}}{N_{\text{consumed}}},$$

where $N_{\text{metabolic}}$ = faecal N output on a protein-free diet;

and $$\text{b.v.} = \frac{N_{\text{absorbed}} - N_{\text{urinary}} + N_{\text{endogenous}}}{N_{\text{absorbed}}},$$

where $N_{\text{endogenous}}$ = urinary N on a protein-free diet.

It can readily be shown that, should d. and b.v. be constant characteristics of dietary proteins, the relationship between dosage level and response should be as illustrated in Fig. 1. The regression coefficients, the slopes of the regression lines shown, would be expressions in *absolute* terms of the digestibilities (Fig. 1a) and the biological values (Fig. 1b) of the proteins concerned.

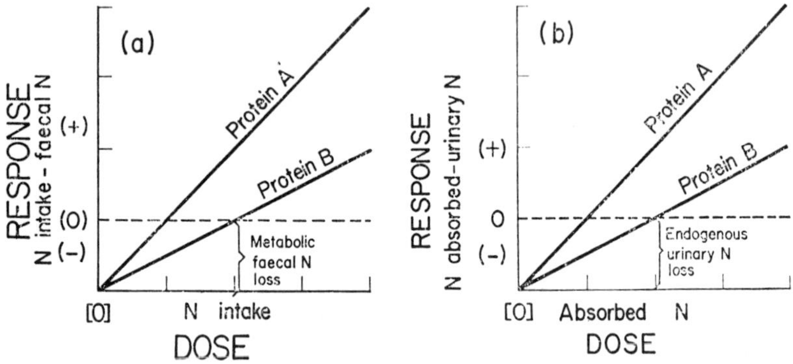

FIG. 1. Dose–response relationships illustrating the concept that every protein can be characterized in absolute terms by its digestibility (a) and its biological value (b)

Should the relationship between an influx of the protein and the response of the animal to this influx—be it measured in terms of nitrogen balance (Allison and Anderson, 1945), gain in body N, body weight or body H_2O (Hegsted *et al.*, 1968) or in any other way—be curvilinear (Fig. 2), it would mean that the proportion of the protein that can be used is dependent on the rate of influx. A relationship of this type would, of course, *not* be in harmony with the concept of a constant protein value expressible in absolute terms. However, if the curves describing the relationship could be shown to be all of a particular "family" irrespective of the protein involved, the protein assayist could express the response to the protein under test *relative* to the response to a "standard". This could be done by adopting protein A in Fig. 2 as a reference, and by either expressing the response to B as a proportion of the response to A at a given point on the influx scale (b/a), or by expressing the area underneath curve B as a proportion of that under curve A. It is clear, however, that it would be impossible to describe digestibilities or biological values in single numerical terms if the response curves obtained with different proteins are not of the same type.

Because of the importance of the nature of the dose–response relationship to the methodology of digestibility and biological value determinations, we investigated the dose–response curve in a number of special

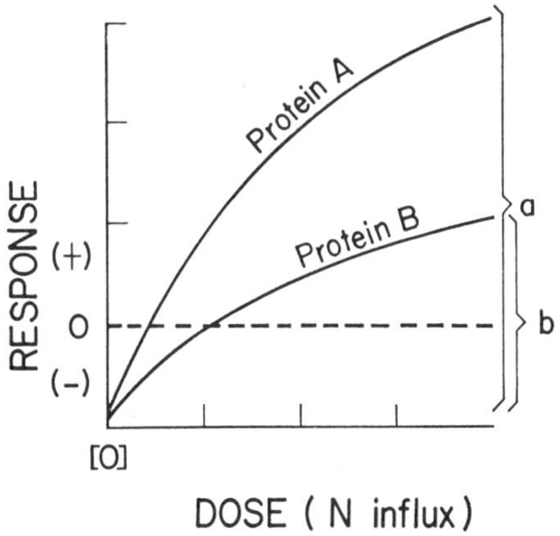

FIG. 2. The conditions under which the nutritive value of a protein could be described in relative rather than absolute terms

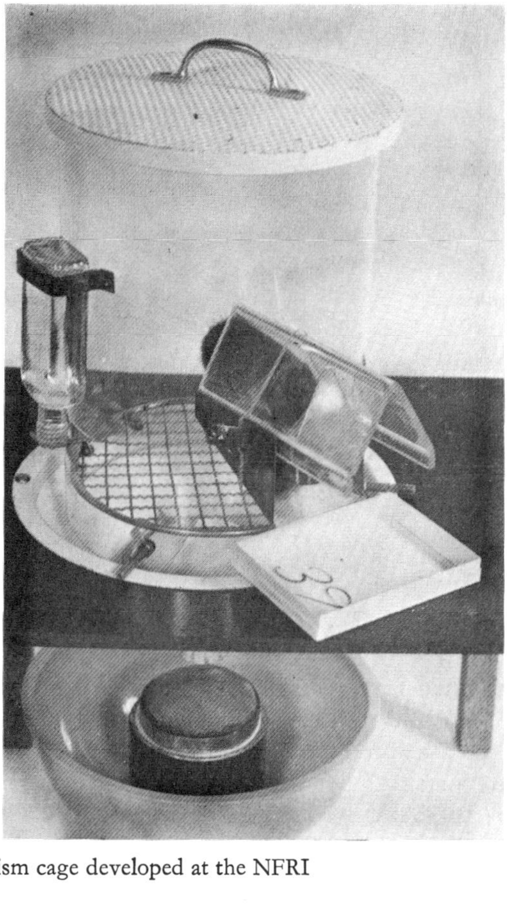

FIG. 3. Metabolism cage developed at the NFRI

cases. The present chapter is an account on the results of these investigations. During the course of this work it appeared, however, that there were certain important side-issues which also needed attention and these will be discussed first.

II. SPECIAL ITEMS OF LABORATORY EQUIPMENT

To meet our need for a reliable metabolism cage, we designed the one shown in Fig. 3 (Dreyer, 1969a). At present we have about 190 of these cages.

As the recovery of excreta from metabolism cages usually requires a great deal of washing, we (Dreyer, 1969a) designed and constructed a cage-washing aid (Fig. 4) which heats the washing liquid to the desired

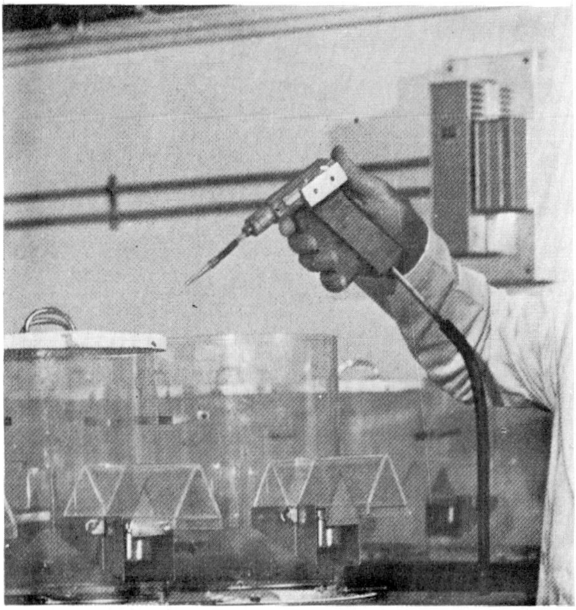

FIG. 4. Cage-washing aid developed at the NFRI

temperature and then forces it along an appropriate length of rubber tubing through a pistol-grip type of outlet.

With the use of the above equipment, it was found that food spillage was seldom more than 0·2 g per 10 days whilst recovery of excreted N was 99–100% (Dreyer, 1969b).

III. A BASIS FOR THE EXPRESSION OF NITROGEN METABOLISM DATA

As urinary N excretion depends to a certain extent upon body size, measurements of the rate of urinary N output are usually expressed in terms of some index of body size. Body weight or a function of body weight—e.g. (body weight in kg)$^{0 \cdot 75}$ (Kleiber, 1947)—is frequently used for this purpose.

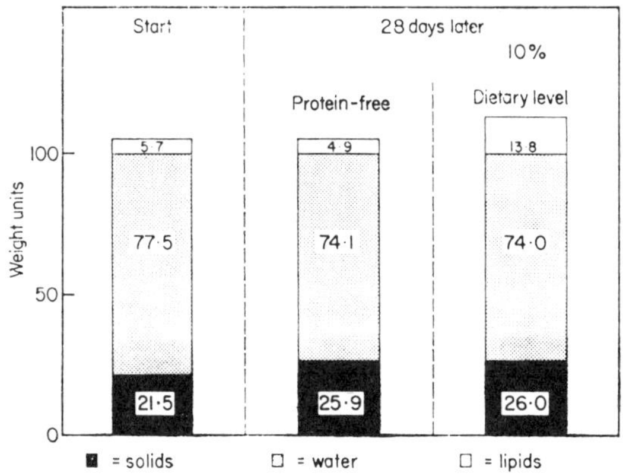

FIG. 5. The effect of age and diet on the fat, water and "solids" content of the body

Body weight is, however, not a fixed entity, since body composition varies according to age and diet, the former having an effect on the solids/water ratio and the latter on body-fat content (Fig. 5). Differences between the urinary N output per unit body weight of two rats could therefore be due to factors such as age and body-fat content (which affect body composition) rather than to differences in protein metabolism. For these reasons we sought an index of body size that was at least relatively independent of dietary conditions.

From Fig. 5 it appears that for rats of the same age, lean weight complies with this requirement. We therefore devised a method by means of which the lean weights of the rats used in our N balance studies could be readily estimated. The figure actually needed was the lean weight at the midpoint in time between the beginning and the end of an 8-day balance period following a 12-day adaptation period. Extensive studies (Dreyer, 1970a) led to the use of the following equation:

$$\left.\begin{array}{r}\text{Lean weight at}\\ \text{middle of collection}\\ \text{period (g) for rats of}\\ \text{about 40 days of age}\end{array}\right\} = \text{body } H_2O \text{ (g)} \times 1{\cdot}343 - \tfrac{1}{2} \text{ N balance (g)} \times 26{\cdot}74$$

It can be seen that the equation is based on the fact that in rats of the same age there is a constant relationship between (a) lean weight and body water and (b) lean weight and N retained. The error involved in using this equation was estimated as less than 2 g per rat.

IV. DURATION OF THE ADAPTATION PERIOD

In the application of N balance methods, digestibility and biological value are conventionally estimated from data obtained in a so-called "balance" or "collection" period at the end of an "adaptation" period. There has never been unanimity on how long the adaptation period should be (cf. Dreyer, 1970b).

We (Dreyer, 1970b) investigated this question according to the plan set out in Fig. 6. We first investigated the average urinary N output per g body N of 5 groups of 15 young, growing rats over four 2-day periods

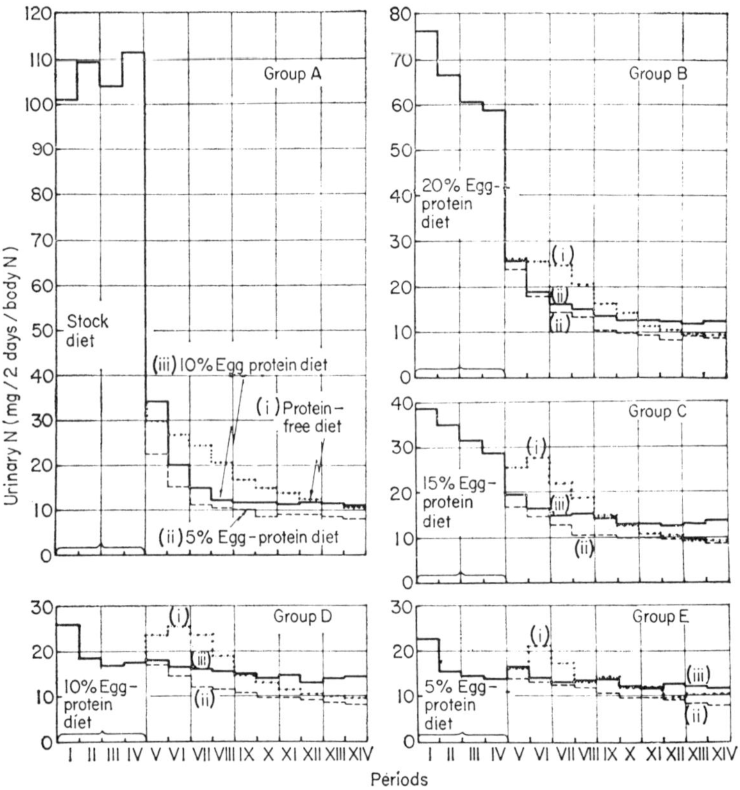

FIG. 6. Course of the urinary N excretion of growing rats given different diets

whilst feeding either a stock diet or experimental diets containing egg protein at certain levels. Each rat group was then subdivided into 3 groups of 5, one being given a protein-free diet, another egg protein at a 5% level and the third egg protein at a 10% level.

Following withdrawal of protein from the diet, the N output of the zero-protein groups during the first 12–14 days tended to be higher than that of the other groups. This finding is of interest, since it implies that exclusion of the preliminary period must yield a biological value for egg protein of more than 1·0. It also implies that the point representing zero N absorption in Fig. 1(b) will fall below the intercept on the y-axis and will therefore be at variance with the general trend of the regression line if no time is allowed for adaptation to the protein-free diet. We therefore considered that for the purpose of our studies the adaptation period should be retained and that it should be not less than 12 days.

It was of interest which of the amino acids in egg protein were responsible for the differences in the courses of the urinary N outputs of the rats described above. In a study of this question we obtained the results shown in Fig. 7. Each line represents the average urinary N output of 7 rats over fourteen 2-day periods. The results, obtained with individual amino acids given at levels equal to those of a 5% egg protein diet, are projected against results obtained in the one case with a 5% egg protein diet and in the other with a protein-free diet.

It will be seen that the excessive urinary N output of the protein-free group during the initial stages of the trial was due mainly to absence from the diet of the sulphur-containing amino acids, although leucine deficiency also appears to have been involved to a minor extent. The N sparing effect of the amino acids concerned manifested itself in a reduction of only the urea excretion, since the non-urea N output remained unchanged. It is, however, clear that there are experimental conditions under which biological values of above 1·0 can be obtained even for single amino acids; in the cases illustrated here the "endogenous" N excretion rate—i.e. the N output of the protein-free group—exceeded the urinary N excretion of the amino acid-supplemented groups mentioned. As this occurred mainly during the initial stages of the experiment, it appears that the duration of the adaptation period is the main factor involved.

V. HOMOGENEITY IN THE RESPONSE OF CERTAIN RAT BREEDS

We investigated the urinary N excretion rates of certain rat breeds under certain dietary conditions to establish which of these breeds would be most uniform in their response to protein feeding.

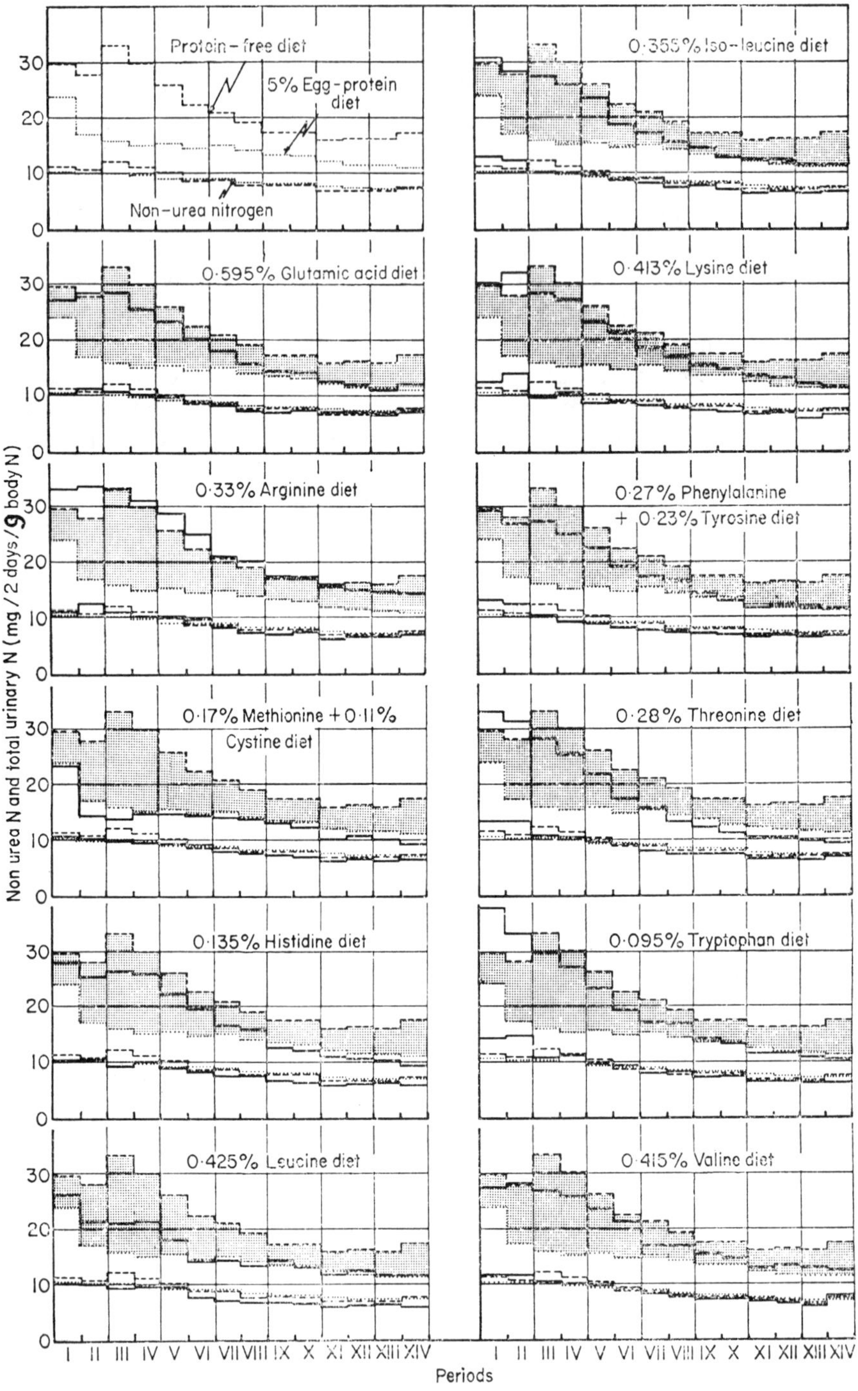

FIG. 7. The effect of giving certain amino acids on the course of the urinary N excretion of growing rats

The protein used was egg protein, given at graded levels in the diet to individual weanling rats; collections of urine and faeces were made during the last 8 days of a 20-day experiment. The rat breeds were: a randomly-bred breed from a Wistar-derived strain which we had had for many years; the offspring of a highly inbred (BD IX) strain obtained from Dr Druckrey of the Chirurgischen Universitätsklinik in Freiburg,

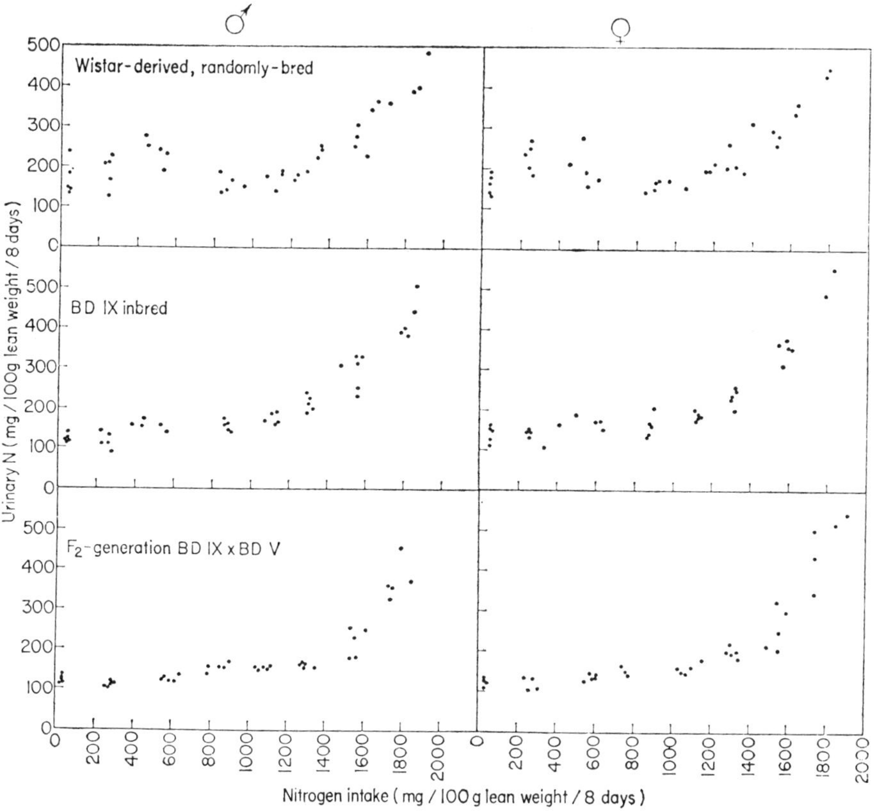

FIG. 8. The relationship between urinary N excretion and N intake for certain rat breeds

Germany (Druckrey *et al.*, 1962); and the F_2-generation of a cross between BD IX and BD V rats, this also being an inbred strain from Dr Druckrey's laboratory.

From the results (Fig. 8) it appears that the BD IX and the F_2-generation rats were less subject to variation in urinary N excretion per 100 g lean weight than the randomly-bred Wistar-derived rats. The F_2-generation rats especially showed a remarkable degree of homogeneity in response. However, as this breed was not available to us in sufficient numbers we used BD IX rats in our studies of the nature of the dose–response relationship.

VI. THE EFFECT OF METABOLIZABLE ENERGY STATUS ON URINARY NITROGEN EXCRETION

Under conditions of inadequate energy intake the body resorts to combustion of dietary protein and sometimes even of body protein as a source of energy. Suboptimal energy intake is a common feature of rat behaviour when the diet fed to the rat is low in protein content or when the protein component of the diet is of poor nutritional quality, so the energy status of the animal should be considered in studies on the relationship between protein intake and retention. We therefore attempted to assess the nature and the extent of the effect of this factor within the context of our particular experimental conditions.

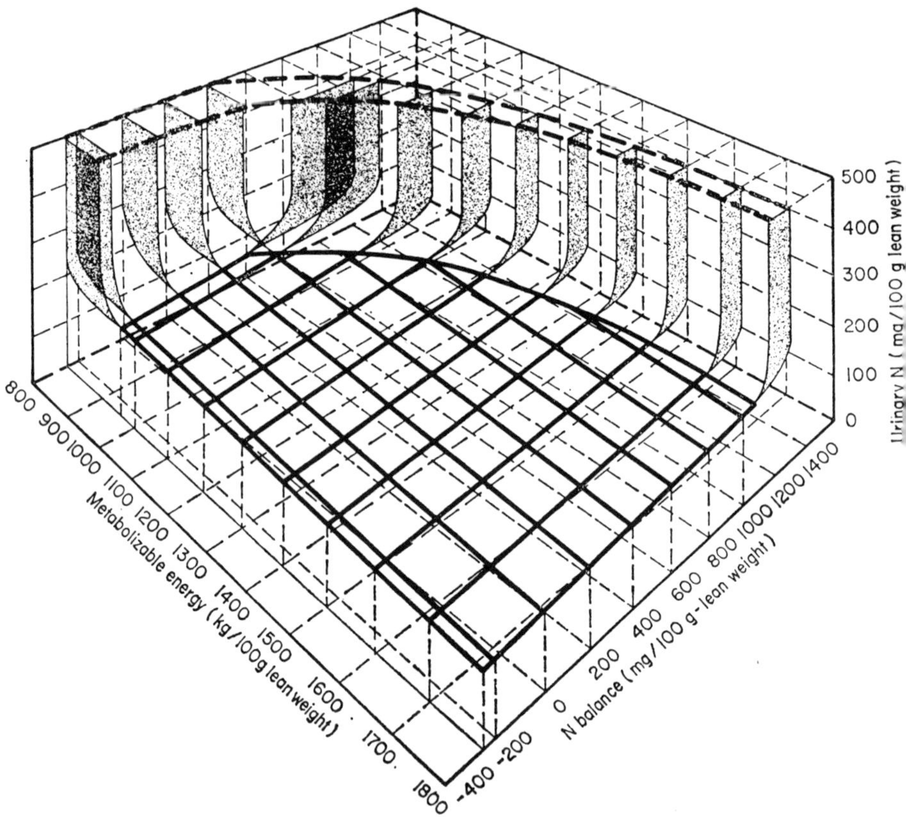

FIG. 9. Idealized relationship between metabolizable energy, N balance and urinary N output with young female rats during the last 8 days of a 20-day experimental period

A large number of weanling rats, 433 females and 424 males, was used in this study. The experiment was carried out at a room temperature of 26°C over a 12-day adaptation + 8-day collection period. Rat-to-rat variations in N balance and energy status were induced by varying over wide ranges the dietary protein contents and the weights of food offered per day. Egg protein was chosen for use in the study because of its relatively small effect on urinary N excretion when fed at suboptimal levels.

Figure 9 is an idealized presentation of the results obtained with the female rats. The index of metabolizable energy status used is the non-protein metabolizable energy consumed (in kJ) plus the energy derived from protein combustion, the latter being urinary N in mg multiplied by 0·133. (This factor is based on the energy value of the nitrogenous compounds in rat urine (Metta and Mitchell, 1954) and the fact that most proteins on complete combustion yield approximately 0·159 kJ/mg N.)

The extent to which a positive N balance could be forced in these rats depended on the metabolizable energy status. We could, however, arbitrarily demarcate an area on the base of the model shown here within which urinary N output was relatively independent of the energy status of the rat. This area represents the conditions which are most suitable for investigation of dose–response relationships, i.e. the conditions under which protein utilization is not affected appreciably by the energy status.

In our studies of absorption–retention relationships we ensured that all the relevant results were obtained from rats falling within this "safe" area.

VII. DOSE–RESPONSE RELATIONSHIPS IN DIGESTIBILITY DETERMINATIONS

The dose–response relationships observed in digestibility trials with 3 different proteins are shown in Fig. 10.

Being essentially linear, and meeting almost at the same point on the y-axis of the graph, the regression lines closely approximate the ideal relationship shown in Fig. 1a. Thus it appeared that the slopes of the regression lines would be fairly good estimates of the digestibilities of the proteins tested.

In a further study we estimated the digestibilities of certain combinations of egg and cooked haricot bean protein (Fig. 11). The values obtained with the combinations of the two proteins were in harmony with those obtained when egg and bean protein were tested separately.

It appears, therefore, that digestibility values are constant characteristics of proteins, lending themselves to determination in absolute terms according to established biometrical procedures.

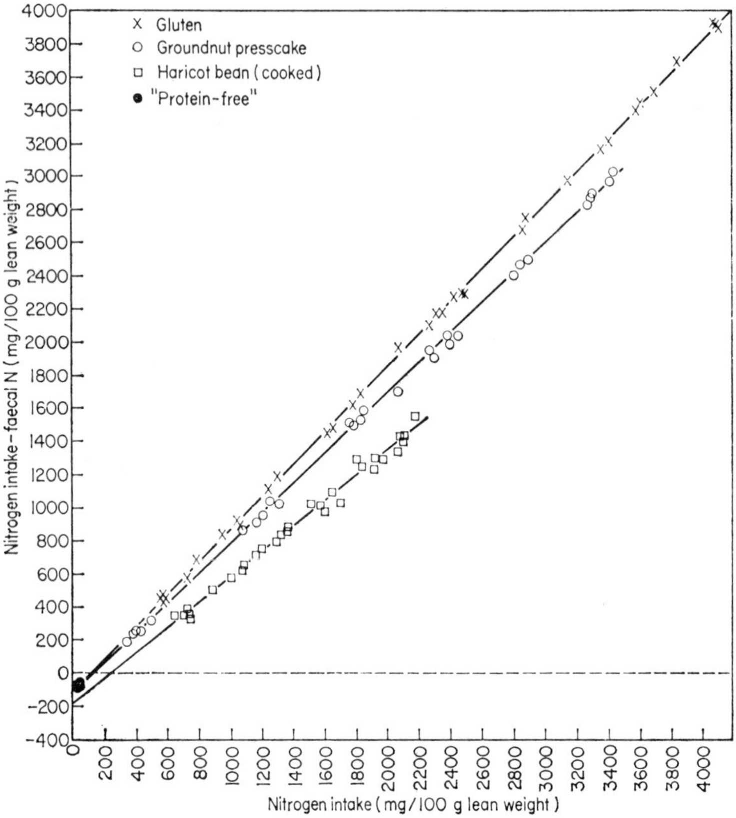

FIG. 10. Relationship between N intake and absorption with young rats given graded levels of gluten, groundnut presscake protein or haricot bean protein

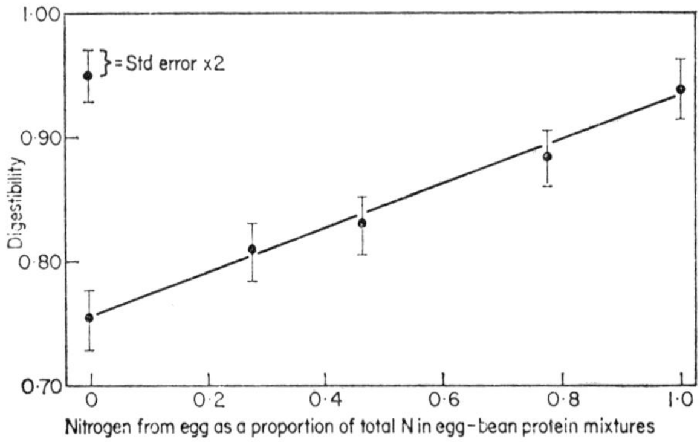

FIG. 11. Digestibility of the protein component of certain mixtures of cooked, defatted whole egg and cooked haricot beans

VIII. DOSE-RESPONSE RELATIONSHIPS IN BIOLOGICAL VALUE DETERMINATIONS

The absorption–retention relationships observed in our studies were by no means as satisfactory as the intake–absorption relationships observed in digestibility determinations. The results obtained in 12 + 8-day trials are shown in Fig. 12.

With egg protein the relationship was found to be linear, i.e. ideal; with casein and soya-bean protein slightly curved regression lines were obtained; and the gluten regression line consisted of two sections, one curved and the other essentially linear. The response of the rats to the absorbed protein thus appeared to be heterogeneous (the response curves were not all of the same "family") and, for this reason, could serve as a basis for describing in a single result the utilization of the absorbed protein only with egg protein. With the other proteins tested utilization

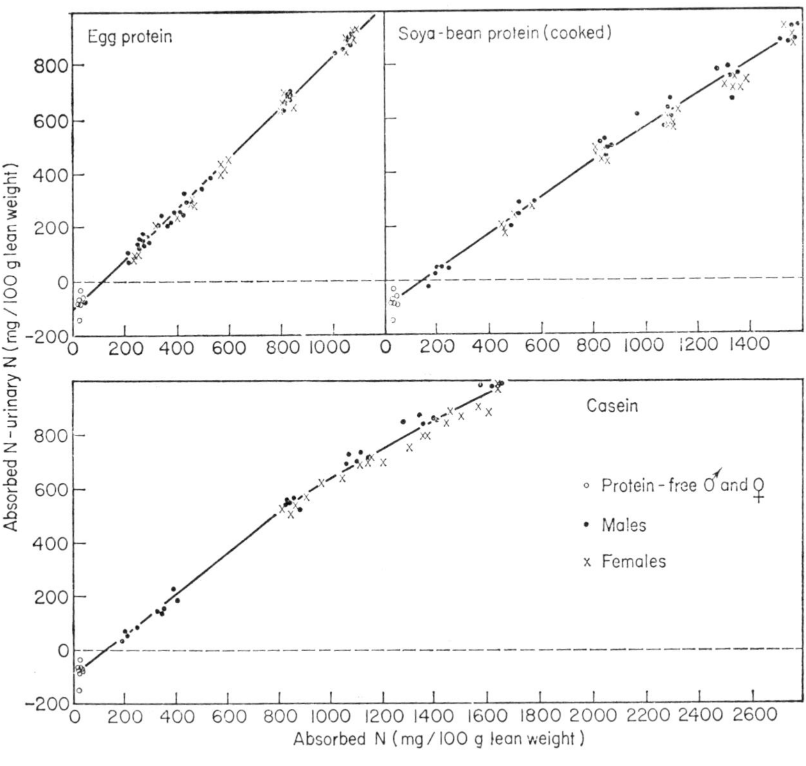

FIG. 12. Nitrogen absorption–retention relationships with young rats during the last 8 days of a 20-day experimental period

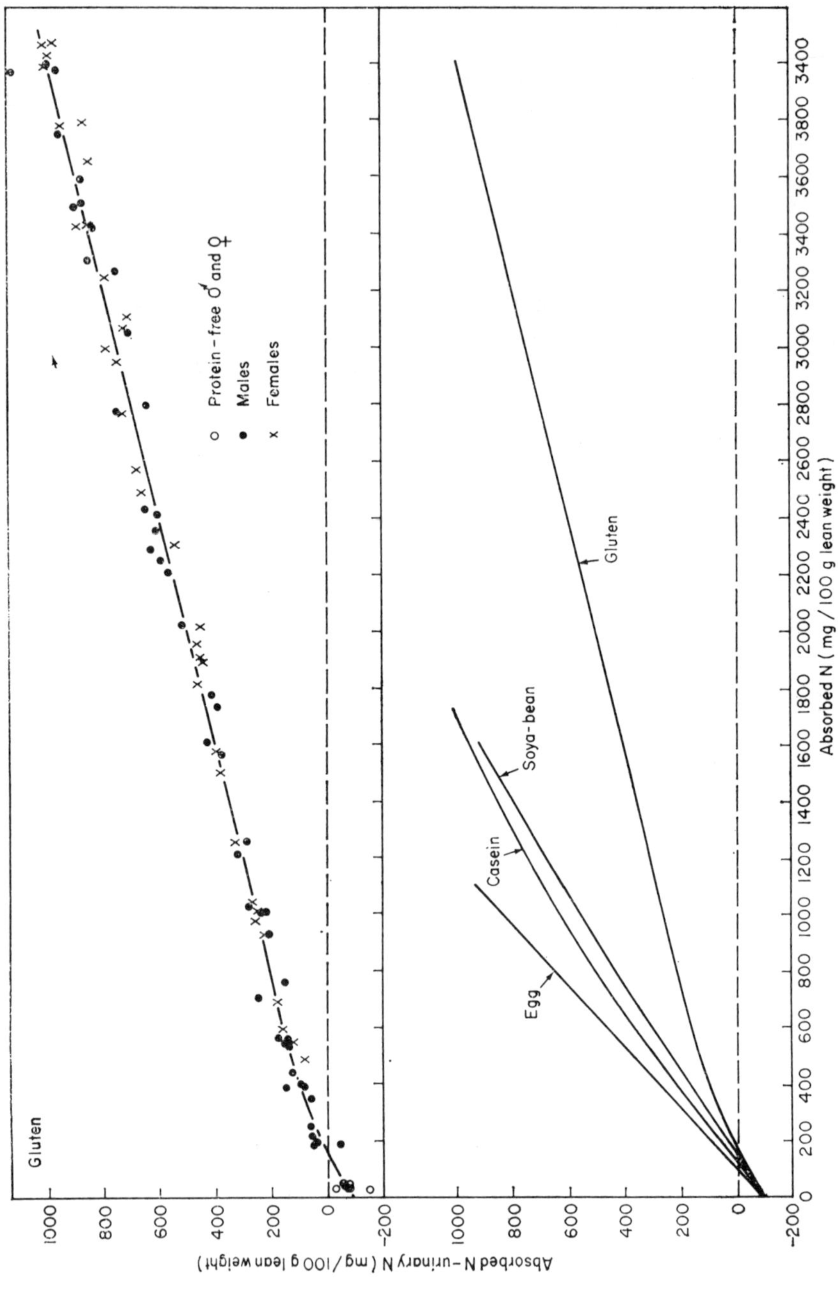
Gluten
Protein-free ♂ and ♀
Males
Females
Absorbed N-urinary N (mg/100 g lean weight)
Absorbed N (mg/100 g lean weight)
Gluten
Soya-bean
Casein
Egg

appeared to depend upon the absorption level, the general tendency being a decrease in the utilization with an increase in the absorption level.

Suspecting that in the above instances the comparatively high utilization rates observed in the lower influx ranges were due to adaptive changes which led to a conservation of limiting amino acids, we carried out another study, this time making the adaptation period very short (4 days). We included two control groups, one receiving a protein-free diet and the other a protein-free diet containing 0·165% L-methionine.

The results (Fig. 13) supported the contention that in the initial stages

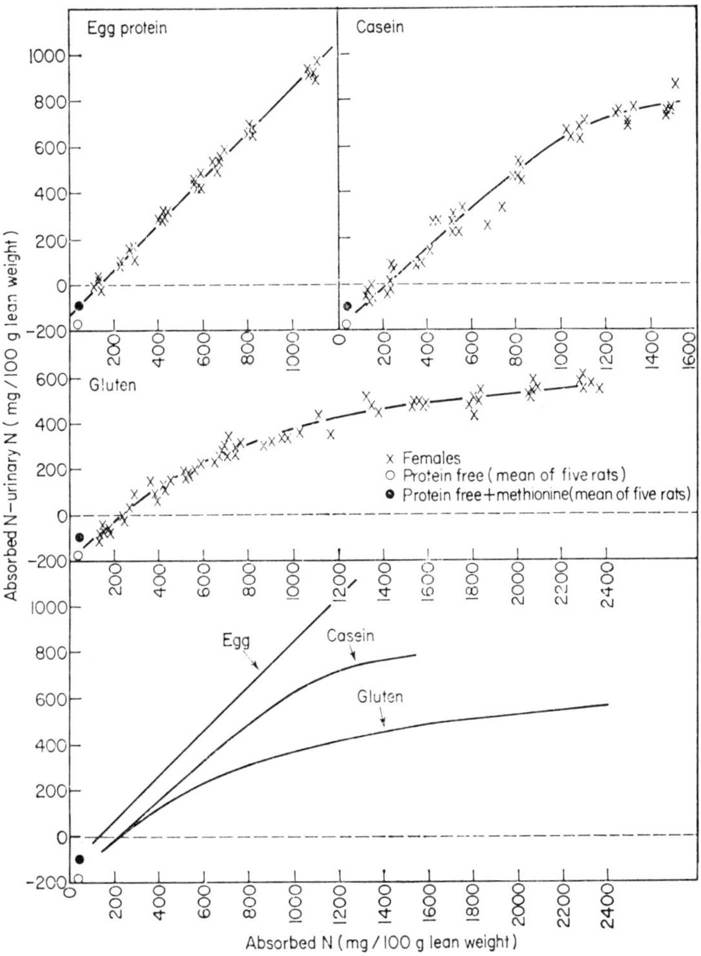

FIG. 13. Nitrogen absorption–retention relationships with young rats during the last 8 days of a 12-day experimental period

of protein depletion methionine has a body N sparing effect. However, a reduction of the adaptation period did not substantially alter the tendency of some of the dose–response relationships to deviate from linearity.

It would therefore appear that whole-body response in the growing rat to an influx of absorbable protein reflects the summation of not one but several "biological values". It appears that there is more than one body compartment which the absorbed protein can fill, that the amino acid demands at a specific feeding level depend upon the compartments being filled at that time, and that this filling is regulated according to prevailing dietary conditions. At low influx levels the predominating protein synthesis presumably entails the filling of a compartment—say collagen synthesis—which does not require as wide a spectrum of amino acids as would synthesis of blood, liver or muscle proteins, for example. With an increase in the influx rate the "lower-order" demands are readily met, even by a poor-quality protein such as gluten. However, with further increases, protein synthesis is extended to the filling of compartments requiring a wider spectrum of amino acids. Hence the drop in the efficiency of utilization of the poorer-quality proteins with an increase in influx rate. Because it is likely that egg protein can be used for the filling of all compartments with equal efficiency there is no drop in the egg protein curve.

The whole-body response of the young, growing rat does not appear to be a suitable criterion for assessment of the biological values of proteins, if our objective is to obtain for each protein one value on which can be based calculations of the weights of the protein needed to meet the assimilable protein requirements of individuals, calculations of the assimilable protein contents of foods, and/or calculations of the assimilable protein produced by countries. On the contrary, it appears that we should continue our search for a less complicated experimental model than the growing rat.

At our Institute we are now planning to investigate the response of the protein-depleted mature rat. We then wish to study the response of certain individual organs such as the liver, the kidneys and skeletal muscle, and also perhaps the response in terms of the rate of synthesis of certain individual high-grade body proteins. The criterion of choice will be the one that yields response curves of the same type for all dietary proteins.

REFERENCES

Allison, J. B. and Anderson, J. A. (1945). *J. Nutr.* **29**, 413–420.
Dreyer, J. J. (1969a). *S. Afr. med. J.* **43**, suppl. 7th June, pp. 3–14.
Dreyer, J. J. (1969b). *S. Afr. med. J.* **43**, suppl. 7th June, pp. 15–20.
Dreyer, J. J. (1970a). *S. Afr. med. J.* **44**, 1411–1414.

DREYER, J. J. (1970b). *S. Afr. med. J.* **44**, 336–361.

DRUCKREY, H., DANNEBERG, P., DISCHLER, W. and STEINHOF, D. (1962). *Arzneimittel-Forsch.* **12**, 911–919.

HEGSTED, D. M., NEFF, R. and WORCESTER, J. (1968). *J. agric. Fd Chem.* **16**, 190–195.

KLEIBER, M. (1947). *Physiol. Rev.* **27**, 511–541.

METTA, V. C. and MITCHELL, H. H. (1954). *J. Nutr.* **52**, 601–611.

MITCHELL, H. H. (1923–4). *J. biol. Chem.* **58**, 873–903.

MITCHELL, H. H. (1943). *J. Anim. Sci.* **2**, 263–277.

MITCHELL, H. H. (1944). *Ind. Engng Chem. analyt. Edn* **16**, 696–700.

MITCHELL, H. H. (1948). *In* "Proteins and Amino Acids in Nutrition" (M. Sahyun, ed.) ch. 2, pp. 46–81. Reinhold, New York.

MITCHELL, H. H. (1962, 1964). *In* "Comparative Nutrition of Man and Domestic Animals", vol. 1, ch. 3; vol. 2, ch. 17. Academic Press, New York.

MITCHELL, H. H. and CARMAN, G. G. (1926). *J. biol. Chem.* **68**, 183–215.

MITCHELL, H. H. and VILLEGAS, V. (1923). *J. Dairy Sci.* **6**, 222–236.

NEVENS, W. B. (1921). *J. Dairy Sci.* **4**, 552–588.

CHAPTER 17

Methods of Protein Evaluation: Assays with Chicks and Rabbits

HANS FISHER

Rutgers University, New Brunswick, New Jersey, USA

I. ASSAYS WITH CHICKS

The application to the chick of the carcass nitrogen retention method as developed by Bender and Miller (1953) with the growing rat is well established (de Muelenaere *et al.*, 1960; Summers and Fisher, 1961). In our laboratory the method is used routinely by selecting from a pool of 7-day-old chicks reared on a conventional starting diet groups containing 4 replicates of 5 chicks each and placing these on the experimental diet together with one group of 4 × 5 chicks placed on an essentially protein-free diet. These experimental diets are given for a period of 2 weeks at the end of which time the chicks are starved overnight, then weighed, killed with chloroform and dried to constant weight. Moisture is determined by difference between the wet and the dry weights. The carcasses of chicks in one of the replicates are finely ground and N determined on a portion of the mixed dried carcass powder. The N content of the carcasses of the remaining 3 replicates is calculated from the moisture content and the water/N ratio as determined for the first replicate. Net protein utilization values are then calculated from the equation given by Bender where

$$\text{n.p.u.} = \frac{B_f - B_k + I_k}{I_f}$$

where B_f and I_f denote carcass N and N intake of birds given the test diet, and B_k and I_k = the carcass N and N intake on the N-free control diet. Table I lists 3-week body weights and n.p.u. values for a number of common and some less common feedstuffs that have been assayed in our laboratory.

It has long been recognized that the level of dietary protein may be an important factor in evaluating protein quality. Thus it has generally been accepted that the level of protein must be kept below the optimum concentration required for rapid growth if meaningful comparative values were to be obtained. By the same token, it has been shown that the efficiency of dietary protein utilization may be influenced by the quality of the protein in question. Velu *et al.* (1971) gave a balanced amino acid mixture over a range of dietary levels and observed protein utilization to be essentially constant over a range equivalent to 9–17% dietary protein (Table II). Summers and Fisher (1961), on the other hand, noted a clear decrease in efficiency of utilization of methionine-supplemented soyabean protein over the same range of dietary protein concentration. These findings suggest that the level of dietary protein may be of lesser importance in the estimation of comparative protein utilization for high-quality protein, although it is of considerable importance with poorer quality protein.

De Muelenaere *et al.* (1965) have suggested that a level of 10% dietary protein is the level of choice in the chick n.p.u. assay since the highest n.p.u. values were obtained with this level for five protein sources tested. Fisher and Griminger (1969) have felt, however, that 10% was an inadequate level to permit proper differentiation of poor-quality proteins with certain amino acid deficiencies.

Table III gives a comparison between the essential amino acid requirements for growth and maintenance of the chicken. It is important to note that in the case of lysine the requirement for growth for this amino acid represents approximately 13% of the total essential amino acid requirement, compared with a requirement of only 4% of the total amino acids for maintenance of the adult chicken. On the other hand, in the case of methionine the growth requirement is 50% lower as a percentage of the total essential amino acid requirement than it is for maintenance of the adult chicken.

For these reasons Fisher and Griminger (1969) considered a level of 10% protein insufficient for a good assay, since it was too close to the maintenance requirement, particularly for proteins severely deficient in lysine. As shown in Table IV, on a low-lysine diet the n.p.u. response to lysine supplementation of 13% dietary protein was 2·5 times as great as the response obtained when lysine was added to a 10% level of dietary protein. In view of these results, and since 13% protein permits sufficient growth beyond the maintenance level, this concentration has been used routinely in our laboratory to evaluate protein quality by the carcass N retention method.

The carbohydrate source also deserves consideration in a discussion of

TABLE I. Three-week weights and n.p.u. values for different proteins given to growing chickens[a]

Protein source	*Measurements*[b]	
	3-week weight	*n.p.u.*
	g	
Isolated soya-bean protein[c] + 0·17% DL-methionine	212 ± 5	0·658 ± 0·016
Soya-bean meal (dehulled)	155 ± 10	0·551
Soya-bean meal (dehulled) + 0·2% DL-methionine	208 ± 7	0·688
Soya-bean meal (not dehulled)	175 ± 8	0·539 ± 0·005
Soya-bean meal (not dehulled) + 0·3% DL-methionine	238 ± 5	0·605 ± 0·031
Linseed meal	139 ± 3	0·360 ± 0·007
Linseed meal + 0·2% DL-methionine + 0·58% L-lysine HCl	184 ± 4	0·389 ± 0·014
Cottonseed meal (expeller)	112 ± 2	0·380 ± 0·006
Cottonseed meal (expeller) + 0·2% DL-methionine + 0·4% L-lysine HCl	188 ± 5	0·401 ± 0·006
Cottonseed meal (solvent extracted)	116 ± 3	0·354 ± 0·011
Cottonseed meal (solvent extracted) + 0·2% DL-methionine + 0·4% L-lysine HCl	184 ± 5	0·383 ± 0·008
Safflower meal	130 ± 4	0·300 ± 0·011
Safflower meal + 0·2% DL-methionine + 0·4% L-lysine HCl	243 ± 7	0·462 ± 0·010
Isolated peanut protein[d]	106 ± 3	0·318 ± 0·012
Isolated peanut protein + 0·2% DL-methionine + 0·4% L-lysine HCl	189 ± 4	0·536 ± 0·014
Rapeseed meal + 0·4% L-lysine HCl	232 ± 6	0·509 ± 0·012
Feather meal	74 ± 1	0·263 ± 0·017
Dried beef[e]	206 ± 8	0·755 ± 0·007
Meat meal		
A	82 ± 2	0·318 ± 0·009
B	88 ± 3	0·360 ± 0·013
C	94 ± 3	0·362 ± 0·015
D	89 ± 2	0·311 ± 0·021
Maize-soya-bean-alfalfa[f]	226 ± 6	0·561 ± 0·002
Maize-soya-bean-alfalfa-fish	229 ± 6	0·647 ± 0·002
Maize-soya-bean-alfalfa-meat	212 ± 4	0·520 ± 0·011

Protein source	Measurements[b]	
	3-week weight	*n.p.u.*
	g	
Whole egg powder		
Inedible, feed grade	276 ± 8	0·787 ± 0·014
Edible, for human consumption	237 ± 9	0·735 ± 0·009
Egg albumen		
Commercial	226 ± 6	0·661 ± 0·017
Laboratory prepared	224 ± 10	0·714 ± 0·021
Menhaden fish meal		
Overheated	167 ± 5	0·463 ± 0·008
Properly processed	234 ± 10	0·632 ± 0·013
Maize gluten	89 ± 2	0·404 ± 0·017
Zein	68 ± 1	0·194 ± 0·016
Zein + amino acids[g]	107 ± 3	0·297 ± 0·009
Gelatin	66 ± 2	0·224 ± 0·006
Casein	120 ± 6	0·418 ± 0·026
Casein + amino acids[h]	275 ± 7	0·599 ± 0·026
Sesame meal	98 ± 3	0·561
Sesame meal + 0·5% L-lysine HCl	198 ± 8	0·627

[a] Taken in part from Summers and Fisher (1962) and Fisher *et al.* (1962)

[b] Average values with their standard error

[c] Assay Protein C-1, Archer-Daniels-Midland Co., Cincinnati, Ohio; used as a standard in these tests

[d] An impulse protein product, Shulton, Inc., New York, N.Y.

[e] Prepared in the laboratory from a lean cut of beef, ground and dried at 60°C in a forced draft oven

[f] The following three rations were designed to simulate the protein combination of a standard 21% starter ration. Each protein-containing component was proportionately reduced to yield a total level of 13%. Dehulled soya-bean meal provided 9·3%, maize 3·4% and lucerne 0·3% of the dietary protein. When fish or meat meal were added, they replaced 1·8% of the soya-bean protein

[g] Zein was provided at the 10% level of protein and supplemented as follows to meet the essential amino acid levels of 13% isolated soya-bean protein: L-arginine 1·11; L-histidine 0·30; L-lysine 1·10; L-tryptophan 0·13; DL-methionine 0·10; DL-threonine 0·48; DL-isoleucine 0·22; DL-valine 0·92; glycine 0·50

[h] 13% casein protein plus L-arginine 0·5%; DL-methionine 0·17% and glycine 0·5%

TABLE II. Dietary protein level and efficiency of protein utilization (n.p.u.)

Soya-bean protein + methionine[a]		*Balanced amino acid mix*[b]	
Protein level (%)	*n.p.u.*	*Amino acid level*[c] (%)	*n.p.u.*
		2·9	0·684
		5·8	0·798
		8·7	0·760
11·8	0·686	11·6	0·755
15·8	0·622	14·5	0·755
18·2	0·583	17·4	0·727
21·4	0·541	20·3	0·665
26·6	0·455	23·2	0·623

[a] From Summers and Fisher (1961)
[b] From Velu *et al.* (1971)
[c] Protein equivalent of amino acid mix

TABLE III. Essential amino acid requirements for growth and maintenance of the chicken

Amino acid	*Growth*		*Maintenance*	
	% of diet[a]	*% of total*	*mg/kg/day*[b]	*% of total*
Arginine	1·00	14	120	18
Histidine	0·30	4	0	0
Lysine	0·95	13	29	4
Leucine	1·20	16	124	19
Isoleucine	0·60	8	72	11
Valine	0·82	11	61	9
Threonine	0·65	9	74	11
Tryptophan	0·15	2	19	3
Methionine	0·70	9	90	14
Phenylalanine	0·95	13	60	9

[a] From Baker *et al.* (1968)
[b] From Leveille *et al.* (1960)

TABLE IV. Effect of protein level on n.p.u. values of a lysine-deficient amino acid mixture[a]

Dietary variables[b]				
Protein equivalence (%)	*Lysine* (%)	*3-week body weight*[c] (g)	*n.p.u.*[d]	% *Change*[e]
10	0·4	63 ± 1	0·426	27·0
10	0·65	96 ± 2	0·541 ± 0·038	
13	0·4·	65 ± 2	0·270 ± 0·018	71·5
13	0·65	98 ± 2	0·463 ± 0·007	

[a] From Fisher and Griminger (1969)
[b] A crystalline amino acid diet was used
[c] Mean ± standard error for triplicate lots of five chicks, or a total of fifteen per treatment
[d] Carcass analyses for n.p.u. were carried out on each of the replicates of five chicks; only two replicates were analysed for the first group since one chick had died in the third replicate
[e] Calculated as the difference between the indicated low lysine (0·4%) group and the corresponding higher lysine (0·65%) group

TABLE V. Effect of different carbohydrates on n.p.u. values for growing rats and chicks given a methionine-supplemented soya-bean protein diet[a]

Carbohydrate[b]	*Net protein utilization*	
	Rat	*Chick*
Dextrin	0·520 ± 0·154[c]	0·386 ± 0·019[d]
Maize starch	0·591 ± 0·027	0·535 ± 0·070
Glucose	0·646 ± 0·070	0·552 ± 0·009
Sucrose	0·578 ± 0·020	0·593 ± 0·013
Maize starch + glucose + dextrin	0·566 ± 0·025	0·629 ± 0·013

[a] From Chalupa and Fisher (1963)
[b] Provided at 76% and 71% of the diet, respectively for rats and chicks for the single carbohydrate sources; the combination of carbohydrates was provided as maize starch 28%, dextrin 5% and glucose 43% (rats) or 38% (chicks)
[c] Mean ± SE for 5 rats
[d] Mean ± SE for quadruplicate groups of 5 chicks

diet composition for n.p.u. assays with chickens. Table V shows that a combination of maize starch, glucose and a small amount of dextrin promoted a significantly higher n.p.u. value than did any single source of carbohydrate tried. Incidentally, the same combination of carbohydrates showed no advantage in a rat evaluation (also shown in Table V). The relatively shorter digestive tract of the chick than that of the rat may play a role in the differential protein utilization of the two species in the presence of different carbohydrates.

In our experience (Fisher and Griminger, 1969) the level of fibre and of maize oil seemed to exert relatively little influence on n.p.u. values in confirmation of the observations of de Muelenaere *et al.* (1965).

The real significance of a good protein evaluation method ultimately

TABLE VI. Effects of proper processing and amino acid supplementation on the n.p.u. of cottonseed meal[a]

Cottonseed meal	*3-week weight* (g)	*n.p.u.*
SAMPLE		
A	112 ± 2[b]	0·380 ± 0·006[b]
A + methionine + lysine	188 ± 5	0·401 ± 0·006
B + methionine + lysine	140 ± 8	0·463
B + methionine + lysine + leucine + isoleucine + threonine	179 ± 7	0·519 ± 0·026
C + methionine + lysine + leucine + isoleucine + threonine	219 ± 5	0·661 ± 0·036

[a] Taken, in part, from Fisher and Quisenberry (1971)
[b] Mean ± SE

resides in its practical application rather than in its theoretical possibilities. The usefulness of the carcass N retention method and its application to the chicken is perhaps best illustrated by pointing to the discovery of unrecognized amino acid deficiencies in cottonseed protein (Fisher, 1965) as a result of observations derived from an n.p.u. evaluation of this protein source (Fisher *et al.*, 1962). As shown in Table VI, the addition of methionine and lysine to cottonseed meal sample A evoked a considerable growth response but only a very small improvement in the n.p.u. value. After much effort to elucidate this observation it was found, as also shown in Table VI, that the further addition of the amino acids leucine, threonine and isoleucine further improved both growth and n.p.u. In fact, with a carefully solvent-extracted processed cottonseed meal (sample C), supplemented with methionine, lysine, leucine, threonine and isoleucine, the n.p.u. value of 0·661 was as good as that obtained with high-quality soya-bean protein or fish meal.

II. AMINO ACID REQUIREMENTS OF RABBITS

Although the demand for information concerning protein quality in rabbit diets has not had the urgency that it has had for the chicken or for other species of economic importance, there has been some concern as to the suitability of certain protein sources used in experimental rabbit diets. Thus, Howard *et al.* (1965), Kritchevsky and Tepper (1968) and most recently Carroll (1971) have all reported abnormally high blood cholesterol levels attributable to the protein portion (casein) of the diet. Since we have

TABLE VII. The percentage composition of a complete purified rabbit diet

		Amino acid mixture[c]	
		Amino acid[d]	*Amount*
Isolated Soya-bean Protein			
(Assay Protein C-1)	20·0	Arginine	0·96
Cellulose	16·0	Histidine	0·55
Maize oil	5·0	Isoleucine	1·04
Mineral mix[a]	6·6	Leucine	1·20
Vitamin mix[b]	0·2	Lysine	1·79
Choline chloride (70% concentrate)	0·1	Methionine	0·36
Antioxidant (Santoquin, 50% concentrate)	0·025	Phenylalanine	0·80
DL-methionine	0·2	Threonine	0·62
Glucose monohydrate	26·0	Tryptophan	0·16
Dextrin	5·0	Valine	0·88
Maize starch	to 100	Glutamic acid	4·21
For pelleting add 5% H_2O		Glycine	2·29

[a] Composition in mg/kg: $CoCl_2{\cdot}6H_2O$, 3·5; $CuSO_4{\cdot}5H_2O$, 34·6; $MnSO_4{\cdot}H_2O$, 31·1; $ZnSO_4$, 169; $Fe[HOCH_2\text{-}(CHOH)_4CO_2]_2$, 706·3; $(NH_4)_6Mo_7O_{24}{\cdot}4H_2O$, 22·7; KI, 10·0

Composition in g/kg; K_2HPO_4, 10; $KHCO_3$, 10; $NaHCO_3$, 8; NaCl, 5; $CaCO_3$, 12·5; $CaHPO_4$, 10; $MgSO_4$, 10

[b] Composition in mg or i.u./kg: Thiamine HCl, 25; riboflavin, 16; Ca pantothenate, 20; pyridoxine HCl, 6; biotin, 0·6; folic acid, 4; menadione, 5; vitamin B_{12}, 0·02; ascorbic acid, 250; nicotinic acid, 150; vitamin A, 10,000 i.u.; vitamin D_3, 600 i.u.; α-tocopheryl acetate, 50 i.u.

[c] In place of isolated soya-bean protein and DL-methionine

[d] Given as the L-isomer

found that the rabbit, unlike other mammals, has an appreciable arginine requirement (Gaman and Fisher, 1970) it is understandable that casein, a protein low in arginine, might prove to be an inadequate sole protein source for this species.

The composition of a complete purified rabbit diet developed in our

TABLE VIII. Changes in body weight of young rabbits given an amino acid—containing diet with single amino acids omitted[a]

Amino acid omitted[b]	*Weight change*[c]	
	% of starting weight	*% of control*
Tryptophan	−14	−213
Methionine[d]	− 8	−192
Histidine	− 2	−110
Leucine	− 5	−149
Lysine	− 4	−113
Threonine	−10	−135
Valine	− 4	−141
Phenylalanine[e]	− 4	−130
Arginine	+ 3	+ 17
Isoleucine	+0·6	+ 8
Glycine	+10	+ 57
None (Control)	+15	+100

[a] From Adamson and Fisher (1971)
[b] All amino acid omissions were adjusted by adding an isonitrogenous amount of glycine, or, when glycine was omitted, of glutamic acid
[c] Groups of five 6-week-old female New Zealand rabbits were each given diets devoid of one of the listed amino acids for 8 days. The average gain in weight $\pm$ SE of rabbits fed the complete diet (control) was 196 $\pm$ 12 g; average starting weight $\pm$ SE was 1393 $\pm$ 32 g
[d] Diet was also free of cystine
[e] Diet was also free of tyrosine

laboratory (Gaman *et al.*, 1970) and found satisfactory for growth, reproduction and lactation of rabbits is given in Table VII. Also shown is the amino acid mixture that was used to study the essential amino acid requirement of growing female rabbits. The qualitative needs of the growing female rabbit are summarized in Table VIII. Omission of arginine and of isoleucine resulted in neither weight loss nor weight gain, whereas omission of glycine resulted in weight gain approximately half that obtained with the complete mixture of amino acids. Omission of any one of the other amino acids found essential caused a sharp loss in body weight.

The results of determining the quantitative needs for the essential amino acids (as yet incomplete) are listed in Table IX and are compared to those of the growing rat and chick. Of particular interest is the relatively high arginine requirement of the rabbit that is of equal magnitude

TABLE IX. Essential amino acid requirements (% of diet) the growing rabbit, rat and chick

Amino acid	*Rabbit*	*Rat*[c]	*Chick*[d]
Arginine	1·00	—	1·00
Histidine	0·45	0·21	0·30
Isoleucine	0·70	0·55	0·60
Leucine	0·90	0·69	1·20
Methionine[a]	0·60	0·49	0·70
Phenylalanine[b]	0·60	0·72	0·95
Threonine	?	0·51	0·65
Tryptophan	?	0·11	0·15
Valine	?	0·56	0·82
Lysine	?	0·90	0·95

[a] In the absence of cystine
[b] In the absence of tyrosine
[c] From Rama Rao *et al.* (1959)
[d] From Baker *et al.* (1968)

to the arginine requirement of the growing chick and contrasts with the semi- or non-essentiality of this amino acid for the growing rat.

It is already apparent that a better understanding of the amino acid requirements of the rabbit will provide important information concerning protein quality for this species, just as it has in the past for the chick and the rat. It is anticipated that the elucidation of the quantitative needs for the remaining essential amino acids in the rabbit will be completed in the near future.

REFERENCES

ADAMSON, I. and FISHER, H. (1971). *Nutr. Rep. int.* **4**, 59–64.

BAKER, D. H., SUGAHARA, M. and SCOTT, H. M. (1968). *Poult. Sci.* **47**, 1376–1377.

BENDER, A. E. and MILLER, D. S. (1953). *Biochem. J.* **53**, vii.

CARROLL, K. K. (1971). *Atherosclerosis* **13**, 67–76.
CHALUPA, W. and FISHER, H. (1963). *J. Nutr.* **81**, 139–146.
DE MUELENAERE, H. J. H., MARTIN, R. S. and MURDOCH, M. G. (1965). *J. Nutr.* **85**, 386–392.
FISHER, H. (1965). *J. Nutr.* **87**, 9–12.
FISHER, H. and GRIMINGER, P. (1969). *J. Sci. Fd Agric.* **20**, 382–384.
FISHER, H. and QUISENBERRY, J. H. (1971). *Poult. Sci.* **50**, 1197–1200.
FISHER, H., SUMMERS, J. D., WESSELS, J. P. H. and SHAPIRO, R. (1962). *J. Sci. Fd Agric.* **13**, 658–662.
GAMAN, E. and FISHER, H. (1970). *Nutr. Rep. int.* **1**, 57–64.
GAMAN, E., FISHER, H. and FEIGENBAUM, A. S. (1970). *Nutr. Rep. int.* **1**, 35–48.
HOWARD, A. N., GRESHAM, G. A., JONES, D. and JENNINGS, I. W. (1965). *J. Atheroscler. Res.* **5**, 330–337.
KRITCHEVSKY, D. and TEPPER, S. A. (1968). *J. Atheroscler. Res.* **8**, 357–369.
LEVEILLE, G. A., SHAPIRO, R. and FISHER, H. (1960). *J. Nutr.* **72**, 8–15.
RAMA RAO, P. B., METTA, V. C. and JOHNSON, B. C. (1959). *J. Nutr.* **69**, 387–391.
SUMMERS, J. D. and FISHER, H. (1961). *J. Nutr.* **75**, 435–442.
SUMMERS, J. D. and FISHER, H. (1962). *J. Sci. Fd Agric.* **13**, 496–500.
VELU, J. G., BAKER, D. H. and SCOTT, H. M. (1971). *J. Nutr.* **101**, 1249–1256.

CHAPTER 18

The Amino Acid Requirements of Rats and Human Beings

D. M. HEGSTED

Harvard School of Public Health, Boston, Massachusetts, USA

I. AMINO ACID REQUIREMENTS

A. Determination

Most of the results on the nutritive quality of proteins have been obtained with young growing rats. There is reason to believe that the nutritional quality of proteins is somehow determined by the content of essential amino acids. A basic question, therefore, is whether the values for the nutritive quality of dietary proteins determined with rats are applicable to man. Since there is no doubt that proteins do differ in nutritive quality and, furthermore, that the protein contents of diets around the world are surprisingly constant, the question of protein quality becomes a central issue in determining protein requirement or assessing the adequacy of diets with regard to protein.

There is little advantage to be gained by simply tabulating the various values for amino acid requirements that have been reported. It is true that confidence is obtained in a certain value if several laboratories come up with approximately the same figure. However, the fact is that different laboratories do come up with different values. It may be useful to consider some of the fundamental problems involved in the determination of amino acid requirements and what they may mean after they are determined. It is quite clear that there are unresolved problems in interpretation that must be considered. Some of these problems are specific to considerations of amino acid requirements; some are more general and relate to nutritional requirements of other nutrients as well.

Most estimates of requirements are based upon inspection of the results. One feeds various levels of a nutrient and by looking at the mean responses of the various groups decides that some level produces a maximum response. The advantages of curve fitting are clear, especially if one can find a linear fit. An example of the advantages and disadvantages are seen in the recent paper on the phenylalanine-tyrosine requirements of young rats by Stockland *et al.* (1971). Figure 1 is redrawn from Fig. 2 of their paper. In two experiments the best straight line was fitted to the points which fell below the maximum response and the requirement was taken as the intersection of this line with a line drawn at the maximum response. It is quite clear, of course, that the true dose–response line is a sigmoid

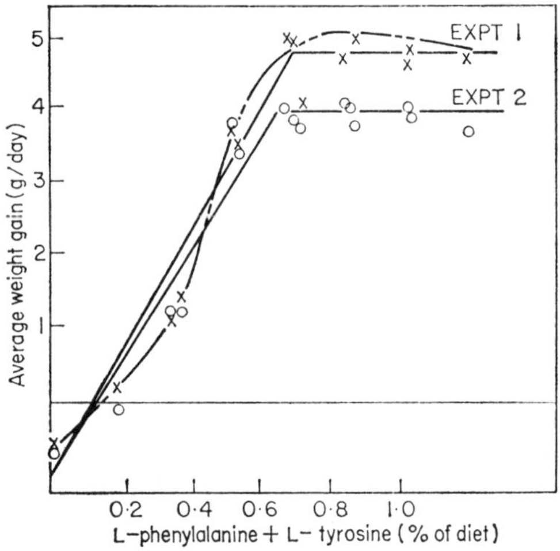

FIG. 1 .Growth response of young rats to phenylalanine. Taken from Stockland *et al.* (1971)

as indicated on the redrawn figure (Fig. 1). This is not pointed out in criticism of the results of Stockland *et al.* (1971). Some years ago when trying to interpret data on the vitamin requirements for growth (Hegsted, 1948), I concluded that this approach was the best available.

Nevertheless, the criticism of the approach is clear as shown in Fig. 2. However one draws the line, this will somewhat underestimate the actual mean requirement. It is a biological phenomenon that efficiency falls as one approaches maximum response. As far as I know, there is no really satisfactory way to determine how much this underestimates the real requirement, especially when there are substantial variations from one experiment to another.

More complex forms of curves have been fitted, of course, which do define a maxima. I do not trust these either because they usually do not fit very well at one part of the curve or another, and I do not understand the meaning of a quadratic curve, for instance, in terms of biological response. Even if one does use such a complex curve, the error of the estimated requirement is difficult or impossible to determine.

Since there is a decreasing efficiency as one approaches the maximum response and when we are talking about requirements we are interested only in the upper end of the curve, one can then consider the use of a log dose–response curve. As is well known, a log dose will often straighten out the top end of the curve and makes some biological sense

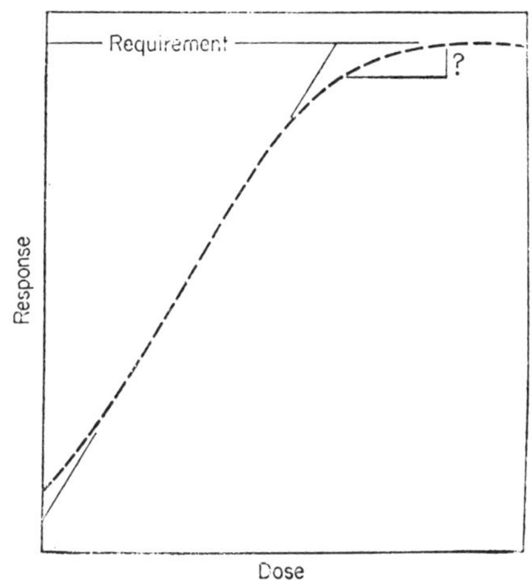

FIG. 2. Example of a dose-response curve

in terms of the diminishing efficiency, e.g. the "law of diminishing returns".

As indicated in Fig. 3, this appears to make the error of the estimate considerably smaller. However, in actual practice, the error becomes extremely large because one is dealing with logarithms. An estimated error of 100% or more is not unusual and often the upper estimate is clearly well above practical dietary limits. If one uses a log dose–response curve, one is likely to have to conclude that the more one feeds the more likely optimum nutrition is to be achieved—not a very useful conclusion.

Finally, in considering the interpretation of the dose–response curves we must be concerned with what we are trying to define. In a typical test, where a protein was fed at several levels to growing rats, the results shown in Fig. 4 were obtained (Hegsted and Neff, 1970). Note that the variance around the line is small at the lower levels of intake but as one approaches the requirement level the spread of the results becomes relatively enormous. It would seem practically certain that the growth of animals which grew rather poorly, relative to other animals at the same intake, was not determined by the amount of protein eaten. Genetic or other uncontrolled factors determined the rate of growth. However, the

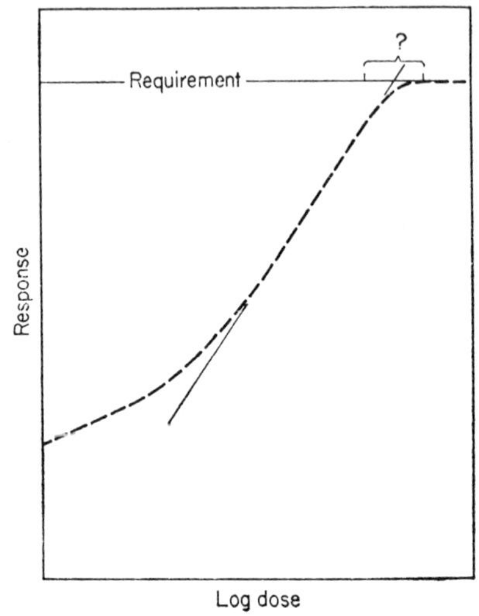

FIG. 3. Example of a log dose–response curve

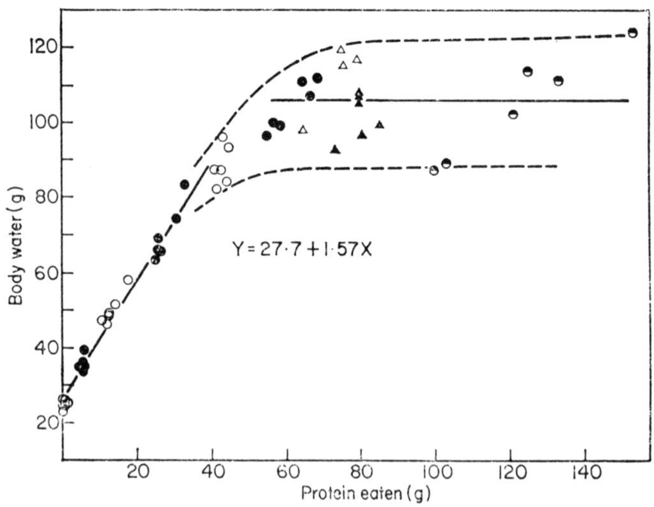

FIG. 4. Response of young rats to various intakes of soya-bean protein. Modified from Hegsted and Neff (1970)

animals that grew very well at an intake of 40 g might be animals with unusually large requirements. They might not have done as well had they been fed less protein. This is difficult to determine in actual practice. However, if one assumes that there are large differences in the requirements of individual animals and that these are only manifest or primarily manifest as one approaches the requirement, then one can draw two lines near the extremes of the results. These give quite different ideas as to the requirement.

B. Variation in Results

It is appropriate to point out here that in studies with animals one may be quite content with a mean value; in animal husbandry one may well be able to calculate a cost/kg to determine the most useful requirement, but in human nutrition we are inevitably concerned with the tail end of distribution curves—those individuals who for some reason or other do have higher requirements than the mean. A deficiency occurring in 2–3% of the population is unacceptable. Thus, in the estimates published by Rose (1957) on adult man and by Holt and Snyderman (1965) on infants, the highest possible estimate was used. The reason for this is clear but it is not a very satisfactory procedure. The upper limits as determined include not only biological variation but methodological and other errors as well. This must be borne in mind when comparing results obtained with man with those from other species.

Thus, it should be emphasized that we have very inadequate procedures for estimating requirements and, partly because of this, most of the reported results of amino acid requirements have had no statistical evaluation. When differing values are reported, there is no way to decide whether they are statistically different or not, let alone why they are different.

As already indicated, it is a relatively useless task to compile tables of amino acid requirements as reported by different authors. The most widely quoted results for the amino acid requirements of young rats are those reported by Rama Rao *et al.* (1959). These workers gave the animals a diet containing 5% casein and then added to this amino acid mixtures which varied in the content of each essential amino acid. The values they chose as representing the requirement for maximum gain in weight are shown in Table I. There is no particular objection to these findings but the results of Pick and Meade (1971) and Stockland *et al.* (1970, 1971) are included in the table to indicate the problems. The results of Pick and Meade (1971) were obtained by feeding a diet containing opaque-2 maize supplemented with amino acids, whereas Stockland *et al.* (1970, 1971) gave a diet with all of the amino acids provided in the free form.

One can present a number of possibilities as to why the results are different, i.e. the basal diet may make a difference, so may the ratio of other amino acids in the diet, and so on. None of these arguments seems very convincing, however, since there appear to be no consistent differences. Thus, Rama Rao *et al.* (1959) and Pick and Meade (1971) agree as to the valine requirement but differ greatly with regard to isoleucine. Stockland *et al.* agree with Rama Rao *et al.* on phenylalanine-tyrosine but derive a lysine value only two-thirds that of Rama Rao *et al.* These are not

TABLE I. Essential amino acid requirements of young rats (% of diet)

Amino acid	*Rama Rao et al. (1959)*	*Pick and Meade (1971)*	*Stockland et al. (1970)*
Histidine	0·21		
Isoleucine	0·55	0·36	
Leucine	0·69		
Lysine	0·90	0·70	0·60
Phenylalanine	0·42		0·38
Phenylalanine + tryptophan	0·72	0·59	0·69
Methionine + cystine	0·50	0·40	
Threonine	0·51	0·43	
Tryptophan	0·11		
Valine	0·56	0·54	
Arginine	0·28		

inconsequential differences but there is no way of guessing which values may be the more correct. We fall back on the need for more research and it is not surprising that people not in the field find this an unsatisfactory reply. Nevertheless, until we know how valid various estimates are or have a great many more results that agree, I do not see the solution. Certainly, there is unlikely to be much validity in simply averaging widely divergent values in the manner in which most food tables have been produced.

II. DIFFICULTIES OF INTERPRETATION

A. Animals

As already indicated, one of the suppositions generally made is that one ought to be able to predict the nutritional quality of proteins from a knowledge of their amino acid content and a comparison of this with amino acid requirements. This seems logical enough but we are not in the clear here either. A number of vexing questions can be raised.

In Fig. 5 are plotted the responses to varying levels of amino acids from the table of Rama Rao *et al.* (1959). No claims are made about the validity of the slopes of these lines. Some seem rather good, being based upon several points. Others are simply the straight lines between two points. Nevertheless, the lines are disturbing, particularly the response line for lysine since this is an amino acid of substantial practical importance. If these findings are correct, then the ratio of the lysine requirement to the requirement of any other amino acid varies greatly with the rate of growth achieved. Stated another way, a protein fed at a level which allowed only little gain might be limiting in one amino acid whereas at a higher level of intake another amino acid might be limiting. This would be equivalent to saying that nutritional quality of a protein is not a

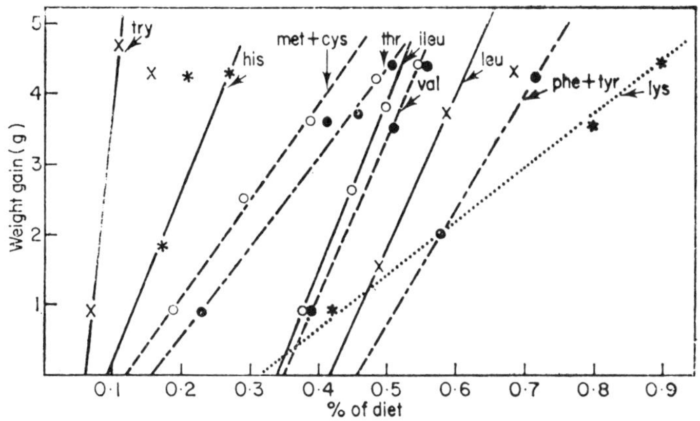

FIG. 5. Growth response of young rats given various levels of essential amino acids. Drawn from results of Rama Rao *et al.* (1959)

characteristic of the protein but dependent upon the conditions under which it is tested.

This concept is, in part, supported by our own results for the amino acid requirements of adult rats (Said and Hegsted, 1969, 1970). No other adequate results for adult rats have been found. Our results were obtained with an amino acid mixture given at a level equivalent to 3·2% protein. Each essential amino acid was varied and intake over a test period was measured. The mean requirement was estimated from the intersection of the regression line with X axis at zero gain and the standard error of that estimate calculated (Fig. 6) (Table II).

First, it is pertinent to point out the substantial variation in response of the individual animals given the same diet that severely limits the accuracy of the estimated requirement.

Second, it is important to point out the great differences in the slopes of the regression lines. A flat regression line gives a much less accurate estimate than a steeper line, other things being equal. Unfortunately, the estimate of the lysine requirement falls in this category. In any event, the standard errors are usually of the order of 10% or worse. It is improbable that these results are inherently worse than most of the other results with which we are dealing, especially those obtained with human subjects.

Third, it is particularly important to point out that when most of the essential amino acids are completely eliminated from the diet, the animals do much better than when fed a protein-free diet. This is to say that when you produce an amino acid mixture with an amino acid score of zero, you do not obtain an n.p.u. or a b.v. of zero. Our findings differ in detail from those of Bender (1961) but the major conclusion is the same. Only with three deficiencies do we obtain the expected result, i.e., deficiencies of threonine, isoleucine and total sulphur amino acids.

TABLE II. Mean estimates of essential amino acid requirements for maintenance of the adult female rat[a]

Essential amino acid	*Mean estimate for maintenance*[b]	
	(mg/day)	% of diet[c]
Histidine·HCl·H_2O	6·5 ± 0·9[d]	0·057
Isoleucine	14·1 ± 1·9	0·123
Leucine	13·0 ± 2·7	0·113
Lysine·HCl	10·2 ± 2·9	0·089
Phenylalanine without tyrosine	15·9 ± 2·0	0·138
Phenylalanine with tyrosine	9·3 ± 1·5	0·081
Tyrosine (difference)	6·6	0·057
Methionine without cystine	13·3 ± 1·8	0·116
Cystine (difference)	10·0	0·087
Methionine with cystine	3·3 ± 0·6	0·029
Threonine	13·8 ± 1·6	0·120
Tryptophan	3·0 ± 0·2	0·026
Valine	14·1 ± 2·2	0·123
Arginine·HCl	0	0

[a] Taken from Said and Hegsted (1970)
[b] Based on change in body water as a response parameter
[c] Food intake of rats whose body water was maintained around initial values as determined by carcass analysis of animals killed on day 1 of each of the three experiments ranged from 8·3 to 15·6 g/day, average 11·5 g/day
[d] Mean ± 2 SE

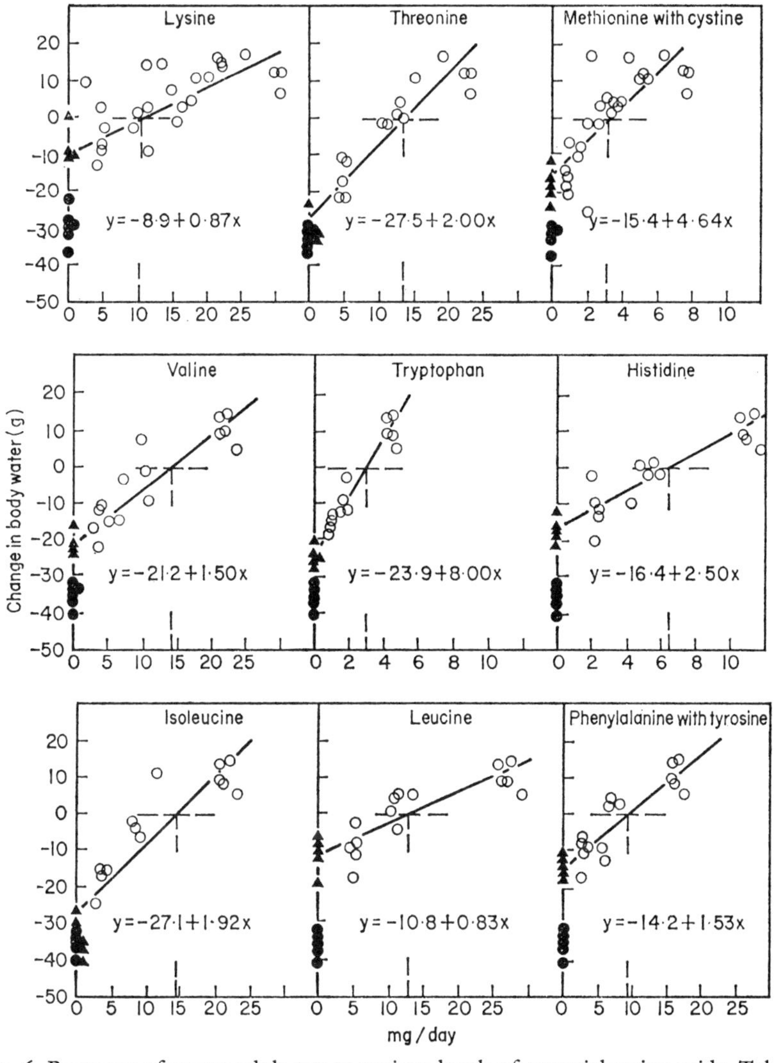

FIG. 6. Response of young adult rats to various levels of essential amino acids. Taken from Said and Hegsted (1970)

It is quite clear that animals have the ability to conserve essential amino acids to varying degrees when they are in short supply by as yet undescribed mechanisms. We can say that it takes longer to become deficient in lysine than threonine, given an equivalent degree of restriction. These differences in metabolism raise serious questions about the methodology for assessing protein quality as well as the methods for estimating requirements. It should be emphasized that because of the differences in the slopes of the dose–response lines, the requirement for those with low slopes is markedly dependent upon criteria of adequacy. For example, if we had assumed that a gain of 10 g in the 6-week period was the appropriate criterion rather than no gain, the requirement for lysine would have been more than doubled—22 rather than 10·2 mg/kg/day. The threonine requirement, on the other hand, would have been increased about 30%—from 13·7 to 18·7 mg/kg/day.

B. Man

All of these problems in the determination of amino acid requirements or the interpretation of the results which are obtained with animals are present, often to an exaggerated extent, in determining the requirements of man.

When we turn to man, we can consider the results with infants obtained by Holt and Snyderman (1965), the more limited findings with school children reported by Nakagawa *et al.* (1960, 1961a,b, 1962, 1965), and the considerably greater number of results with adult men and women. These results have been reviewed, interpreted and reinterpreted in all recent reports on protein requirements (Food and Agriculture Organization, 1957; Food and Nutrition Board, 1959; World Health Organization, 1965), without necessarily reaching the same conclusions.

Several points ought to be made. One is that the original results of Rose (1957) and Rose and Wixom (1955) are rather poor as quantitative results go. This is not said in criticism of the pioneering work which certainly established the order of magnitude of the requirements of the different amino acids. However, too much has been made of the actual values he recorded. An inspection of the original results, the few points available, the wide variations between individuals that were observed, etc. will convince anyone that this is true.

The results with women obtained by Leverton *et al.* (1956) are much better quantitative results. The design is better. These results do not indicate any real difference in the requirements of men and women when compared with the actual values reported by Rose *et al.* (1954), certainly not if differences in body weight are taken into account. The differences in the conclusions of the two groups were due simply to the different ways in which the experimental findings were interpreted.

I believe that our own reinterpretation of the results presented by Leverton, Rose and others (Hegsted, 1963) still represents the best estimates of the average requirement of the adult. An example of the treatment is shown in Fig. 7. Since most of the results were obtained at relatively high intakes approaching the requirement level, log dose–response lines were used which appear to fit the results better than simple dose–response lines. Moreover, the values recorded by Rose (open circles) although not included in the calculation of the line, do not appear to be particularly aberrant. The mean estimates arrived at by these calculations using the original values are shown in Table III.

As previously indicated, the values for some amino acids appear particularly poor and, unfortunately, some of these are those which are generally believed to be of special importance in practical nutrition—lysine and the sulphur amino acids.

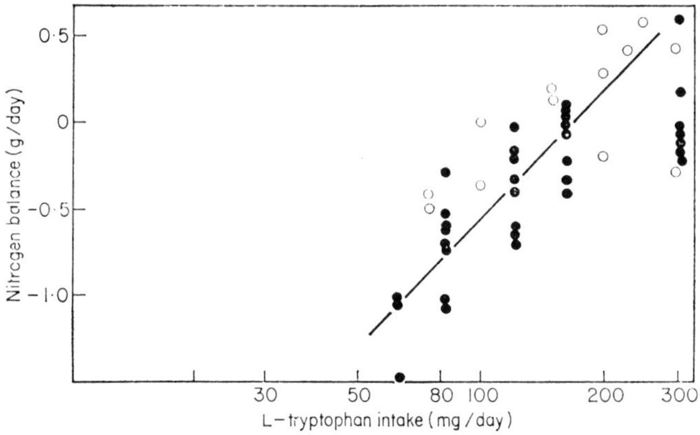

FIG. 7. Nitrogen balance in adult human subjects at different levels of tryptophan intake (Hegsted, 1963). Results with men, open circles; results with women, closed circles

TABLE III. Calculated amino acid requirements (mg/day)

Amino acid	*Required*	*Limits*	*Female*[a]	*Male*[a]
Tryptophan	168	146– 193	157	250
Phenylalanine	258	215– 310	220	300
Threonine	375	270– 515	305	500
Isoleucine	550	280–1065	450	700
Lysine	545	355– 835	500	800
Methionine	700	250–1950	550	1100
Methionine + cystine	194	164– 230	180	200
Valine	622	550– 705	650	800
Leucine	727	560– 940	620	1100

[a] Estimate made by original authors

III. FACTORS INFLUENCING AMINO ACID REQUIREMENTS

Without considering either in detail, some attention should be given to two papers which raise considerable doubt about the validity of all of the published findings on amino acid requirements. It may be that until these observations are explained, we should simply hold in abeyance the interpretation of the results available on amino acid needs.

The first is the paper of Kies *et al.* (1965), results from which are shown in Fig. 8. In this study all subjects received 6 g of N per day supplied by maize protein. To this basal diet varying amounts of "non-specific N"—glycine and ammonium citrate—were added. It appears quite clear that the balance improved as the level of "non-specific N" was increased. One could conclude, then, that there were plenty of essential amino acids in the maize at 6 g of total N, but the total N intake was borderline or insufficient. Snyderman *et al.* (1962) concluded that the

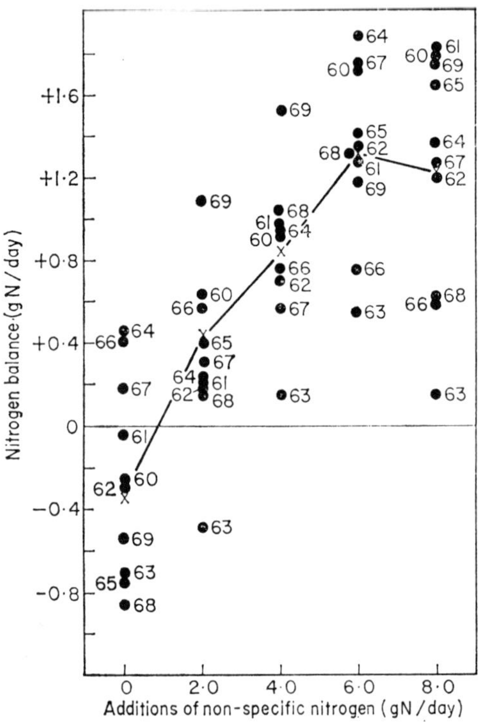

FIG. 8. Nitrogen balance with additions of "non-specific nitrogen" to a basal diet containing 6 g of N supplied by maize protein. Taken from Kies *et al.* (1965).

essential amino acid content was not the factor which determined the requirement for milk protein in infants and these findings confirm that observation, but with a rather poor quality protein such as maize.

In contrast to this conclusion is that of Romo and Linkswiler (1969) who kept the total N intake constant but increased the proportion of essential amino acids in the mixture. Whether they used an amino acid mix that approximated that of maize protein or of egg protein (Fig. 9), the efficiency of utilization rose as the proportion of essential amino acid N increased. With a total intake of slightly more than 6 g of N, the average individual achieved balance when somewhat less than 40% of the total N

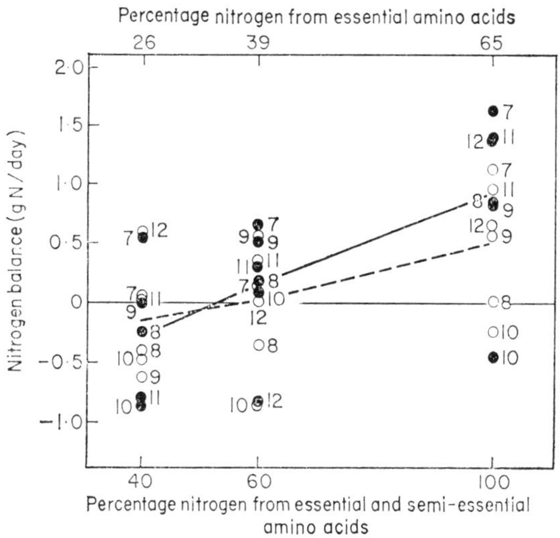

FIG. 9. The effect of changing the ratio of essential to non-essential amino acids. All subjects received the same intake of total N. Taken from Romo and Linkswiler (1969)

came from essential amino acids and it did not seem to make much difference whether the pattern of maize or of egg was used. Both of these papers contrast rather sharply with the paper of Rose and Wixom (1955) who obtained N balance with an intake of only 3·5 g of N per day and substantial other evidence that the requirement of egg protein is of this order of magnitude (Hegsted, 1968; Irwin and Hegsted, 1971a).

It should be emphasized that when we are using the balance technique or growth or changes in tissue N to estimate amino acid requirements, we are measuring the efficiency of utilization of the total N consumed and how it is influenced by variations in a particular amino acid. The results discussed above seem to show we cannot consider amino acid requirements in isolation. The efficiency of utilization of the dietary N is also influenced by the total N intake. Thus, the traditional approach—keeping the total N intake high so that it is not a limiting factor—is different from the practical conditions under which we want to assess the possible importance of amino acid deficiencies. Presumably, the conditions used by Rose, Leverton, Holt and others led to estimates that may be too low to be realistic under practical conditions. The discrepancy between estimates of total protein requirements and total essential amino acid requirements has been commented upon many times in the past.

It should be noted, of course, that the results of Romo and Linkswiler do not necessarily indicate that the determining factor was the ratio of essential to non-essential N. It could have been any one component of the essential or non-essential N mixture that was varied.

In a short review it is clearly impossible to discuss all the relevant literature, most of which has been summarized by Irwin and Hegsted (1971b). However, I might mention that the papers of Clark *et al.* (1957, 1960) on lysine requirements indicate a range of requirements of 400–1200 mg/day, a discouragingly wide range in itself, whereas the results of Fisher *et al.* (1969) indicate that the requirement under their conditions might be as low as 50 mg/day.

As a practical example of amino acid imbalance, the work should be mentioned of the Hyderabad laboratories showing that high leucine intakes appear to be an aetiological factor in pellagra and that isoleucine requirements are apparently elevated under these conditions (Gopalan, 1968). Moreover, results obtained from measuring changes in serum amino acids as criteria of requirements (Young *et al.*, 1971) have not been discussed. This method has the disadvantage that it is even less direct evidence of abnormality than is a change of N balance. On the other hand, we should all be aware that N balance is a very crude tool indeed. This intake–output method tells us nothing about what is going on inside the body. Performance can be severely compromised under conditions of approximate N balance (Ausman and Hegsted, unpublished results).

Recent estimates (FAO, 1973) of the best probable requirements for infants, school children, and adults are shown in Table IV. The figures for infants were derived largely from Holt's values modified when these estimates seemed out of line with intakes obtained from breast feeding or adequate baby foods (Fomon, 1961). Values for children were derived primarily from the reports of Nakagawa *et al.* and the adult values seem sensible compromises based largely upon the results of Rose and Leverton *et al.* These results indicate a considerable degree of uniformity of the "pattern" of amino acids, i.e., the ratio of one to another. There is also, of course, a general similarity in the pattern of requirements for young and adult rats.

The most striking conclusion one reaches from the values in Table IV is that the requirement of essential amino acids relative to the total N requirement falls with age but at considerably more rapid rates than does the total protein requirement. According to these estimates the total essential amino acid needs constitute nearly 50% of the total protein requirement of the young infant but fall to only 15% in the adult. The first value is similar to that found in highest quality proteins; the latter value is below that of any commonly available protein. If these conclusions are correct, then protein quality is of little or no significance in adults.

TABLE IV. Concentration of amino acids mg/g of protein required when protein is supplied in an amount to meet the requirements[a,b]

Amino acid	*Infant*	*Preschool age (2–5 years) scoring pattern*	*School age*	*Adult*
Histidine	26	—	—	—
Isoleucine	46	40	25	18
Leucine	93	70	44	25
Lysine	66	57	53	22
Methionine + Cystine	42	42	25	24
Phenylalanine + Tyrosine	86	77	25	24
Threonine	43	40	31	13
Tryptophan	17	10	4	6
Valine	55	50	30	18
E/T	47	38	24	15

[a] Taken from FAO (1973)
[b] Average protein requirement (g/kg/day): Infant 1·60; 2–5 years 1·00; 10–12 years 0·90; 0·55

It is tempting to ascribe such differences to variation in the rate of growth. We should feel some scepticism about this conclusion. It has often been pointed out that the rate of growth in the human species after the first years of life is very slow compared to most species and compared to the actual body size. A child of 10 years of age is expected to weigh about 30 kg and be gaining about 10 g per day, a daily increment of about 0·3%. It is not apparent why rates of growth of this order of magnitude should nearly double the essential amino acid per gram of protein, especially when the total protein intake per unit weight is also nearly doubled.

One might conclude that these differences are largely a matter of the way the experimental findings have been interpreted (see above) but my own feeling is that the growing animal may well be a different metabolic creature from the adult and we should be searching for flaws in the so-called "factorial approach" to estimating protein and amino acid needs.

One can summarize the current status in this field by observing that it is perfectly clear that there are very apparent similarities in the "pattern" of the amino acid requirements of rats and man (Table V). The relative

TABLE V. Comparisons of requirements/g dietary protein

Amino acid	*A* *Infant*	*B* *Adult*	*A/B*	*C* *Growing rat*	*D* *Adult rat*	*C/D*
Histidine	18			21	14	1·5
Isoleucine	44	18	2·4	55	31	1·8
Leucine	94	25	3·8	70	35	2·0
Lysine	64	22	2·9	90	21	4·3
Methionine	18	6	3·0	—	7	
Methionine + cystine	39	24	1·6	50	29	1·7
Phenylalanine + tyrosine	71	25	2·8	72	34	2·1
Threonine	55	13	4·2	50	30	1·7
Tryptophan	11	6	1·8	11	7	1·6
Valine	58	18	3·2	55	31	1·8

requirements of the various amino acids is similar in the two species, as is the fall in requirement as growth rate decreases. However, we should note that the discrepancies that still exist are large enough to prevent our concluding that the rat, either growing or adult, is an entirely adequate biological model for man. Attempts to generalize across species when the results are still inadequate or controversial may actually obscure the important differences between species that we need to know. The amino acid requirements of the rat, after all, are of little consequence unless they tell us something significant about the amino acid needs of man or other species important to man.

REFERENCES

BENDER, A. E. (1961). *In* "Progress in Meeting Protein Needs of Infants and Preschool Children": proc. symp. 1960 (L. Voris, ed.) pp. 407–424. *Publs natn. Res. Coun., Wash.* no. 843.

CLARK, H. E., YANG, S. P., WALTON, W. and MERTZ, E. T. (1960). *J. Nutr.* **71**, 229–234.

CLARK, H. E., MERTZ, E. T., KWONG, E. H., HOWE, J. M. and DELONG, D. C. (1957). *J. Nutr.* **62**, 71–82.
FAO (1957). "Protein Requirements." *F.A.O. nutr. Stud.* no. 16.
FAO/WHO (1973). "Energy and Protein Requirements", *F.A.O. Nutr. Mtg Rep. Ser.* no. 52.
FISHER, H., BRUSH, M. K. and GRIMINGER, P. (1969). *Am. J. clin. Nutr.* **22**, 1190–1196.
FOMON, S. J. (1961). *Pediatrics* **28**, 347–361.
FOOD AND NUTRITION BOARD (1959). "Evaluation of Protein Nutrition." *Publs natn. Res. Coun., Wash.* no. 711.
GOPALAN, C. (1968). *Nutr. Rev.* **26**, 323–326.
HEGSTED, D. M. (1948). *J. Nutr.* **35**, 399–409.
HEGSTED, D. M. (1963). *Fedn Proc. Fedn Am. Socs exp. Biol.* **22**, 1424–1430.
HEGSTED, D. M. (1968). *Am. J. clin. Nutr.* **21**, 352–357.
HEGSTED, D. M. and NEFF, R. (1970). *J. Nutr.* **100**, 1173–1179.
HOLT, L. E., JR. and SNYDERMAN, S. E. (1965). *Nutr. Abstr. Rev.* **35**, 1–13.
IRWIN, M. S. and HEGSTED, D. M. (1971a). *J. Nutr.* **101**, 385–430.
IRWIN, M. S. and HEGSTED, D. M. (1971b). *J. Nutr.* **101**, 539–566.
KIES, C., WILLIAMS, E. and FOX, H. M. (1965). *J. Nutr.* **86**, 357–361.
LEVERTON, R. M., JOHNSON, N., PAZUR, J. and ELLISON, J. (1956). *J. Nutr.* **58**, 219–229.
NAKAGAWA, I., TAKAHASHI, T. and SUZUKI, T. (1960). *J. Nutr.* **71**, 176–181.
NAKAGAWA, I., TAKAHASHI, T. and SUZUKI, T. (1961a). *J. Nutr.* **73**, 186–190.
NAKAGAWA, I., TAKAHASHI, T. and SUZUKI, T. (1961b). *J. Nutr.* **74**, 401–407.
NAKAGAWA, I., TAKAHASHI, T., SUZUKI, T. and KOBAYASHI, K. (1962). *J. Nutr.* **77**, 61–68.
NAKAGAWA, I., TAKAHASHI, T., SUZUKI, T. and KOBAYASHI, K. (1965). *J. Nutr.* **86**, 333–336.
PICK, R. T. and MEADE, R. J. (1971). *J. Nutr.* **101**, 1241–1248.
RAMA RAO, P. B., METTA, V. C. and JOHNSON, B. C. (1959). *J. Nutr.* **69**, 387–391.
ROMO, G. S. and LINKSWILER, H. (1969). *J. Nutr.* **97**, 147–153.
ROSE, W. C. (1957). *Nutr. Abstr. Rev.* **27**, 631–647.
ROSE, W. C. and WIXOM, R. L. (1955). *J. biol. Chem.* **217**, 997–1004.
ROSE, W. C., LAMBERT, G. F. and COON, M. J. (1954). *J. biol. Chem.* **211**, 815–827.
SAID, A. K. and HEGSTED, D. M. (1969). *J. Nutr.* **99**, 474–480.
SAID, A. K. and HEGSTED, D. M. (1970). *J. Nutr.* **100**, 1363–1375.
SNYDERMAN, S. E., HOLT, L. E., JR, DANCIS, J., ROITMAN, R., BOYER, A. and BOLES, M. E. (1962). *J. Nutr.* **78**, 57–72.
STOCKLAND, W. L., MEADE, R. J. and MELLIERE, A. L. (1970). *J. Nutr.* **100**, 925–933.
STOCKLAND, W. L., LAI, Y. F., MEADE, R. J., SOWERS, J. E. and OESTEMER, G. (1971). *J. Nutr.* **101**, 177–184.
WHO (1965). "Protein Requirements." *Tech. Rep. Ser. Wld Hlth Org.* no. 301.
YOUNG, V. R., HUSSIEN, M. A., MURRAY, E. and SCRIMSHAW, N. S. (1971). *J. Nutr.* **101**, 45–59.

CHAPTER 19

The Usefulness of Results with Human Beings in Standardizing Rat Assays

RICARDO BRESSANI, F. VITERI AND L. G. ELÍAS

Institute of Nutrition of Central America and Panama (INCAP)
Guatemala

I. INTRODUCTION

At present there is little agreement among research workers about the choice or selection of a single protein assay technique with experimental animals that will satisfy the requirements of everyone. It is even more difficult to select protein assay techniques with human subjects that are suitable for standardizing animal assays.

Although the subject is difficult for various reasons one cannot refuse the opportunity to discuss the usefulness of evaluating protein quality with human subjects. The problem of the world's protein supplies is of great importance and so is the cost of evaluating proteins with human subjects. If experimental conditions are well standardized, the values resulting from animal assays are closely similar to those from assays with human subjects. It is also important to have a clear understanding of the objective of protein assays, as distinct from the application of assay techniques to evaluate the nutritive value of the protein in foods. This chapter considers the relative merits of three protein quality assays commonly used with human subjects. It also attempts to point to the similarities between results when the same methods are used with experimental animals and human subjects.

II. THE PURPOSE OF PROTEIN QUALITY ASSAYS

Before discussing the value and use of protein quality figures derived from young and adult human beings to standardize rat assays, it is necessary to review briefly three aspects which apply to all species as well as to all available methods of protein quality evaluation.

First, it is accepted that the primary function of dietary proteins is to furnish a mixture of amino acids of the proper pattern and some additional nitrogen for the synthesis and maintenance of tissue proteins (Allison and Fitzpatrick, 1960; Allison, 1955). The relative efficiency of a protein in making the required amino acid pattern available to the animal will determine the magnitude of measurable biological responses. According to this concept, practically all methods of protein quality evaluation are directly or indirectly measuring the relative efficiency of protein sources in satisfying essential amino acid requirements.

Most of the methods used today in evaluating protein quality are concerned with the comparison of biological responses obtained under carefully controlled experimental conditions (Pellett, 1963).

The usefulness of any particular method chosen for the assay of protein quality will depend on successfully ensuring that, under the experimental conditions employed, protein is the only factor limiting the response chosen to be measured. This implies that the subjects must not constitute a variable; a condition easily attained with experimental animals but difficult with human subjects.

The second generally accepted aspect concerns the purpose of protein quality assays. This is to classify biologically the essential amino acid balance of proteins as a whole in relation to well-identified standards. In this sense the result of an assay represents a biological confirmation of the essential amino acid content of the protein and allows one to predict the usefulness of the protein in meeting nutrient needs alone or as a component of diets. It identifies the protein as good, intermediate or poor, just as protein content indicates whether the material corresponds to a protein isolate, legume or animal protein, or cereal protein (Block and Mitchell, 1946–7).

Thus, biological evaluation of protein quality has various applications:

(a) To monitor processing techniques that are used in food preparation or preservation (Mauron, 1961; Braham *et al.*, 1965).

(b) to measure the effectiveness of a protein source in supplying the nutrients needed for specific physiological functions, such as protein repletion, reproduction, production and growth (Allison, 1964; Chan and Waterlow, 1966).

(c) Recently, protein quality evaluation techniques have been found valuable for monitoring changes in protein quality brought about by breeding improved varieties of cereal grains, particularly since chemical methods do not give an entirely satisfactory assessment (Bressani *et al.*, 1971; Knipfel, 1969; Olivares, unpublished results).

(d) The methods have also been extremely useful in establishing optimum levels of protein and of amino acid supplementation of deficient proteins, and in studies of amino acid interrelationships (Rosenberg, 1959; Rosenberg and Culik, 1957; Bressani *et al.*, 1968).

(e) Protein quality assays are also valuable in assessing the nutritive value of the protein in diets as consumed both by man and by animals (Braham *et al.*, 1965; Tagle, 1971). Although such determinations might be thought to be the only objective of the various assays, interpretation of the results obtained with diets may be better understood and explained if knowledge is available about the quality of individual components.

(f) Finally, protein quality assay techniques can also be used to estimate the minimum needs for amino acids and protein *per se* (Chan and Waterlow, 1966; Bricker *et al.*, 1945; Smuts, 1935).

The third aspect that should be recognized is that all protein quality assay techniques, whether applied to experimental animals or to man, are interrelated and are affected by the same group of factors. For example, protein intake affects in the same manner Protein Efficiency Ratio (PER) and Net Protein Utilization (n.p.u.) (Braham *et al.*, 1967; Bressani *et al.*, 1965) in the rat, and Nitrogen Balance (NB) and biological value (b.v.) in man (Bressani and Viteri, 1970); an energy, mineral or vitamin deficit in the diet decreases the determined values in both species (Allison, 1958; Campbell, 1963; Hegsted and Haffenneffer, 1949). The age, sex and physiological state of the subject also affect the results obtained by the various techniques (Pellett, 1963; Campbell, 1963).

If these statements are accepted, then it is difficult to draw on results with human subjects to standardize animal assay techniques, since if the results obtained with the latter come from well-controlled studies and are analysed within the set of conditions used, the values between methods within species, and between species within methods, should be consistent.

III. PROTEIN ASSAY METHODS WITH HUMAN SUBJECTS

The methods most commonly used in protein evaluation research with human subjects are the classical biological value procedure in its simplified form, nitrogen balance (NB) and nitrogen balance index (NBI). From the results obtained, other calculations expressing protein quality have been made, such as net protein utilization and percentage N retention. Nitrogen balance methods have also been used to assess the nutritive value of proteins, and this has led to confusion and lack of agreement when the values obtained are considered as being the same as those indicating protein quality. There is a basic difference: in nutritive value, both protein concentration and protein quality are taken into consideration. Nutritive value provides the best estimate of the usefulness of a protein but the use of these values without knowledge of the quality of the protein may give results that indicate N retention, but with inefficient utilization of the amino acids.

A. Biological Value

Biological value has been defined as the amount of the absorbed protein (N) retained in the body to meet its needs for that nutrient for specific physiological functions. As originally developed, its measurement was used to determine the efficiency of a protein food in repleting the protein reserves of the depleted organism (Thomas, 1909; Mitchell, 1923–4; Mitchell and Carman, 1926). The technique requires that the experimental subjects be fed on a protein-free diet to measure metabolic faecal and endogenous urinary N. These values are then used to correct faecal and urinary N losses when the subjects are given the protein under study. From the results obtained, it is possible to calculate the true digestibility of the protein. The method also requires that protein intake, during the protein feeding periods, be such as to give a slightly negative N balance, or N equilibrium. Endogenous values can also be obtained from different trials, by using a N-free diet given to supply an adequate intake of energy.

The method is affected by the level of protein intake, the measured values being lower as protein intake increases, though the extent of change is a function of the amino acid composition of the protein under study (Henry and Kon, 1957). The age of the subject is another factor affecting biological value. Adult subjects yield higher values than young subjects; however, there is also an interaction with the amino acid composition of the protein and this is more evident with the poorer-quality proteins (Henry and Kon, 1957). The energy intake also affects biological value, as does the state of protein depletion of the individual (Allison, 1955, 1958).

When biological values are determined with human subjects under well-standardized and defined conditions the results are in good accord with those determined with experimental animals. Thus Truswell and Brock (1962) studied the protein quality of maize proteins fed to malnourished, protein-depleted adults (Table I). They found that the biological value of

TABLE I. Biological value of maize meal[a]

Subject	*Nitrogen* (g/day)		*Mean biological value*
	Intake	*Balance*	
P.N.	7·414	+0·487	0·42
M.P.	9·238	+0·697	0·43
K.S.	9·500	+0·015	0·34
P.N.	4·046	−0·137	0·54
M.P.	5·092	−0·081	0·55
I.A.	3·812	+0·014	0·63

[a] Taken from Truswell and Brock (1962)

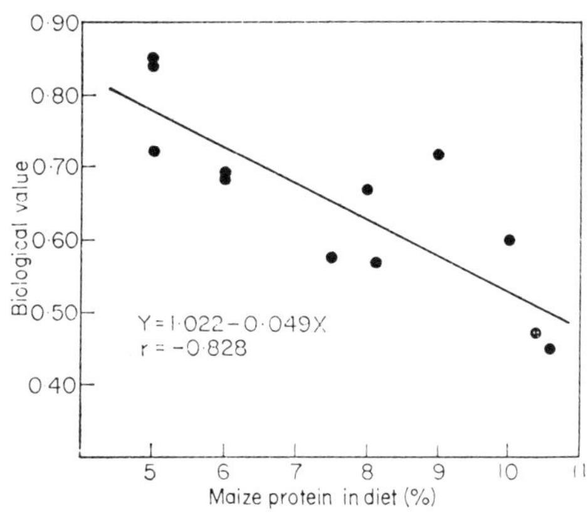

FIG. 1. Biological value of maize proteins at various levels of intake by adult rats

maize was 0·45 when the protein–energy ratio was 0·09, whereas when the protein–energy ratio was only 0·05, the value increased to 0·57. It is noteworthy that protein intake affected the value in the same way as had been found with experimental animals. Figure 1 shows the biological value of maize proteins determined by various authors during the past 40 years (Bressani, 1972). It can be seen that as protein intake increases, biological value decreases, and that the values for the rat are very similar to the values for adult human subjects receiving comparable levels of protein intake.

Similar conclusions can be drawn from other carefully conducted studies in which the biological values of egg, milk and other proteins have been determined with adult human subjects and with adult rats.

When biological value is measured with young, growing human subjects, the value represents the capacity of the protein both to provide the essential amino acids to promote growth and to build up the protein reserves of the body. There is, therefore, no possibility of distinguishing between the two functions. An example of biological value measured with young human subjects is shown in Fig. 2 (Bressani *et al.*, unpublished

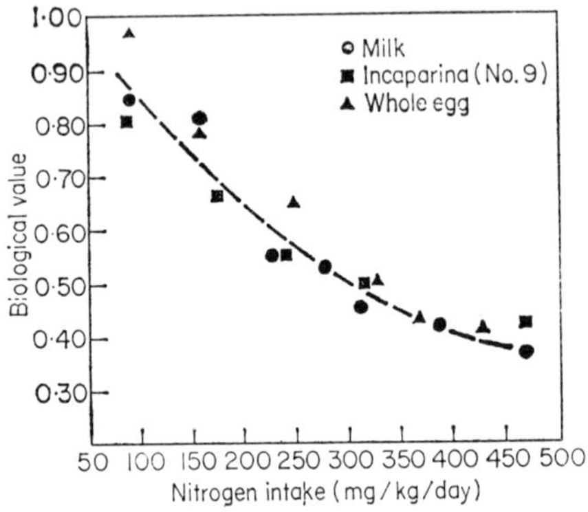

FIG. 2. Effect of N intake on biological value for children

results). In this experiment groups of children were given decreasing levels of various protein sources, including egg, milk and a protein-rich food based on cottonseed and maize. The endogenous urinary and metabolic faecal N values used were those obtained when the subjects were given a protein-free diet.

The results show decreasing biological values with increasing N intake. Values for egg are somewhat higher than those for milk protein, with those for the vegetable protein slightly lower. The results of Forbes *et al.* (1958), who fed young, growing rats with increasing levels of egg, casein and groundnut flour, are shown in Fig. 3, although some of the proteins differed from ours. The regression equations for each protein are also shown. Except with egg protein at the 4% and 8% levels, the biological value decreased as the protein concentration increased above 4%. The analysis of these results revealed that the slopes of the regression lines differed significantly. Thus, not only does the biological value of protein depend on its concentration in the diet but the quantitative relationship between proteins depends on the level at which they are compared.

The effect of age on protein quality measurements with human subjects is not as evident as it has been shown to be with experimental animals, mainly because only a small number of experiments has been carried out. Table II shows some results with both adults and children.

TABLE II. Biological value of proteins from various sources as determined with children and adult human beings

Protein source	Biological value			
	Children	*Reference*	*Adult*	*Reference*
Whole egg	0·97	Bressani *et al.* (unpublished results)	0·92	Young *et al.* (1971)
	0·90	De Maeyer and Vanderborght (1960)	0·94	Hawley *et al.* (1948)
Milk	0·84	Bressani *et al.* (unpublished results)	0·74	Bricker *et al.* (1945)
	0·82	Parthasarathy *et al.* (1964)		
Maize, common	0·32	Bressani (1972)	0·46	Kies *et al.* (1965)
			0·45	Truswell and Brock (1962)
			0·57	Truswell and Brock (1962)
Maize, opaque-2	0·80	Bressani (1972)	0·80	Young *et al.* (1971)
Soya-bean flour	0·61	De Maeyer and Vanderborght (1960)	0·41	Bricker *et al.* (1945)
Rice	0·65	Parthasarathy *et al.* (1964)		

If the limited number of results permit an evaluation, it could be decided that there is no difference in biological value of the high-quality proteins for adult and young human subjects. However, the poorer-quality proteins have lower values for children than for adults. This aspect is of particular importance because the poorer-quality proteins are more widely available

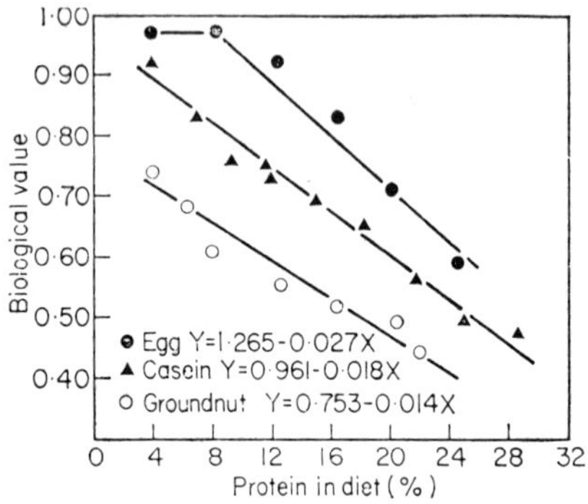

FIG. 3. Effect of protein intake on biological value for rats

in the world than the better-quality proteins, and because children are more susceptible to protein deficiency than adults.

The point to be made from these results is that when the method used to evaluate protein quality is carried out under the proper experimental conditions, the values obtained with different species confirm each other, and with human subjects, the results follow the trends established with experimental animals. For this reason, it is difficult to suggest changes that might be introduced into animal assays to improve their usefulness.

B. Nitrogen Balance

1. *Determination*

A method that is extensively used to evaluate protein quality in man is the N-balance technique. It is essentially the same as determining biological value with the exception that endogenous N losses are not considered. The figures calculated from the excretions of N in faeces and urine and from the N intake represent apparent values for protein digestibility and biological value.

Allison (1955) indicated that N balance can be used as a measure of dietary protein quality for the individual tested, since the value represents the sum of the gains and losses of all tissue proteins of the body. Nitrogen balance has been defined as the amount of ingested N retained in the body, and is represented by the formula $NB = N_I - N_F - N_V$; where NB is N balance; N_I, N intake; N_F, faecal N and N_V, urinary N.

Nitrogen balance may be thought of as the final outcome of the dynamic catabolic and anabolic metabolism of N. Since it represents the end-point at a fixed time, it does not indicate what changes are taking place within the body.

Allison (1955) has indicated that it is possible to be in a positive N balance with a loss of N occurring from some tissues; for example, under conditions of stress, although some tissues may be maintained at the expense of others, an overall positive balance is still possible.

Likewise, maintenance of N equilibrium (NB $= 0$) does not mean that every tissue is being maintained, just as the intake of sufficient N to maintain N equilibrium in the adult does not necessarily imply the fulfilment of N requirements. Nitrogen equilibrium can shift through metabolic adaptation, so that it is possible to maintain an individual in a depleted state.

Nitrogen balance, like biological value, responds to several variables. One of the most important is N intake, as seen in representative results in Table III. These results were obtained from children 25–69 months old, weighing 9·9–18·33 kg, given skim milk or whole egg protein (Bressani *et al.*, unpublished results). It is obvious that as N intake decreased, urinary N also decreased, with a parallel decrease in N balance. This indicates, therefore, that when absolute N-retention values are used to evaluate the quality of proteins, the study must be carried out at a fixed level of N intake.

As with other techniques of evaluating protein quality, applied either to experimental animals or to man, N balance is not capable of detecting small differences in quality, as implied by essential amino acid content, when total N intake is high. An example is shown in Table IV. In this case, children were given the same amount of various proteins at intakes slightly above 2·0 g of protein/kg body-wt/day, and at constant energy intakes of 420 kJ/kg body-wt/day (Bressani *et al.*, unpublished results). In the examples shown, N balance was essentially the same for all proteins tested, whether of animal or of vegetable origin, as are INCAP Vegetable Mixture 15, based on cottonseed, soya-bean, and maize flour; INCAP Vegetable Mixture 9, based on cottonseed and maize flour; and INCAP Vegetable Mixture 14, based on soya-bean and maize flour. The results also show that the vegetable proteins yield higher amounts of faecal nitrogen, suggesting a lower digestibilities than those of animal proteins. In spite of this, similar amounts of retained N were obtained from all proteins, suggesting that the amino acid balance of the absorbed N was as good as that from the proteins of animal origin.

Therefore, when the N-balance method is utilized to evaluate protein quality, not only is it essential to keep N intake constant but it is also

TABLE III. Effect of decreasing nitrogen intake on nitrogen balance in children[a]

Nitrogen (mg/kg/day)				
Intake	*Faecal*	*Urine*	*Absorbed*	*Retained*
MILK PROTEINS				
477 ± 7·5[b]	65 ± 6·8[b]	313 ± 13·7[b]	412 ± 11·6[b]	99 ± 10·3[b]
386 ± 5·6	45 ± 3·0	258 ± 11·0	342 ± 4·8	83 ± 11·3
303 ± 6·4	48 ± 3·8	185 ± 7·7	255 ± 6·9	69 ± 10·4
225 ± 3·4	42 ± 4·1	132 ± 3·6	184 ± 5·9	52 ± 5·5
164 ± 2·6	36 ± 2·7	74 ± 4·8	128 ± 4·2	54 ± 6·3
95 ± 1·2	29 ± 1·0	50 ± 3·0	66 ± 1·1	15 ± 3·5
0	23 ± 1·7	46 ± 4·2	—	—
WHOLE EGG PROTEINS				
385 ± 7·9	42 ± 3·3	262 ± 3·4	343 ± 6·0	80 ± 5·9
328 ± 4·6	40 ± 2·6	214 ± 6·7	288 ± 5·2	75 ± 6·5
239 ± 5·5	27 ± 1·9	142 ± 4·1	212 ± 5·6	69 ± 6·4
160 ± 6·1	25 ± 1·4	93 ± 6·2	134 ± 6·2	41 ± 6·6
76 ± 4·4	19 ± 2·5	63 ± 3·7	57 ± 6·0	−6 ± 7·2
37	23	54	14	−40
0	17 ± 3·2	59 ± 3·0	—	—

[a] Taken from Bressani *et al.* (unpublished results)
[b] Standard error

TABLE IV. Nitrogen balance in children given high N intakes[a]

	Nitrogen (mg/kg/day)				
Protein source	*Intake*	*Faecal*	*Urine*	*Absorbed*	*Retained*
Skim milk	386	45	258	342	83
Whole egg	385	42	262	343	80
INCAP 15	398	89	216	309	93
INCAP 9	388	110	201	277	77
INCAP 14	347	85	168	262	94

[a] Taken from Bressani *et al.* (unpublished results)

necessary to carry out the tests at N intakes which will maximize the differences in quality. In animal testing 9–10% protein diets are used, since it was found that at this level quality differences became more evident. Little work has been done on this aspect in children; however, results of some studies (Bressani *et al.*, unpublished results) are shown in Table V. To determine the level of N intake at which the greatest differences in N-balance values were obtained, the results at intakes of 81–360 mg of N were grouped as shown in the Table, and were studied statistically.

The analysis indicated that highly significant differences in N-balance

TABLE V. Average nitrogen balance at various levels of nitrogen intake (children)[a]

Protein foods tested	*Nitrogen intake range* 310–360	230–251	156–174	81–114
	Nitrogen balance (mg/kg/day)			
Milk	62	50	54	8
Cottonseed–maize mix	64	40	26	−4
Soya-bean–maize mix	86	65	38	0
CSF–SBF–maize mix	59	51	24	−5
Soya-bean textured food	82	49	9	−10
Whole egg	80	80	49	—
F	1·51	5·85**	11·06**	1·84
LSD (0·01)[b]	45	22	21	20
No. observations	31	31	32	22

** Highly significant
[a] Taken from Bressani and Viteri (1970)
[b] LSD: Least Significant Difference

values can be detected among different proteins with children given intakes of 156–251 mg N/kg body-wt/day.

The procedure for the N-balance technique with children is different from that with adults. A young body has greater requirements for essential amino acid N, mainly for growth and maintenance purposes. On the other hand, an adult subject who is not pregnant or lactating or under any unusual stress condition, requires only enough essential amino acid N for maintenance. Therefore, when the N-balance method is used in adult subjects to measure the protein quality of different sources, the subjects must first be placed in a state of negative N balance. Once this has been achieved, the proteins under study are given to the individual at low levels, usually not more than 10 g per day. Following this procedure, Kies and Fox (1970), for example, were able to measure the relative nutritive values of wheat and Triticale as shown in Table VI. Wheat protein gave lower N-balance values at either level of protein intake than did Triticale grain. Since the values were obtained at low levels of N intake, the results can be used to calculate biological value and true protein digestibility.

TABLE VI. Nitrogen balance with adult man given two levels of protein from wheat and triticale[a]

Cereal grain	*Protein intake* (g N/day)	*Mean nitrogen balance* (g N/day)
Wheat grain	4	−0·62
Triticale	4	−0·44
Wheat grain	6	−0·16
Triticale	6	+0·01

[a] Taken from Kies and Fox (1970)

An example of the influence of energy intake on N balance is shown in Fig. 4 taken from work by Clark *et al.* (1960). The subject in the study received 1500 mg lysine and 9 g N per day. There was no apparent difference in N retention as energy intake was reduced from 18·2 MJ/day to 14·9 MJ/day, but further reduction caused a downward trend, and a negative balance was reached when the subject received 11·5 MJ/day.

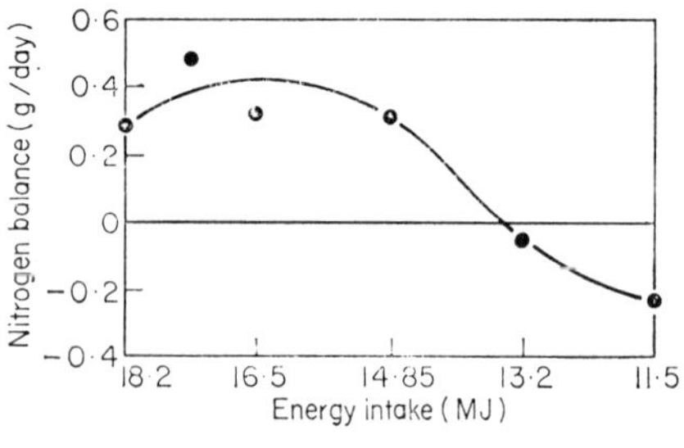

FIG. 4. Effect of energy intake on N balance of human subjects at constant N and lysine intakes

As indicated previously, protein quality assays measure the relative efficiency of proteins in supplying the essential amino acid needs of the test animal. The relative efficiency is dependent upon the most limiting amino acid in the protein. Thus, high correlations are obtained between the value obtained for protein quality and the level of the limiting amino acid in the protein. For example, Fig. 5 shows the quite high correlation

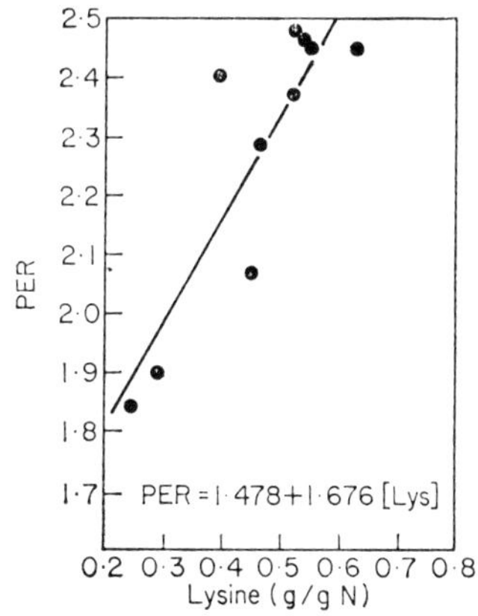

FIG. 5. Relationship between protein efficiency ratio and the lysine content of maize supplemented with various protein concentrates

obtained between PER measured with weanling rats and the lysine content of maize supplemented with 4–8% levels of various protein sources (Bressani and Marenco, 1963). Similarly, N balance also correlated highly with lysine content in studies with children (Viteri *et al.*, unpublished results) who were given diets containing various protein sources differing in protein quality (Fig. 6). Good correlations were also obtained in tests with rats. These results emphasize again the similarities between results with different species, suggesting that the methods are

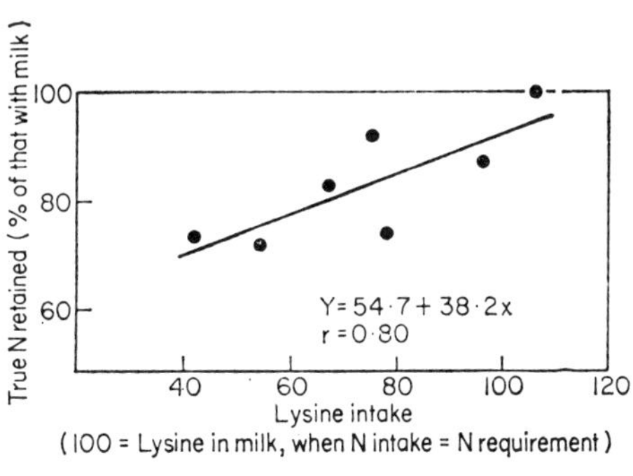

FIG. 6. The relationship between the nitrogen balance of preschool children and the lysine content of their diet

measuring the relative efficiency of the provision of an adequate amino acid pattern to the test animal.

2. *Application of Nitrogen-balance Method*

The N-balance procedure carried out under standardized conditions has provided useful information for the assessment of the quality of dietary protein, and about protein metabolism in general.

TABLE VII. Nitrogen balance of children given various protein sources at essentially the same nitrogen intake[a]

Protein source	*Nitrogen* (mg/kg/day)				
	Intake	*Faecal*	*Urine*	*Absorbed*	*Retained*
Milk	225	42	132	184	52
Whole egg	239	27	142	212	69
Cottonseed–maize	251	81	127	170	43
Soya-bean–maize	230	69	96	161	65
Cottonseed–soya-bean–maize	234	54	131	178	48
Opaque-2 maize	238	68	107	170	63
Common maize	238	58	190	180	−10
Soya-bean, textured food	231	42	140	190	49
Rolled oats	251	49	164	202	38
White rice	235	38	157	197	40

[a] Taken from Bressani and Viteri (1970)

The examples in Table VII illustrate the assessment of the protein quality of various protein sources given to young children (Bressani and Viteri, 1970; Bressani *et al.*, unpublished results). The results show differences in quality as indicated by the N-retention values. Figures were higher for animal sources, some vegetable protein mixtures, and opaque-2 maize than for the other sources tested.

A second application shown in Table VIII is the amino acid supplementation of maize for children and adults (Bressani, unpublished results). The results show the poor quality of common maize proteins, even at high N intakes, and also the improvement obtained when they are supplemented with lysine and tryptophan. Similar results were obtained with experimental animals with this protein source and with other sources with both species.

Nitrogen balance is also a sensitive technique for measuring amino acid imbalance. Table IX summarizes results with children (Bressani, 1971a)

TABLE VIII. Effects on nitrogen balance of adults and children of amino acid supplements to cereal grains

Cereal grain	*Nitrogen intake*	*Nitrogen balance*	*Subjects*	*Reference*
Maize	461 mg/kg/day	+10 mg/kg/day	Children	Bressani (1972)
Maize + Lys + Try	464 mg/kg/day	+86 mg/kg/day		
Maize	0·9 g protein/kg/day	+0·538 g/day	Adults	Truswell and Brock (1962)
Maize + Lys + Try		+1·035 g/day		
Maize	8 g N/day	+0·50 g/day	Adults	Kies *et al.* (1965)
Maize + Lys + Try	8 g N/day	+0·74 g/day		

and with dogs (Bressani, 1963) demonstrating this effect. With children, the addition of methionine decreased N balance when maize was supplemented with lysine, tryptophan, or lysine, tryptophan and isoleucine. With dogs the response to methionine addition was also a decrease in N balance, an effect which appeared to be corrected by the further addition of threonine.

The N-balance method has also been used to study the minimum ratio of dietary essential amino acid to total N in various proteins, amino acid supplementation and requirements, stress and diet, the influence of non-specific N intake on the adequacy of cereal proteins, evaluation of amino acid patterns, and for other purposes (Bressani and Viteri, 1970; Bressani, 1971b).

TABLE IX. Effect of amino acid imbalance on nitrogen balance with children and dogs given maize protein[a]

Diet	*Nitrogen* (mg/kg/day)		
	Intake	*Absorbed*	*Retained*
CHILDREN			
Maize + Lys + Try	470	336	112
Maize + Lys + Try + Met	462	316	83
Maize	471	354	39
Maize	453	330	−8
Maize + Lys + Try	463	334	76
Maize + Lys + Try + Ile	475	376	108
Maize + Lys + Try + Met	464	379	90
DOGS			
Maize + Lys + Try	1111	844	318
Maize + Lys + Try + Met	975	717	222
Maize + Lys + Try + Met + Thr	969	773	310

[a] Taken from Bressani (1963) and Bressani *et al.* (1971a)

C. Nitrogen Balance Index

Allison and Anderson (1945) showed that with adult dogs under highly standardized conditions the relationship between absorbed N and N balance was linear in the region of negative N balance; the linearity extended over into the region of positive balance but became obviously curvilinear further on. The empirical equation for the linear portion of the relationship between absorbed N (N_A) and NB shown in Fig. 7 is: $NB = -a + bN_A$, where the slope b gives a measure of the biological value b.v. and a is the total excretion of N on a protein-free diet (i.e. the sum of endogenous urinary and metabolic faecal N).

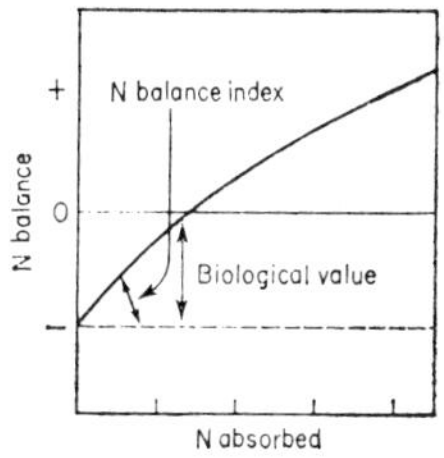

FIG. 7. Nitrogen balance index

Hoffman and McNeil (1949) have used this method with adult human subjects (Fig. 8). It can be seen that, in the region of negative and slightly positive NB, the relation between N_A and NB is a straight line but that intakes of N above 100 mg/kg/day give a curvilinear response. The N-

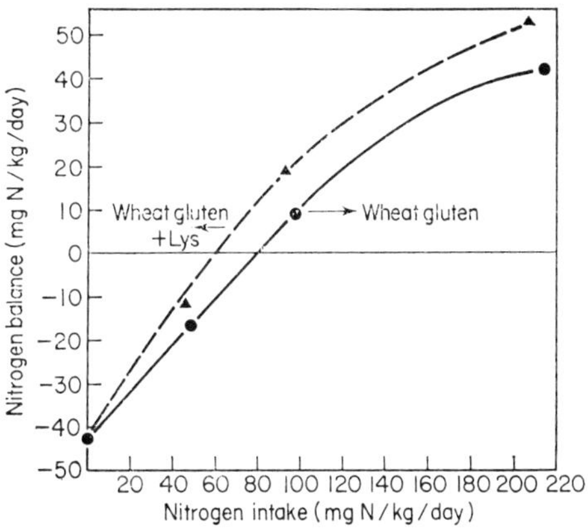

FIG. 8. Nitrogen balance index for wheat gluten and for wheat gluten + lysine with adult human subjects

balance index is 0·53 for wheat gluten, and 0·67 for wheat gluten supplemented with lysine. The respective N requirements for N equilibrium for wheat gluten and wheat gluten plus lysine are 81 and 64 mg/kg/day. Bricker *et al.* (1945) used this technique to establish protein requirements of adult human subjects. Table X summarizes their regression equations which describe the relationships between N intake and N balance.

According to these authors each regression coefficient is the product of the true protein digestibility and biological value. From their results they were able to calculate the true protein digestibility, its biological value, the amount of N required for N equilibrium and the protein required per day from each source.

The technique has also been used with young children. An example is shown in Fig. 9 (Bressani and Viteri, 1970; Viteri and Alvarado, 1971) in which are plotted N-retention values against N intake and absorbed N for two experiments in which children who were fully protein repleted, after having had severe protein malnutrition, received whole egg or a vegetable protein mixture as the only source of N. It is apparent that N retention in the case of egg protein breaks from a steep slope to a flat one at about 200 mg/kg/day intake, and at about 180 mg N/kg/day of absorbed N

TABLE X. Relationship between nitrogen intake and nitrogen balance with different diets given to adults[a]

Protein source	*Regression equation*
Milk	$Y = -1{\cdot}924 + 0{\cdot}697\ X$
Soya-bean flour	$Y = -1{\cdot}719 + 0{\cdot}598\ X$
Soya-bean flour + White flour	$Y = -1{\cdot}757 + 0{\cdot}520\ X$
White flour	$Y = -1{\cdot}917 + 0{\cdot}402\ X$
Mixed foods	$Y = -1{\cdot}831 + 0{\cdot}586\ X$

[a] Taken from Bricker *et al.* (1945)

(points E and F). Furthermore, the slope at low intakes is steeper for this protein than for the vegetable protein mixture (protein M). As a consequence, N equilibrium is reached with lower levels of N intakes and N absorbed with whole egg than with protein M (points C and C_1, and D and D_1). The slopes of the plots of retained N against absorbed N indicate the biological value and differentiate the two proteins tested. Figure 10 shows the high reproducibility of this method with fully recovered children under strict experimental conditions (Bressani and Viteri, 1970; Viteri and Alvarado, 1971). The standard deviation about the calculated regression line is no greater than 3 mg of N retained/kg/day at intakes of 50–200 mg/kg/day.

The N-balance index method probably represents one of the best techniques available for determining the nutritive value of proteins. The protein under study must be given at levels of intake below and slightly above those resulting in N equilibrium, where there is a straight-line

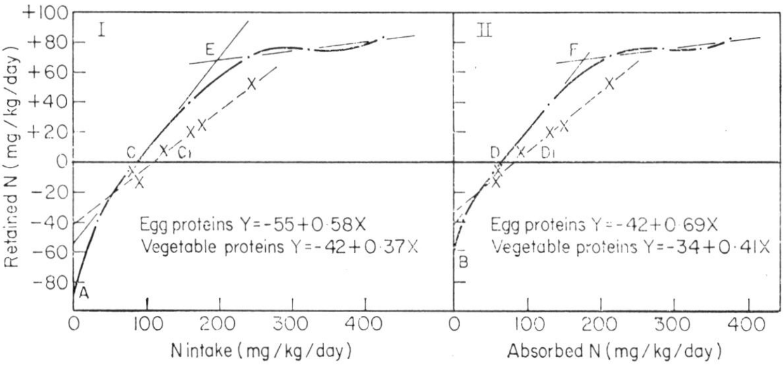

FIG. 9. Relationships between the retained N and (I) N intake and (II) absorbed N for egg proteins (•——•) and a vegetable protein mixture (×——×) with children

relationship between absorbed N and N balance, so that the regression equations may be calculated. It is not necessary to feed N-free diets. One disadvantage of the method is the time needed to obtain N retention values at three or four levels of N intake.

When the technique was carried out under equivalent conditions with men and experimental animals, good agreement was found between the results for the same protein. Results using the method with rats and with children in our laboratory were in good agreement for various protein sources of animal and vegetable origin (Fig. 11). The graph was prepared by plotting the regression coefficients of N retention on absorbed N against the regression coefficients of weight gained on protein intake.

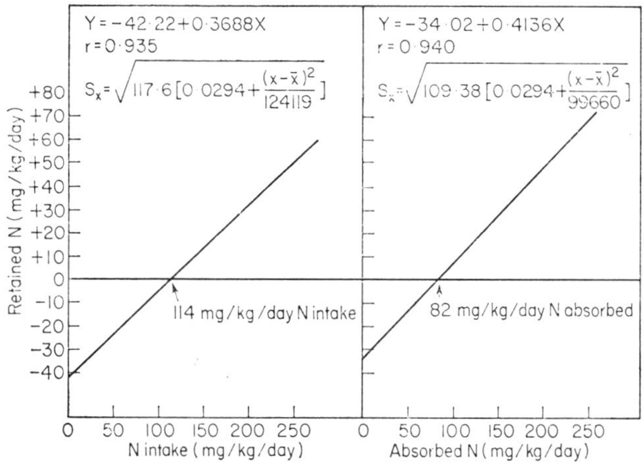

FIG. 10. The reproducibility of N-balance index determined with children

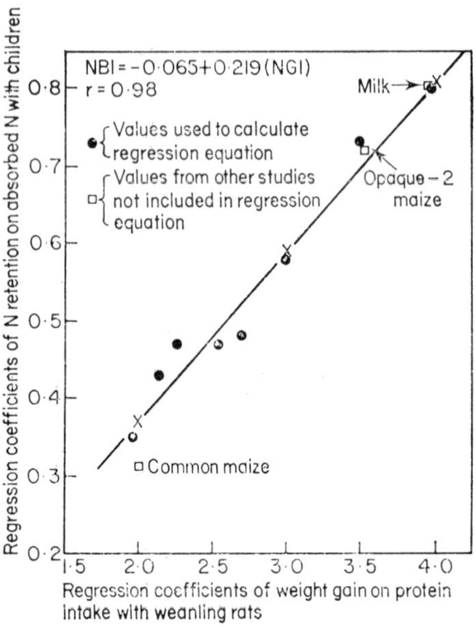

FIG. 11. Correlation between N-growth index (NGI) with rats and N-balance index (NBI) with children

These same proteins were evaluated by n.p.u. and PER assays. Preliminary analysis suggests that these two values also show a good correlation with the N-balance index values for children. The graph also shows that values from other independent studies fall on the regression line.

IV. NUTRITIVE VALUE OF PROTEINS

As indicated earlier in this paper there are two ways used to evaluate the potential of a protein to meet the needs of essential amino acids. The first has already been discussed and is the classical way to study protein quality. The second does not really measure protein quality, but measures the capacity of a protein to meet amino acid needs when sufficient amounts of it are ingested. This is called the nutritive value of the protein. Although for practical purposes this approach may be satisfactory, it has the disadvantage that the utilization of the N ingested is very inefficient, resulting in significant losses of N through faeces and urine, since the generally accepted principles of amino acid balance and limiting amino acid are completely disregarded.

Although N balance correlates highly with lysine content, nutritive value determined by N balance does not. This has caused much debate on the value of N balance and lack of correlation between results with man and with animals.

The difference between true protein quality and nutritive value of a protein, or apparent protein quality, is shown graphically in a simplified form in Fig. 12. The left side of the diagram shows that protein quality is strictly dependent on the pattern of amino acids, with the limiting amino acid controlling the true quality of the protein. On the right side, all amino acids in the protein meet minimum needs; however, these are obtained with a significant loss of N, represented by the levels of amino acids above the requirement line.

Nutritive value of proteins should therefore be obtained not by feeding high intakes of the protein and measuring the effect by N balance, but by

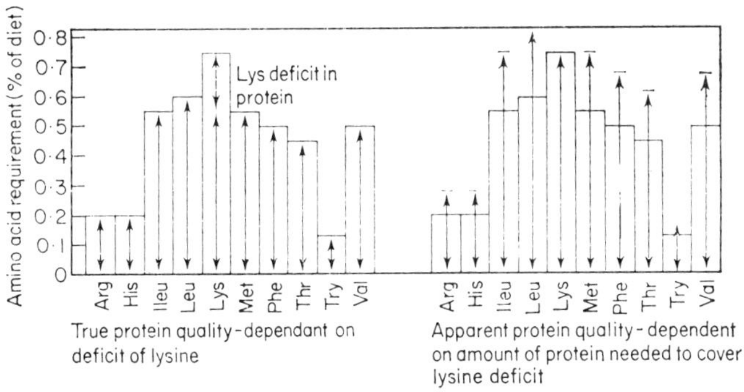

FIG. 12. Difference between true and apparent quality of protein

correcting the value obtained by the true quality of the protein. This is best done by the N-balance index value, which is not obtained at a fixed level of intake, but rather at various levels, as was shown in the preceding section.

As was pointed out, the misuse of N balance to predict protein quality or to measure protein needs has caused concern with respect to protein quality values assessed in experimental animals or in human subjects. For example Clark *et al.* (1971) compared the nutritive value of the protein of a high- and of a low-protein rice (Table XI). Both rice samples gave positive N balances, although the high-protein variety gave higher N balances. This was not due to a better quality in the high-protein rice, but rather to the fact that intake of essential amino acids was higher. Although the conclusions and interpretation of the results are correct this does not mean that the high-protein rice (BPI) has the higher quality protein. The same high-protein rice was evaluated in rats using the N-growth index (Bressani *et al.*, 1971). The results with this rice and those with other varieties are

TABLE XI. Mean nitrogen balance of adult human subjects given a low- and high-protein rice[a]

	Nitrogen (g/day)			
Diet given	*Intake*	*Urine*	*Faeces*	*Balance*
480 g BPI Rice	12·06	8·00	2·65	1·41
480 g BB Rice	6·72	4·92	1·55	0·24
480 g BB Rice + Nitrogen	12·06	9·92	1·66	0·48
320 g BB Rice + Nitrogen	6·72	5·87	1·41	−0·58

[a] Taken from Clark *et al.* (1971)

TABLE XII. Protein quality of rice varieties differing in protein content[a]

Rice variety or protein	*Protein content* (g/100 g)	*Regression of weight gain on protein intake*	*Protein quality, relative to casein* = 1	*Lysine in Rice* (g/16·8 g N)
INTAN	5·7	Y = −14·05 + 3·49 X	1·1	4·27
IR 8	7·3	Y = −14·35 + 3·25 X	1·0	3·77
IR 8	9·7	Y = −15·46 + 3·04 X	0·91	3·69
Casein	87·7	Y = −14·44 + 3·23 X	1·0	—
BPI	14·3	Y = −11·1 + 2·78 X	0·72	3·35
Casein	87·7	Y = −10·7 + 3·63 X	1·0	—

[a] Taken from Bressani *et al.* (1971b)

shown in Table XII, from which it is evident that the high-protein rice showed the lowest protein quality. Furthermore, the values obtained correlated very well with the lysine content of the rice varieties tested.

From this discussion it would appear that the N-balance index is a good method of evaluating protein quality as well as the nutritive value of a protein with human subjects. The corresponding method with experimental animals is the N-growth index. The technique is essentially the same, except that in the experimental animal weight gain rather than N balance is measured. These methods have an advantage over others in that the value representing protein quality is dynamic in nature, since it represents the changes in weight gain or N balance with rate of change of protein intake. Furthermore, this method provides additional information on the protein tested which is not given by any of the other methods available for protein quality evaluation.

Although it is elegant and impressive to evaluate protein quality with human subjects, it is likely that further comparative tests using these techniques with experimental animals and man will give results that correlate well.

REFERENCES

Allison, J. B. (1955). *Physiol. Rev.* **35**, 664–700.

Allison, J. B. (1958). *Ann. N.Y. Acad. Sci.* **69**, 1009–1024.

Allison, J. B. (1964). *In* "Mammalian Protein Metabolism" (H. B. Munro and J. B. Allison, eds) Vol. II, pp. 41–86. Academic Press, New York.

Allison, J. B. and Anderson, J. A. (1945). *J. Nutr.* **29**, 413–420.

Allison, J. B. and Fitzpatrick, W. H. (1960). *In* "Dietary Proteins in Health and Disease". C. C. Thomas, Springfield, Ill.

Block, R. J. and Mitchell, H. H. (1946–7). *Nutr. Abstr. Rev.* **16**, 249–278.

Braham, J. E., Bressani, R., Zaghi, S. de and Flores, M. (1965). *J. agric. Fd Chem.* **13**, 594–597.

Braham, J. E., Elías, L. G. and Bressani, R. (1965). *J. Fd Sci.* **30**, 531–537.

Braham, J. E., Elías, L. G., Zaghi, S. de and Bressani, R. (1967). *Nutritio Dieta* **9**, 99–111.

Bressani, R. (1963). *J. Nutr.* **79**, 389–394.

Bressani, R. (1971a). *In* "Amino Acid Fortification of Protein Foods" pp. 184–204 (N. S. Scrimshaw and A. M. Altschul, eds). MIT Press, Cambridge, Mass.

Bressani, R. (1971b). *In* "Recursos Proteínicos en América Latina" (M. Béhar and R. Bressani, eds) p. 21. INCAP, Guatemala, C.A.

Bressani, R. (1972). *In* "Proceedings of the Conference on Improvement of the Nutritive Value of Maize". INCAP, Guatemala, C.A.

Bressani, R., Braham, J. E., Elías, L. G. and Zaghi, S. de (1965). *Nutritio Dieta* **7**, 161–174.

Bressani, R., Elías, L. G. and Braham, J. E. (1968). *Archos lat.-am. Nutr.* **18**, 123–134.

Bressani, R., Elías, L. G. and Juliano, B. O. (1971). *J. agric. Fd Chem.* **19**, 1028–1034.

Bressani, R. and Marenco, E. (1963). *J. agric. Chem.* **11**, 517–522.

Bressani, R. and Viteri, F. (1970). *In* "Proc. III Int. Congr. Fd Sci. Technol. (SOS/70)" p. 344. Washington, D.C.

Bricker, M., Mitchell, H. H. and Kinsman, G. M. (1945). *J. Nutr.* **30**, 269–283.

Campbell, J. A. (1963). *In* "Methodology of Protein Evaluation", Publ. 21, American University of Beirut. Beirut, Lebanon.

Chan, H. and Waterlow, J. C. (1966). *Br. J. Nutr.* **20**, 775–782.

Clark, H. E., Howe, J. M. and Chung-Ja Lee (1971). *Am. J. clin. Nutr.* **24**, 324–328.

Clark, H. E., Yang, S. P., Reitz, L. L. and Mertz, E. T. (1960). *J. Nutr.* **72**, 87–92.

DeMaeyer, E. M. and Vanderborght, H. L. (1961). *In* "Progress in Meeting Protein Needs of Infants and Preschool Children": proc. symp. 1960, (L. Voris ed.) pp. 143–155. *Publs natn. Res. Coun., Wash.* no. 843.

Forbes, R. M., Vaughan, L. and Yohe, M. (1958). *J. Nutr.* **64**, 291–302.

Hawley, E. E., Murlin, J. R., Nasset, E. S. and Szymanski, T. A. (1948). *J. Nutr.* **36**, 153–169.

Hegsted, D. M. and Haffenneffer, V. K. (1949). *Am. J. Physiol.* **157**, 141–148.

Henry, K. M. and Kon, S. K. (1957). *Br. J. Nutr.* **11**, 305–313.

Hoffman, W. S. and McNeil, G. C. (1949). *J. Nutr.* **38**, 331–343.

Kies, C. and Fox, H. M. (1970). *Cereal Chem.* **47**, 671–678.

Kies, C., Williams, E. and Fox, H. M. (1965). *J. Nutr.* **86**, 350–356.

Knipfel, J. E. (1969). *Cereal Chem.* **46**, 313–317.

Mauron, J. (1961). *In* "Progress in Meeting Protein Needs of Infants and Preschool Children": proc. symp. 1960, (L. Voris, ed.) pp. 425–442. *Publs natn. Res. Coun., Wash.* no. 843.

Mitchell, H. H. (1923–4). *J. biol. Chem.* **58**, 873–903.

Mitchell, H. H. and Carmen, G. G. (1926). *J. biol. Chem.* **68**, 183–215.

Murlin, J. R., Marshall, M. E. and Kochakian, C. D. (1941). *J. Nutr.* **22**, 573–588.

Parthasarathy, H. N., Kantha, J., Daniel, V. A., Doraiswamy, T. R., Sankaran, A. H., Narayana Rao, M., Swaminathan, M., Sreenivasan, A., and Subrahmanyan, V. (1964). *Can. J. Biochem.* **42**, 385–393.

Pellett, P. L. (ed.) (1963). "Evaluation of Protein Quality". p. 311. *Publs natn. Res. Coun., Wash.* no. 1100.

Rosenberg, H. R. (1959). *J. agric. Fd Chem.* **7**, 316–321.

Rosenberg, H. R., and Culik, R. (1957). *J. Nutr.* **63**, 477–487.

Smuts, D. B. (1935). *J. Nutr.* **9**, 403–433.

Tagle, M. A. (1971). *In* "Recursos Proteínicos en América Latina" (M. Béhar and R. Bressani, eds). INCAP Pub. L–1, pp. 78–109.

Thomas, K. (1909). *Physiol. Abstr.* 219–302.

Truswell, A. S. and Brock, J. F. (1962). *Am. J. clin. Nutr.* **10**, 142–152.

Viteri, F. and Alvarado, J. (1971). *In* "Recursos Proteínicos en América Latina" (M. Béhar and R. Bressani, eds). INCAP pub. L–1, p. 53.

Young, V. R., Ozalp, I., Cholakos, B. V., and Scrimshaw, N. S. (1971). *J. Nutr.* **101**, 1475–1482.

CHAPTER 20

The Levels of Blood Amino Acids and Blood Urea as Indicators of Protein Quality

BJØRN O. EGGUM

Institute of Animal Science, Copenhagen, Denmark

I. INTRODUCTION

The use of plasma amino acid and plasma urea levels as indices of dietary protein quality is discussed in this paper. Several authors have considered whether there is any relationship between the amino acid composition of the protein eaten and the pattern of free amino acids appearing in the plasma during absorption, but relatively few studies have been made of the value of measurements of blood urea as a means of assessing protein quality. This does not necessarily mean that the latter technique is less useful for the purpose.

II. PLASMA AMINO ACID LEVELS AS INDICATORS OF DIETARY PROTEIN QUALITY

One might expect increases in the plasma levels of free amino acids that would reflect the relative amounts of these amino acids in the protein undergoing digestion. On this basis, amino acids present in abundance in the diet should cause the largest increases. This relationship has been confirmed by several workers who have compared the levels of amino acids in portal blood during absorption with the amino acid content of the diet (Denton and Elvehjem, 1954; Goldberg and Guggenheim, 1962; McLaughlan *et al.*, 1963; Pion *et al.*, 1964; Nielsen, 1965; Buraczewski *et al.*, 1967; Erbersdobler, 1969; Andah and Chamberlain, 1971). On the other hand, some investigators have failed to establish a relationship between the relative abundance of dietary amino acids and their increase in plasma during the absorptive period. Thus Levenson *et al.* (1959) and Nasset *et al.* (1963) found no relationship between the amino acid composition of the diet and the free amino acid levels in the blood of dogs. The same was observed by Eggum (1966) with 10 different diets fed to pigs. The free amino acid composition in the plasma of blood taken from the vena cava 2 h after feeding did not reflect the amino acid composition of the diets. However, it must be remembered that the liver affected the amino acid patterns in these samples.

There may be several reasons for the discrepancies observed, one of them being the differences in availability of the individual amino acids within the same protein. However, it was shown that such differences could not explain the results. Part of the answer may lie in differences in the rate of absorption of the individual amino acids. It was demonstrated by Delhumeau *et al.* (1962) that the rate of absorption of lysine was only 63% the rate for cystine. Furthermore, the availability of individual amino acids in the proteins tested varied considerably. The amino acids in fish meal were approximately 95% available whereas in barley the availability was only about 80% (Eggum, 1966). This difference must necessarily affect the amino acid pattern in blood plasma, and make it difficult always to obtain a direct relationship between amino acids in feed and plasma.

The results of these analyses are shown in Table I. As the biological values of the samples given in Table I were measured, comparisons could be made between these values and the amino acid composition of the diets and blood plasma. These comparisons showed no relationship between biological values and plasma amino acids whereas biological value was related to the amino acid composition of the diets. However, this work could be criticized because blood samples were taken only once (2 h after feeding) during the absorptive period. On the other hand, several workers (Denton *et al.*, 1953; Nielsen, 1965; Erbersdobler, 1969; Stockland *et al.*, 1971) have shown that free amino acids in the plasma reach peak levels about 2 h after feeding.

It has been reported by some (Lebedeva and Nuriakhmetova, 1964; Nielsen, 1965) that the state of excitement of the experimental animals markedly affects plasma levels of individual amino acids, and great care was taken by Eggum (1966) to avoid such effects during blood sampling.

Zimmerman and Scott (1965) reported that there was a definite relationship between plasma amino acid levels in chicks and the amino acid adequacy of the diet. The first limiting amino acid remained at a very low level in the blood irrespective of the severity of the amino acid deficiency. They suggested that this observation helps to explain why, in some in-

TABLE I. A comparison of amino acids in diet (g/16 g N) with free amino acids in plasma (mg/100 ml plasma)[a]

	Fish meal	*Soya-bean meal*	*Sunflower meal*	*Groundnut meal*	*Barley*	*Oats*	*Wheat*	*Rye*	*Skim milk powder + oats*	*Soya-bean meal + oats*
Aspartic acid	10·8	12·9	10·3	11·8	7·0	8·7	5·3	7·3	7·4	8·5
	0·8	0·9	0·4	0·7	0·9	0·3	0·3	0·5	0·4	0·2
Threonine	5·0	4·4	4·1	2·7	3·6	3·6	3·0	3·3	3·5	3·2
	3·3	5·3	5·0	1·8	4·9	3·4	2·7	1·1	7·8	4·5
Serine	4·7	4·5	4·5	4·6	4·2	5·0	4·7	4·2	4·7	4·3
	5·1	7·0	3·4	6·5	2·2	3·6	6·4	3·8	3·8	4·0
Glutamic acid	14·9	21·7	24·0	19·9	25·1	22·1	35·8	23·6	21·4	18·8
	5·8	3·5	1·6	3·0	2·2	1·7	2·8	3·4	3·8	2·3
Glycine	6·8	4·6	5·9	5·7	4·5	5·5	4·2	4·6	3·1	4·1
	15·8	8·5	7·3	9·5	9·4	8·6	12·1	8·3	5·2	6·0
Alanine	7·0	4·7	4·4	3·7	4·6	4·9	3·8	4·5	3·8	4·1
	7·1	6·4	5·0	5·0	5·7	5·4	6·3	8·4	6·7	6·7
Valine	5·8	5·2	5·1	3·9	5·3	5·1	4·6	4·6	5·6	4·9
	4·6	4·6	5·5	3·4	2·9	3·8	3·0	2·7	3·5	3·3
Isoleucine	4·8	4·9	4·7	3·5	3·7	4·0	3·4	3·1	4·4	3·9
	2·3	3·1	3·0	2·2	1·2	1·5	1·9	1·8	2·0	2·0
Leucine	7·9	8·1	6·6	6·2	7·1	7·1	6·8	5·9	8·2	6·8
	2·0	2·8	2·3	2·1	1·2	1·5	1·8	1·0	2·0	1·5
Tyrosine	3·1	3·7	3·1	4·2	3·7	3·5	3·1	2·9	3·9	2·8
	1·2	3·1	2·4	3·2	1·2	2·6	1·8	2·0	3·4	2·2
Phenylalanine	5·2	5·1	4·9	4·9	4·9	4·9	4·4	4·4	4·5	4·5
	0·8	1·9	1·8	2·2	1·2	1·3	1·8	1·6	1·9	1·7
Lysine	7·9	6·4	3·5	3·2	3·7	4·0	2·6	3·7	4·9	4·3
	6·2	5·6	4·0	4·1	1·7	2·4	3·0	2·9	3·2	4·6
Histidine	2·2	2·5	2·9	2·1	2·2	2·2	2·3	2·3	2·1	2·4
	0·9	2·0	1·6	1·5	1·3	1·6	1·8	1·3	1·4	1·3
Arginine	5·8	7·5	8·0	8·4	5·4	6·1	4·7	5·7	4·2	5·9
	2·7	2·8	2·2	1·9	1·2	1·1	1·4	1·7	2·3	2·9

[a] Upper figures refer to the diets and the lower to the plasma

stances, supplementing diets with the first limiting amino acid has failed to increase the concentration of this amino acid in the plasma (Richardson *et al.*, 1953; Owings and Balloun, 1961). According to these workers, no increase would be anticipated until the dietary level exceeded that needed for maximum growth.

Furthermore, Zimmerman and Scott (1965) and Kihlberg (1970) showed that the presence of an amino acid in the diet, in excess of that required for maximum weight gain, consistently resulted in a rapid accumulation of that amino acid in the plasma. This accumulation appeared to proceed linearly, even though, as was the case for lysine and valine, the highest dietary level given was more than twice that required for maximum weight gain. It was of interest that severe deficiencies of either lysine or arginine in the diet markedly increased plasma threonine. According to Zimmerman and Scott (1965) this did not appear to be unique for threonine since many of the other amino acids also behaved in this manner, but to a lesser degree.

Smith and Scott (1965) showed that supplementing intact proteins with their first limiting amino acid tended to reduce the concentration of other amino acids in the plasma. This effect probably reflected an improved utilization of plasma amino acids for protein synthesis. However, if a dietary protein is low in a specific amino acid that is essential for the animal ingesting it, catabolism of body tissue proteins will be necessary. In spite of this Dean and Scott (1966) used free amino acid concentrations in blood plasma of chicks to detect deficiencies and excesses of dietary amino acids. Giving diets containing suboptimal amounts of either lysine or valine resulted in a marked lowering of the limiting amino acid and an increase in most of the other amino acids in plasma. A dietary excess of lysine resulted in a striking increase in plasma lysine and relatively small changes in other amino acids. Similar observations were made by Stockland *et al.* (1970) with pigs: supplementing the limiting amino acids in meat and bone meal diets with crystalline amino acids reduced the plasma levels of amino acids that were not included in the supplement and increased the plasma levels of the amino acids that were supplemented, but to a relatively smaller extent than might have been expected from the increase in dietary levels. These results were probably due to the same cause as discussed by Smith and Scott (1965) and Dean and Scott (1966), i.e. improved amino acid balance with amino acid supplementation which stimulated rate of weight gain and caused removal of amino acids from the plasma for protein synthesis.

Stockland and Meade (1970) reported that giving rats meat and bone meals supplemented with all the amino acids in which they were deficient either reduced the levels of the plasma free essential amino acids or increased them to a relatively smaller extent than might have been expected from the increased dietary levels. This suggests, as indicated by Stockland and Meade, an increased removal of amino acids from the plasma for tissue protein synthesis as average daily weight gain increased.

The findings of Stockland and Meade (1970) are in accord with those of Pawlak and Pion (1968), who compared the levels of free amino acids in plasma with those in muscle of rats given graded levels of amino acids. Free lysine in blood and muscle increased with that in the diet, but the increases were greater in the muscular tissue. The free lysine level in muscle of rats given a diet supplemented with lysine was 27 times greater than that in animals eating wheat not supplemented with lysine, whereas the highest value found in blood was only 7 times the lowest. In tissue a large increase was found when the requirement of the animal was met. The levels of the other amino acids changed little, except for threonine which accumulated in blood and particularly in muscle when lysine was deficient. These findings agree with these of Zimmerman and Scott (1965). Pawlak and Pion suggested that the particularly large increase in lysine in muscle when the requirement for lysine was met shows that measurement of this concentration could be a particularly sensitive method for estimating the degree to which the requirement of this amino acid had been met. Later work by Pion and Pawlak (1969) demonstrated that the same procedure could also be used for threonine (cf. Chapter 21). Moreover, it can be seen from these studies that a relationship exists between the concentrations of both lysine and threonine in the tissues and the amounts absorbed in the digestive tract when the dietary supply is not sufficient to meet the requirements of the animal.

However, Andah and Chamberlain (1971) failed to produce significant positive linear regressions between several plasma and dietary amino acids when increasing amounts of fish meal were given to pigs receiving a barley diet. These were phenylalanine, methionine, arginine and tryptophan. This work is in agreement with the results of Tasaki and Ohno (1971) with chicks given increasing amounts of casein. But there was a highly significant correlation between the body weight gain and the total plasma essential amino acids.

Such direct relationships of diet to blood amino acid levels are also obscured by differences in the rates of removal of amino acids from the plasma to meet the requirements of the tissues. Moreover, amino acids may be metabolized within the epithelium of the small intestine. Finch and Hird (1960) observed that arginine was converted in appreciable amounts to ornithine and that transamination of glutamic and aspartic acids with pyruvate also resulted in low recoveries of these amino acids from the mucosal cells, significant amounts of alanine being formed. These observations agree with those of Neame and Wiseman (1957, 1958), Nielsen (1965) and Eggum (1966). High contents of glutamic and aspartic acids in the diets given were not reflected in the plasma, whereas the concentrations of alanine and glycine were unexpectedly high. Furthermore, a significant proportion of the amino acids liberated in the intestinal lumen is incorporated into the proteins of the mucosal cells (Schlüssel, 1959; Dawson and Holdsworth, 1962). According to Gitler (1964) only during the initial periods after protein ingestion (60 min or less) would the amino acids released originate mainly from exogenous proteins. Subsequently breakdown of endogenous protein also occurs.

Although the plasma amino acid method may provide valuable information regarding the nutritional status, limiting amino acids and amino acid requirements, no one—as Gitler (1964) commented—has yet presented convincing evidence that there are unique advantages in using plasma amino acid levels for ranking the relative quality of various food and feed proteins. Moreover, in this discussion several other factors that might obscure the results have not been considered. These include, for example, the influence of energy-yielding nutrients, the effect of dietary carbohydrates, hormones, amino acid antagonism and toxicity and so on. With this in mind it is not surprising that little success has attended attempts to find correlations between intestinal release of amino acids and changes in these amino acids in portal blood.

III. PLASMA UREA LEVELS AS INDICATORS OF DIETARY PROTEIN QUALITY

In experiments with growing rats and pigs, Münchow and Bergner (1968) found a very high negative correlation between the biological value of the feed and the blood urea level. The correlation coefficients were 0·99 and 0·96 for rats and pigs, respectively. Münchow and Bergner (1968) found that the blood urea level increased with the protein content of the diet. In their experiments the urea level increased by 2·4 units each time the rats were supplied with another 10 mg N/day, and they concluded that blood urea level depended on both the quality and the quantity of the protein supplied in the diet. Fonnesbeck and Symons (1969), in experiments with horses, also showed that the blood urea level depended on the quality and quantity of protein in the diet. Pastuszewska (1967) obtained similar results with suckling pigs. This relationship is consistent with the demonstration that an increase in dietary protein content caused a decline in biological value (Barnes *et al.*, 1946; Nehring and Haesler, 1954; Forbes *et al.*, 1958). Kornegay *et al.* (1964) found, as expected, that the inclusion of large quantities of urea in the diet caused an increase in the blood urea level. In experiments with rats, Kumta and Harper (1961) demonstrated that an amino acid imbalance raised the blood urea level, and that this level could be reduced by restoring the balance. The urea level reached a maximum 3 h after feeding. A similar dependence of blood urea level on time after feeding was found by Anderson and Edney (1969) in experiments with dogs given a diet containing 8·5% protein. However, they did not find a clearly-defined maximum, but rather a steady increase up to 3 h and thereafter an almost constant level over the following 2 h. When the diet contained 5·0% protein the maximum level of urea in blood was reached 2 h after feeding.

From this it appears that at least three factors influence the urea level: the quality and content of protein in the diet and the time after feeding. By standardizing the technique it is possible to eliminate the effects of both protein content and time after feeding (Eggum, 1970). Thus, the protein quality should be the decisive factor influencing blood urea level.

A. Effect of Protein Level

Groups of five Wistar male rats weighing approximately 75 g were used in a series of experiments in which the preliminary period lasted 4 days and the balance period 5 days. Each animal received 150 mg N and 10 g dry matter each day throughout the preliminary and the balance periods. The N content was adjusted by using a N-free mixture consisting mainly of autoclaved potato starch, soya-bean oil and minerals.

All blood samples were taken from the cervical vein at the end of the experiment, between 10.00 and 11.00 h. Any food or water left in the cage from the previous day was removed at 06.00 h, i.e. 4–5 h before the blood samples were taken.

Seventeen groups, each of five rats, were given graded quantities of casein supplemented with 1% methionine. The crude protein content ($N \times 6{\cdot}25$) of the diet was increased from 5% to 30% of the dry matter.

The relationship between protein content of the diet and blood urea level is shown in Fig. 1. The regression equation is:

Blood urea (mg/100 ml) = 6·98 + 1·07 [crude protein (%)]

$$r = 0{\cdot}95; \quad s = 2{\cdot}77; \quad s_b = 0{\cdot}09,$$

where s = deviation from regression and s_b = deviation of the regression coefficient.

The regression coefficient is significantly different from zero, as a t test showed ($P < 0{\cdot}001$). Thus urea content increases when the protein content in the diet increases. This is in agreement with other findings and must be taken into account if the blood urea levels are to be used as a measure of the protein quality. Accordingly, all the experiments on the

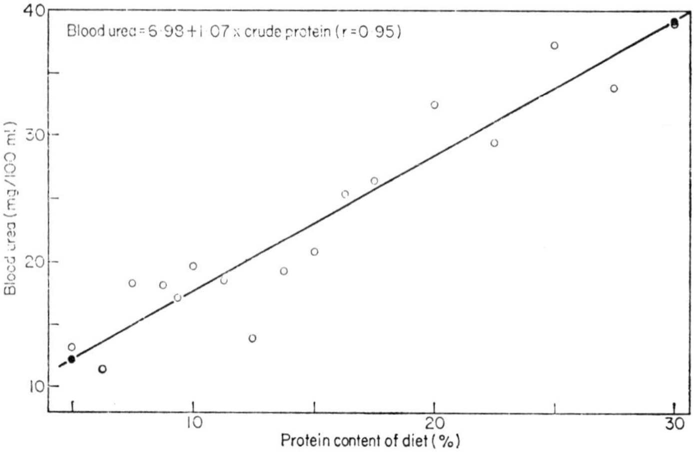

FIG. 1. Variation in blood urea level of rats with the dietary protein content

effect of protein quality were carried out using diets containing the same protein level.

B. Effects of Time after Ingestion

Blood samples were taken from a pig (68 kg) immediately before feeding and then at hourly intervals after feeding; the blood was taken from a portal vein catheter. The test meal consisted of 1·5 kg barley and 0·1 kg casein.

The results from this experiment are shown in Fig. 2.

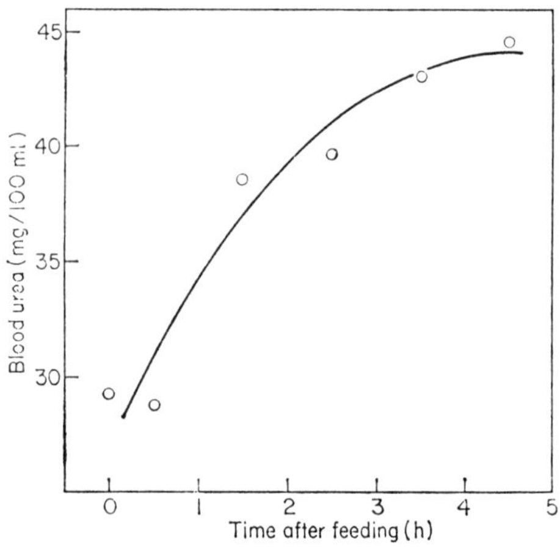

FIG. 2. Variation in blood urea level of a pig with time after feeding

It can be seen that the blood urea level in the pig depended on the time interval after feeding. With the diet used, barley and casein, it appeared that at least 3–4 h might elapse before the blood urea level became constant and this suggested that 4–5 h after feeding would be the most suitable time to take blood samples in a standardized test.

C. Effect of Protein Quality

In a further experiment, the relationship of the blood urea level to the protein quality of the diet was investigated. One group of five rats was used for experiments with each of forty-two feeding-stuffs. These included cereals, oilcake extracts, offal, fish meal, dried grass products and concentrates for pigs, poultry and ruminants. The experimental technique was as described above, and all animals received 150 mg N and 10 g dry matter/day.

The results of the experiment are shown in Fig. 3. It is clear that there was a direct relationship between blood urea level and the biological value of the protein in the diet. The regression equation is:

$$\text{b.v.} = 0{\cdot}9454 - 0{\cdot}015 \times \text{blood urea (mg/100 ml)};$$

$$s = 4{\cdot}96; \quad s_b = 0{\cdot}08; \quad r = -0{\cdot}95.$$

The regression coefficient differs significantly from zero ($P < 0{\cdot}001$). Thus the equation shows that the level of blood urea decreases with increasing quality of the protein in the diet. This relationship agrees very well with the findings of Münchow and Bergner (1968), and with recent work with Indian feedstuffs by Prabhu (1971) who obtained a correlation

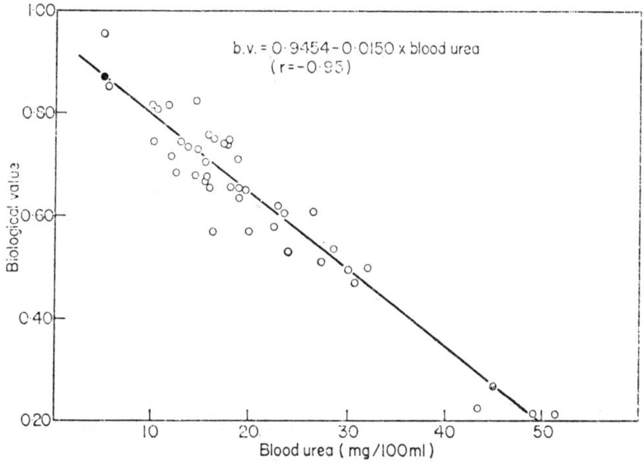

FIG. 3. Relationship between the blood urea level of rats and the biological value of the dietary protein

coefficient of −0·93 between the blood urea level and the biological value of the protein of the diet.

Bergner *et al.* (1971) have re-examined the method under practical conditions with growing pigs and concluded that, under strictly standardized conditions, measurement of blood urea levels could be used to estimate protein quality of practical rations.

D. Conclusions

The results of these experiments confirm the thesis that blood urea increases as the protein content of the diet increases (Münchow and Bergner, 1968; Fonnesbeck and Symons, 1969; Pastuszewska, 1967). The significant relationship between the biological value of the diet and blood urea levels is in accordance with the findings of Münchow and Bergner (1968). It appears that a determination of the blood urea level could be a rapid and efficient method for evaluating protein quality. However, the experimental conditions must be standardized, especially in relation to the protein content of the diet and to the time after feeding at which blood samples are taken.

REFERENCES

Andah, D. O. and Chamberlain, A. G. (1971). *Proc. Nutr. Soc.* **30**, 11A.

Anderson, R. S. and Edney, A. T. B. (1969). *Vet. Rec.* **84**, 348–349.

Barnes, R. H., Bates, M. J. and Maack, J. E. (1946). *J. Nutr.* **32**, 535–548.

Bergner, H., Münchow, H. and Reischuck, M. (1971). *Arch. Tierernähr.* **21**, 133–140.

Buraczewski, S., Porter, J. W. G., Westgarth, D. R. and Williams, A. P. (1967). *Proc. Nutr. Soc.* **26**, viii–ix.

Dawson, R. and Holdsworth, E. S. (1962). *Br. J. Nutr.* **16**, 13–25.

Dean, W. F. and Scott, H. M. (1966). *J. Nutr.* **88**, 75–83.

Delhumeau, G., Velez Pratt, G. and Gitler, C. (1962). *J. Nutr.* **77**, 52–60.

Denton, A. E. and Elvehjem, C. A. (1954). *J. biol. Chem.* **206**, 449–454.

Denton, A. E., Gershoff, S. N. and Elvehjem, C. A. (1953). *J. biol. Chem.* **204**, 731–735.

Eggum, B. O. (1966). *Z. Tierphysiol. Tierernähr. Futtermittelk.* **22**, 32–38.

Eggum, B. O. (1970). *Br. J. Nutr.* **24**, 983–988.

Erbersdobler, H. (1969). *Z. Tierphysiol. Tierernähr. Futtermittelk.* **25**, 119–121.

Finch, L. R. and Hird, F. J. R. (1960). *Biochim. biophys. Acta* **43**, 278–287.

Fonnesbeck, P. V. and Symons, L. D. (1969). *J. Anim. Sci.* **28**, 216–219.

Forbes, R. M., Vaughan, L. and Yohe, M. (1958). *J. Nutr.* **64**, 291–302.

Gitler, C. (1964). *In* "Mammalian Protein Metabolism" (H. N. Munro and J. B. Allison, eds), Vol. 1, pp. 35–69. Academic Press, New York.

Goldberg, A. and Guggenheim, K. (1962). *Biochem. J.* **83**, 129–135.

KIHLBERG, R. (1970). *In* "Evaluation of Novel Protein Products": proc. symp. 1968 (A. E. Bender *et al.* eds), pp. 149–158. Pergamon Press, Oxford.
KORNEGAY, E. T., MILLER, E. R., ULLREY, D. E. and HOEFER, J. A. (1964). *J. Anim. Sci.* **23**, 688–693.
KUMTA, U. S. and HARPER, A. E. (1961). *J. Nutr.* **74**, 139–147.
LEBEDEVA, Z. N. and NURIAKHMETOVA, Z. YU. (1964). *Vop. Pitan.* **23** (4), 23–26.
LEVENSON, S. M., ROSEN, H. and UPJOHN, H. L. (1959). *Proc. Soc. exp. Biol. Med.* **101**, 178–180.
McLAUGHLAN, J. M., NOEL, F. J., MORRISON, A. B. and CAMPBELL, J. A. (1963). *Can. J. Biochem. Physiol.* **41**, 191–199.
MÜNCHOW, H. and BERGNER, H. (1968). *Arch. Tierernähr.* **18**, 222–228.
NASSET, E. S., GANAPATHY, S. N. and GOLDSMITH, D. P. J. (1963). *J. Nutr.* **81**, 343–347.
NEAME, K. D. and WISEMAN, G. (1957). *J. Physiol., Lond.* **135**, 442–450.
NEAME, K. D. and WISEMAN, G. (1958). *J. Physiol., Lond.* **140**, 148–155.
NEHRING, K. and HAESLER, E. (1954). *Arch. Tierernähr.*, Suppl. no. 5, 110–126.
NIELSEN, J. J. (1965). Licentiate Thesis. The Royal Veterinary and Agricultural College, Copenhagen.
OWINGS, W. J. and BALLOUN, S. L. (1961). *Poult. Sci.* **40**, 1718–1730.
PASTUSZEWSKA, B. (1967). *Roczn. Nauk roln.*, Ser. B. **89**, 503–509.
PAWLAK, M. and PION, R. (1968). *Annls Biol. anim. Biochim. Biophys.* **8**, 517–530.
PION, R., FAUCONNEAU, G. and RÉRAT, A. (1964). *Annls Biol. anim. Biochim. Biophys.* **4**, 383–402.
PION, R. and PAWLAK, M. (1969). *Wiss. Z. Univ. Rostock* **18**, 117.
PRABHU, G. A. (1971). Personal Communication.
RICHARDSON, L. R., BLAYLOCK, L. G. and LYMAN, C. M. (1953). *J. Nutr.* **51**, 515–522.
SCHLÜSSEL, H. (1959). *Clinica chim. Acta* **4**, 748–751.
SMITH, R. E. and SCOTT, H. M. (1965). *J. Nutr.* **86**, 45–50.
STOCKLAND, W. L. and MEADE, R. J. (1970). *J. Anim. Sci.* **31**, 1156–1167.
STOCKLAND, W. L., MEADE, R. J. and NORDSTROM, J. W. (1970). *J. Anim. Sci.* **31**, 1142–1155.
STOCKLAND, W. L., MEADE, R. J., TUMBLESON, M. E. and PALM, B. W. (1971). *J. Anim. Sci.* **32**, 1143–1152.
TASAKI, I. and OHNO, T. (1971). *J. Nutr.* **101**, 1225–1231.
ZIMMERMAN, R. A. and SCOTT, H. M. (1965). *J. Nutr.* **87**, 13–18.

CHAPTER 21

The Relationships between the Levels of Free Amino Acids in Blood and Muscle and the Nutritive Value of Proteins

R. PION

Centre de Recherches Zootechniques et Vétérinaires, 63-Saint-Genes-Champanelle, France

I. INTRODUCTION

The products of digestion of dietary proteins are carried by the blood to the tissues mainly as free amino acids (Dawson and Porter, 1962). Their levels in blood are the results of the differences between the uptake by the tissues and the amounts coming from the diet or of endogenous origin, and may reflect the differences between the needs and the dietary supplies. Many workers, such as Longenecker and Hause (1959) with dogs, Morrison *et al.* (1961) with rats and Zimmerman and Scott (1965) with chicks, found a relationship between the levels of free amino acids in the blood and the amino acid composition of the diet.

As far as growing animals are concerned, the muscle is the tissue that has the largest need for amino acids, and it takes them from the blood; furthermore the concentration of each amino acid reflects at each time the difference between supply and uptake for protein synthesis. Harper and Rogers (1965) found that dietary amino acid imbalances affected free amino acid levels in muscle more than in blood and Pawlak and Pion (1967) showed that the differences between the levels of lysine in the muscle of rats receiving a balanced diet or a diet low in lysine were greater than those in the blood. Subsequently we have studied in more detail the relationship between the levels of lysine, threonine, isoleucine and methionine in the diet and those in blood and muscle in an attempt to develop a sensitive test to estimate the amounts of amino acids being absorbed from the digestive tract and hence the availability of dietary amino acids.

II. EXPERIMENTAL METHODS

The experimental diets were isonitrogenous (12% crude protein) and isoenergetic (19 000 kJ/kg dry matter). In the experiments concerning lysine and in some concerning threonine they contained wheat supplemented with DL-methionine, L-tryptophan, and different proportions of L-lysine HCl and L-threonine (Table I). In other experiments, free amino acids (Table II) and wheat starch were used instead of wheat; these amino acid mixtures contained enough essential amino acids to meet all the requirements except of the one under study, and had a non-essential amino acid pattern similar to that of the wheat proteins. The energy level

TABLE I. Amino acids in wheat diets (g/kg dry matter)

	From wheat	*Added*	*Total*
Aspartic acid	5·55		5·55
Threonine[a]	3·1	0–3·0	3·1–6·1
Serine	5·45		5·45
Glutamic acid	38·8		38·8
Proline	11·35		11·35
Glycine	4·6		4·6
Alanine	4·2		4·2
Valine	5·6		5·6
Cystine	2·9		2·9
Methionine	1·75	1·2	2·95
Isoleucine	4·4		4·4
Leucine	7·9		7·9
Tyrosine	3·6		3·6
Phenylalanine	5·4		5·4
Lysine[b]	2·9	0–14·4	2·9–17·3
Histidine	2·65		2·65
Arginine	5·45		5·45
Tryptophan		0·6	

[a] 5·4 in lysine experiments
[b] 8·5 in threonine experiments

TABLE II. Amino acids in semi-synthetic diets (g/kg dry matter)

L-Aspartic acid	5·9	DL-Methionine[c]	3·2
L-Threonine[a]	4·5	L-Isoleucine[d]	5
L-Serine	5·8	L-Leucine	8·3
L-Glutamine	20·5	L-Tyrosine	3·8
L-Glutamic acid	20·5	L-Phenylalanine	5·7
L-Proline	12	L-Lysine HCl	11
Glycine	4·8	L-Histidine HCl H_2O	3·8
L-Alanine	4·4	L-Arginine HCl	7
L-Valine	5·9	L-Tryptophan	1·7
L-Cystine[b]	3·0		

[a] 2·25 to 5·8 in threonine experiment
[b] 2·0 or 3·0 in methionine experiment
[c] 0·5 to 9·0 in methionine experiment
[d] 2·0 to 6·0 in isoleucine experiment

TABLE III. Mineral content of diets (per kg dry matter)

Ca	10 g	Mn	30 mg
P	3 g	Zn	10 mg
Na	2 g	F	5 mg
Fe	30 mg	I	150 μg
Cu	5 mg	Co	150 μg

TABLE IV. Vitamin content of diets (per kg dry matter)

B_{12} (Cyanocobalamin)	0·05 mg
Folic acid	1 mg
Vitamin E	100 mg
Vitamin K	2 mg
Thiamine hydrochloride	10 mg
Nicotinic acid	30 mg
Pyridoxine hydrochloride	10 mg
Riboflavin	15 mg
Calcium pantothenate	50 mg
Inositol	300 mg
Para-aminobenzoic acid	100 mg
Ascorbic acid	100 mg
Biotin	0·2 mg
Choline chloride	100 mg
Vitamin A	4000 i.u.
Vitamin D_2	2000 i.u.

of the diets was adjusted with peanut oil. The vitamin and mineral contents of the diets are shown in Tables III and IV.

The rats, eight in each group, weighed 110 g at the beginning of the experiments. They were reared in individual cages and were given the semi-liquid experimental diets *ad libitum* for two weeks. Their food intake and weight gains were recorded. At the end of the experiment the animals were killed in the morning, without prior starvation, and samples of blood and of hind limb muscle were taken.

Blood samples were immediately mixed with cold ethanol and muscles were frozen in liquid nitrogen. All samples were stored at −15°C. Free amino acids were extracted from blood with 84% ethanol, and from muscle with 1% picric acid as described elsewhere (Pawlak and Pion, 1968a), and estimated by ion-exchange column chromatography using an automatic amino acid analyser.

III. RESULTS

A. Mean Values in Blood and Muscle (Table V)

The free amino acid levels in the blood and muscle of rats receiving the balanced wheat diet are shown in Table V. The concentrations of most

TABLE V. Level of free amino acids (mg/100 g) in blood and muscle of rats receiving a balanced wheat diet[a]

	Blood	*Muscle*
Aspartic acid	0·5	5·2
Threonine	5·1	20·5
Serine + glutamine	12·1	84·0
Glutamic acid	2·5	42·4
Glycine	2·1	34·2
Alanine	3·6	29·1
Valine	1·0	0·9
Methionine	0·8	0·6
Isoleucine	0·5	0·3
Leucine	0·9	0·7
Tyrosine	0·9	1·2
Phenylalanine	0·8	0·7
Ornithine	0·5	1·2
Lysine	4·3	11·7
Histidine	0·8	3·8
Arginine	1·8	3·5

[a] Average daily weight gain 7·15 g

of the non-essential amino acids were ten to thirty times higher in muscle than in blood. The levels of some essential amino acids—valine, methionine, isoleucine, leucine and phenylalanine—were similar in the two tissues, whereas the amounts of the others—lysine, threonine, histidine and arginine—were higher in muscle than in blood. Cystine was generally present only in very small amounts, and could not be estimated. Tryptophan was present in some extracts, but was not quantitatively recovered from the tissues. Muscle extracts contained large amounts of some compounds which are not tabulated, such as carnosine, anserine and taurine.

B. Lysine Experiments (Table VI; Pawlak and Pion, 1968a)

1. *Growth and Food Consumption*

The average daily weight gain ranged from 5·8 g to 7·25 g with diets containing adequate levels of lysine. The growth rates of rats receiving

TABLE VI. Levels of free lysine in rat blood and muscle[a]

Lysine in diet (g/kg dry matter)	*Gain/rat* (g/day)	*Feed* (g/day)	*Lysine* (mg/100 g)	
			Blood	*Muscle*
Expt I: Wheat diet				
4·2	4·2	18·3	1·3	2·7
5·5	5·7	18·4	2·3	3·6
6·7	5·8	17·6	2·7	4·1
8·0	5·9	16·9	3·8	8·5
Expt II: Wheat diet				
2·9	3·3	16·2	1·3	1·8
5·5	6·0	16·9	2·4	4·6
9·3	6·5	17·2	5·9	22·6
10·3	7·0	17·8	6·4	22·9
Expt III: Wheat diet				
7·7	6·7	17·7	3·9	10·7
8·5	7·15	18·8	4·3	11·7
11·7	7·0	18·4	6·0	21·7
12·5	7·25	18·0	9·2	27·9
Expt IV: Wheat diet				
8·5	5·8	15·9	4·5	9·6
17·3	6·0	16·0	9·9	50·1

[a] Pawlak and Pion (1968a)

slightly lysine-deficient diets (containing more than 60–70% of the requirement) were slightly lower than those of the control rats which received a balanced diet and were reared at the same time.

Lysine deficiencies of more than 50% of the requirement resulted in considerably lower growth rates. A large excess of lysine (up to twice the requirement) did not affect either the growth rate or the food consumption.

There was some variability in growth rate between experiments, and the growth rates obtained with different diets could be compared only if they were obtained in the same experiment.

2. *Free Lysine in Blood and Muscle*

The free lysine level in blood increased slowly when the lysine content of the ingested food was raised from 2·9 g/kg of dry matter (unsupplemented wheat) to 8·5 g/kg of dry matter. A further increase of 10% in lysine eaten produced a rise of 30% in the free lysine level in the blood. There was no further increase when the lysine content of the diet was higher than 12·5 g/kg of dry matter.

The differences in free lysine concentration between muscle samples were larger than those which occurred in the blood. The free lysine level in muscle increased gradually for lower dietary levels and rose sharply when the lysine content of the diet was higher than 8·5 g/kg of dry matter. It increased twofold when the dietary level was raised by 10%. In contrast to what occurred in the blood, there was an accumulation of free lysine in the muscle of animals given the diet richest in lysine.

The magnitude of the changes in the lysine level in muscle indicates that its estimation may be a very sensitive method for measuring the available lysine content of foods.

C. Threonine (Table VII; Pawlak and Pion, 1968b)

Both wheat and amino acid diets were used in these experiments because wheat proteins are not sufficiently low in threonine to give a markedly threonine-deficient diet.

1. *Growth and Food Consumption*

The growth rate was depressed by 1 g/day when the diet contained only 60% of the requirement with both types of meals, but the feed consumption was only slightly changed. When the dietary threonine was only 40% of the requirement, the food intake was lowered by 30%, and the average daily weight gain was 1 g, only one-sixth of the growth rate of the animals given the balanced diets.

TABLE VII. Level of free threonine in rat blood and muscle[a]

Threonine in diet (g/kg dry matter)	*Gain/rat* (g/day)	*Feed* (g/day)	*Threonine* (mg/100 g)	
			Blood	*Muscle*
Expt I: Wheat diet				
3·2	5·3	17·2	0·8	2·3
3·7	6·3	17·9	1·3	4·9
4·2	6·1	16·7	1·5	5·4
4·7	6·7	17·3	2·4	—
5·5	7·15	18·6	5·1	20·5
Expt II: Wheat diet				
3·45	5·3	17	0·8	2·7
3·95	6·1	17·7	1·0	3·7
4·45	5·8	16·7	2·4	9·0
4·95	5·8	16·0	3·2	11·4
5·2	5·9	16·6	4·1	13·9
5·7	5·8	15·95	5·2	18·5
6·2	6·15	16·9	7·6	22·4
Expt III: Crystalline amino acid diets				
2·25	1·2	11·5	0·6	1·8
2·5	2·6	13·9	0·65	2·3
2·75	3·1	14·3	0·8	2·3
3·0	3·0	13·6	0·7	1·8
3·25	4·7	14·95	1·2	4·0
5·8	5·5	15·8	9·8	27·6
Expt IV: Crystalline amino acid diets				
3·7	5·5	15·8	1·2	4·3
4·2	5·8	15·1	2·0	7·6
5·0	5·4	14·7	17·9	

[a] Pawlak and Pion (1968b)

2. *Free Threonine in Blood and Muscle*

The changes in the levels of free threonine in blood and muscle in relation to threonine intake were slightly different from those found with lysine. The levels were higher in muscle than in blood, but the relative increases were the same in the two tissues, and generally larger than those that occurred with lysine. The free threonine concentration in both tissues increased slowly with threonine intakes lower than 4·2 g/kg dry matter, and rose sharply with higher intakes. The level of threonine in the muscle of animals given a diet containing 4·45 g/kg of dry matter was twice that of rats given a diet containing only 4·2 g/kg of dry matter. As with lysine, a sharp rise in blood and muscle concentrations was obtained at intakes lower than the estimated requirements of the animals.

With lower dietary threonine levels, the free threonine levels in blood and muscle did not depend on whether the diet contained wheat or crystalline threonine. With higher threonine intakes, the free threonine levels in blood and muscle were higher in the animals given the crystalline amino acid diets.

This difference was greatly reduced if the free amino acid levels were related to an approximate estimate of digestible threonine (dietary threonine × apparent digestibility of nitrogen) instead of to total threonine.

As with lysine, determination of the level of free threonine in muscle appeared to be a very sensitive test for the estimation of the availability of dietary threonine.

D. Isoleucine (Table VIII; Pawlak and Pion, 1971)

The crystalline amino acid diets contained 2–6 g of isoleucine per kg of dry matter, supplying from 36–110% of the estimated requirement.

TABLE VIII. Level of free isoleucine in rat blood and muscle[a]

Isoleucine in diet (g/kg dry matter)		*Gain/rat* (g/day)	*Feed* (g/day)	*Isoleucine* (mg/100 g)	
				Blood	*Muscle*
Expt I	2·0	0·4	8·7	0·53	0·85
	3·0	3·0	11·9	0·47	1·08
Expt II	2·25	0·8	9·9	0·37	0·40
	2·50	1·3	9·7	0·35	0·58
	2·75	2·2	10·8	—	0·63
	3·25	2·8	11·2	0·75	0·79
	3·50	4·0	12·9	0·49	0·72
Expt III	4·0	4·5	14·1	0·43	0·52
	4·25	3·85	12·1	0·60	0·48
	4·50	4·60	14·3	0·65	0·60
Expt IV	4·75	4·25	13·0	0·79	0·82
	5·0	5·8	15·0	0·80	0·70
	5·25	5·6	14·5	0·75	0·87
	5·50	5·45	14·0	0·65	0·77
	5·75	6·20	14·6	0·85	0·94
	6·0	5·70	14·2	0·79	0·94

[a] Pawlak and Pion (1971)

1. *Growth Rate and Food Consumption*

Food consumption and weight gains were very low when the diets were highly deficient in isoleucine. Growth rates were decreased by 35% and 25% respectively, and food intakes by 15% and 5%, when the diets contained 60% and 80% of the estimated isoleucine requirement. Greatest weight gains were observed when the isoleucine level of the diet was 90% or more of the requirement.

2. *Free Amino Acids in Blood and Muscle*

The free isoleucine levels in the blood and muscle of rats given the highly deficient diets were low; they increased slowly with the dietary levels. Isoleucine did not accumulate in the muscle once the requirement was satisfied, as did threonine and lysine. The total non-essential amino acids increased and the total essential amino acids decreased as the isoleucine content of the diet increased.

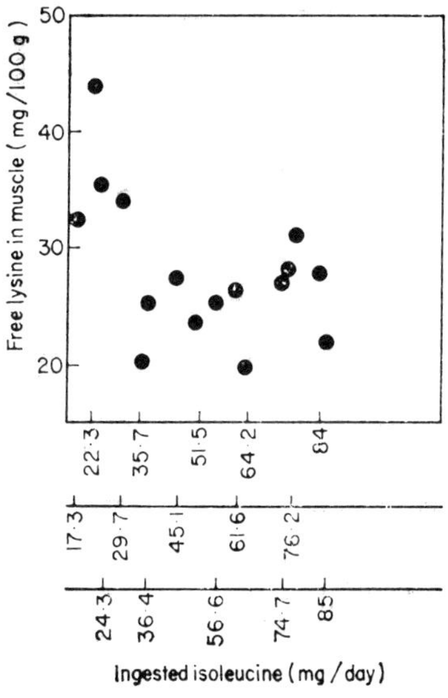

FIG. 1. Relation between free lysine in muscle and ingested isoleucine

There was a negative correlation between free threonine in muscle and the level of isoleucine in the diet, and the lysine level in muscle was very high when the intake of isoleucine was very low (Figs 1–4).

It is less easy to estimate deficiencies of dietary isoleucine than of lysine or threonine; however, they can be inferred from the simultaneous examination of growth, food intake and concentrations of essential amino acids (especially threonine and isoleucine) in muscle and blood.

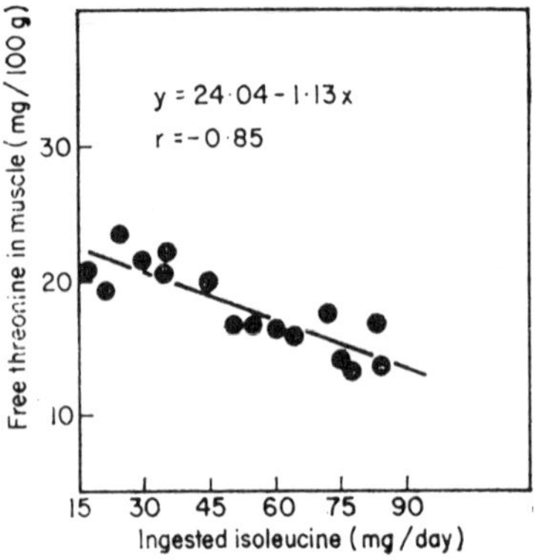

FIG. 2. Relation between free threonine in muscle and ingested isoleucine

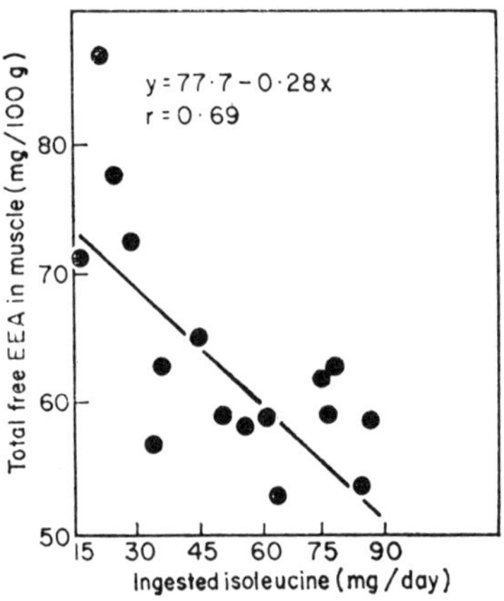

FIG. 3. Relation between the sum of the free essential amino acids in muscle and ingested isoleucine

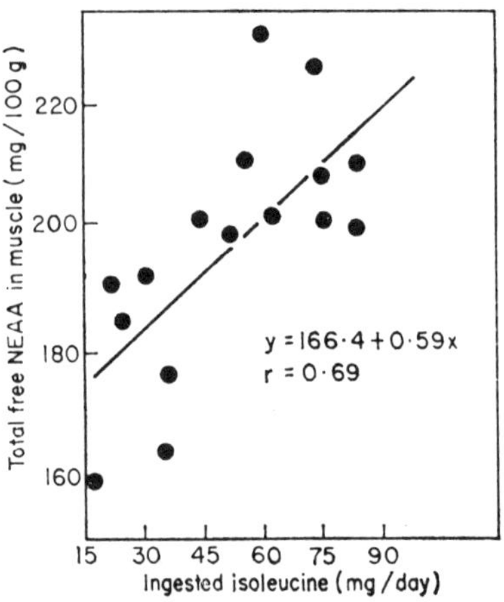

FIG. 4. Relation between the sum of free non-essential amino acids in muscle and ingested isoleucine

E. Methionine (Table IX)

TABLE IX. Level of free methionine in rat blood and muscle[a]

	Methionine in diet (g/kg dry matter)	*Methionine + cystine in diet* (g/kg dry matter)	*Gain/rat* (g/day)	*Feed* (g/day)	*Methionine* (mg/100 g)	
					Blood	*Muscle*
Expt I	1·7	4·7	5·85	16·7	1·0	1·8
	2·2	5·2	6·3	18·3	1·2	1·8
	2·7	5·7	6·3	17·35	1·3	2·4
	3·2	6·2	6·1	17·1	1·2	
	9·0	12·0	5·9	17·7	1·4	1·8
Expt II	1·0	3·0	0·9	11·6	0·5	0·5
	1·5	3·5	3·7	13·6	0·8	0·9
	2·0	4·0	3·9	12·8		0·9
	2·5	4·5	4·2	14·4	1·1	1·2
	3·0	5·0	4·9	14·3	1·1	0·9
	0·5	3·5	−1·0	8·05	0·6	1·0
	1·0	4·0	0·35	9·85	0·6	0·7
	3·2	6·2	5·3	15·0	1·2	1·6
	6·0	9·0	5·4	14·7	1·4	1·8
	8·0	11·0	5·8	15·25	1·6	2·0

[a] Pawlak and Pion (unpublished results)

The amounts of methionine provided in the two experiments ranged from 0·5–9 g/kg of dry matter, and the cystine level was 2 or 3 g/kg of dry matter.

1. *Growth and Food Consumption*

The mean weight gains of the animals receiving the highly deficient diets were very low, or negative. Highest growth rates were obtained with diets containing 3 g cystine per kg of dry matter and 2·2 or more g methionine per kg of dry matter, or 2 g of cystine and 3 or more g of methionine.

2. *Free Amino Acids in Blood and Muscle*

The free cystine levels in blood and muscle were always very low, and could not be accurately estimated. The free methionine levels were low when the diets were deficient in sulphur amino acids, and generally increased with their dietary level. Muscle methionine levels were similar to blood methionine levels when intakes of methionine were low, but increased more quickly with increasing dietary levels. Thus, as with lysine and threonine, muscle level appeared to represent a more sensitive test than blood level, though the response was much smaller.

IV. DISCUSSION

A. Experimental Period

It was necessary to use a relatively short period for several reasons: we needed to use rapidly growing young animals with high amino acid requirements, for the least number of days sufficient to adapt them to a new type of diet.

B. Feeding Procedure

The animals were given food *ad libitum* instead of being trained to eat meals in a short period, and they were allowed to eat during the whole day and particularly the whole night. This method led to relatively constant amino acid levels, and allowed greater food intakes and higher growth rates than single meals. On the other hand, some differences occurred in food intake from day to day and from one animal to another, and this led to some variability in the free amino acid content of the tissues.

C. Crude Protein Level in the Diets

In all the experiments we supplied dietary levels of amino acids sufficient to allow optimal growth, but perhaps slightly too low for maximum nitrogen retention. We have made other trials to evaluate the influence of the protein level in the diets on the free amino acid contents of blood and muscle, using diets containing wheat or sunflower meal supplemented with amino acids (Pawlak and Pion, 1968c, 1970b). Slightly decreasing the nitrogen content of the diet was partially compensated by an increase in food intake, but the net effect was to enhance amino acid deficiencies.

The results obtained with high protein levels in the diet showed that the blood and muscle levels of one amino acid were related to the dietary amounts of the others which must be supplied in sufficient quantities to permit a high rate of protein synthesis. Thus it was necessary to consider the proportions of amino acids in the diet as well as their concentrations.

V. STUDY OF AMINO ACID AVAILABILITY IN FEEDSTUFFS

Although the levels of free amino acids in muscle were generally a better criterion than the levels in blood, estimations were made in both tissues.

The feed under study was used as far as possible as the sole protein source and it was supplemented with amino acids in order to correct any deficiencies. Supplementation with several amino acids was thought preferable to using a higher protein level, since it was possible to avoid a large excess of some amino acids. The vitamin mixture used was the same for all diets, but the mineral mixture was calculated taking into account the mineral content of the feedstuff. The energy content of the diet or, better, the digestible energy content, was adjusted to an adequate level by the addition of wheat starch and peanut oil. The feeding technique was the same as in the amino acid experiments, and the free amino acid levels in blood and muscle were compared with the results obtained previously. The results of experiments with wheat and sunflower have already been published (Pawlak and Pion, 1970a,b), and other feedstuffs are now being studied.

VI. APPLICATION TO OTHER ANIMALS

It is difficult to obtain representative samples of muscle for estimation of free amino acids from living animals, and the animals slaughtered for meat production are generally not young enough to give good results. So it is easier to use free amino acid levels in blood to study amino acid availability for pigs, or to determine products of digestion in ruminant animals.

The chick is an animal of economic interest that can also be used as a test animal for protein evaluation using muscle or blood amino acid levels. Richardson *et al.* (1965) found with chicks killed after an 18 h fast a relationship between free amino acid levels in muscle and the level of dietary protein and lysine. Larbier *et al.* (1971a) studied the influence of the lysine and methionine content of the diet on free amino acids in the muscle of growing chicks. They did not find any direct relationship between muscle free amino acids and the corresponding dietary levels when the animals were fed *ad libitum*, but they were able to demonstrate the effects of lysine and methionine deficiencies when the animals were given single meals. The difference between these results and those we obtained with rats may perhaps result from the high protein content of the diet used with chicks (21·4% crude protein) or from the starvation before slaughter. In further experiments, Larbier and Yvoré (1971) found that coccidiosis affected the level of free amino acids in muscle, and Larbier *et al.* (1971b) applied this method to the study of the influence on protein quality of drying and storage of maize. They demonstrated effects of drying methods that did not affect, or affected only slightly, the weight gain.

REFERENCES

DAWSON, R. and PORTER, J. W. G. (1962). *Br. J. Nutr.* **16**, 27–38.

HARPER, A. E. and ROGERS, Q. R. (1965). *Proc. Nutr. Soc.* **24**, 173–190.

LARBIER, M. and YVORÉ, P. (1971). *C.r. hebd. Séanc. Acad. Sci., Paris, Sér. D* **273**, 1228–1230.

LARBIER, M., GUILLAUME, J. and BLUM, J. C. (1971a). *Nutr. Rep. int.* **3**, 273–276.

LARBIER, M., GUILLAUME, J. and CALET, C. (1971b). *Annls Zootech.* **20** (Suppl.), 653–661.

LONGENECKER, J. B. and HAUSE, N. L. (1959). *Archs Biochem. Biophys.* **84**, 46–59.

MORRISON, A. B., MIDDLETON, E. J. and MCLAUGHLAN, J. M. (1961). *Can. J. Biochem. Physiol.* **39**, 1675–1680.

PAWLAK, M. and PION, R. (1967). *C.r. hebd. Séanc. Acad. Sci., Paris, Sér. D* **264**, 380–382.

PAWLAK, M. and PION, R. (1968a). *Annls Biol. anim. Biochim. Biophys.* **8**, 517–530.

PAWLAK, M. and PION, R. (1968b). *C.r. hebd. Séanc. Acad. Sci., Paris, Sér. D* **266**, 1993–1995.

PAWLAK, M. and PION, R. (1968c). *Annls Biol. anim. Biochim. Biophys.* **8**, 457–459.

PAWLAK, M. and PION, R. (1970a). *Annls Biol. anim. Biochim. Biophys.* **10**, 171–174.

PAWLAK, M. and PION, R. (1970b). *Annls Biol. anim. Biochim. Biophys.* **10**, 317–322.

PAWLAK, M. and PION, R. (1971). *Annls Biol. anim. Biochim. Biophys.* **11**, 505–510.

RICHARDSON, L. R., CANNON, M. L. and WEBB, B. D. (1965). *Poult. Sci.* **44**, 248–257.

ZIMMERMAN, R. A. and SCOTT, H. M. (1965). *J. Nutr.* **87**, 13–18.

CHAPTER 22

The Use of Ileal Content Analysis to Assess the Digestibility of Amino Acids

K. J. CARPENTER

Department of Applied Biology, University of Cambridge, England

I. THE FORMULATION OF PRACTICAL DIETS

The method of protein evaluation using ileal digestibility may, of course, have wider interests, but the immediate application of the work is in poultry nutrition. Chicks are capable of very rapid growth. From hatching they can double their weight six times in 8 weeks, going from 35 g to about 2 kg. This rate of growth requires a diet of over 20% protein content, or an n.d.-p : e of 0·18 in the early stages (as compared with values of 0·04–0·08 for human beings at different stages of life). Although cereals, costing approximately £30/ton, form the most economical source of energy in such diets, their 10% protein content is quite inadequate. The high-protein foods available for balancing the diets are all more expensive at £50–100/ton. Nevertheless, it is still economic to feed the chicks so that they grow at their maximal rate. There is, therefore, a considerable incentive for the poultry industry to find the most economical way of supplying the amino acids needed to support this very rapid growth. There is strong competition between feed-compounding companies, as also between the suppliers of various types of high-protein feedstuffs (of both animal and vegetable origin) and of synthetic amino acids.

It is interesting that the people actually concerned with this work of formulating economic diets to meet exacting requirements do not make use of the concepts of "protein efficiency ratio" or "net protein utilization". The reason is that such values are not additive, and any balanced diet has to be made up of a mixture of several ingredients each contributing useful protein. Instead, each of the essential amino acids that might possibly be limiting is considered as a separate nutrient. Usually these are taken as lysine, methionine, "methionine plus cystine" and tryptophan, with separate limits set for each. Calculations are then made, using electronic computers, as to which combination of ingredients will provide all the required nutrients at minimum cost, and experience has shown that these "flexible formulae", varying according to the fluctuation of ingredient prices, are extremely successful. Questions of choice for the birds do not arise: they eat a single well-mixed powder (or pellet) and differences in flavour or palatability seem negligible so long as certain materials are avoided.

Apart from deciding on requirement levels for each nutrient, the computer has to be provided with data for the potency of each ingredient as a source of all the likely limiting nutrients. Ordinary amino acid analysis provides an *upper* limit for the provision of these nutrients in a food, but many of the ingredients are heat-processed (e.g. oilseed meals and meat meals) so that it is necessary to consider whether or not the amino acids can be considered equally available from every ingredient. Under practical conditions there is normally no time for testing of every batch of material before use and it becomes necessary to assume an average "availability factor" for each particular type of material. But commercial buyers use quality control tests on batches of material from different sources that they have already purchased, so as to build up a historical record of which sources have been supplying better—or worse—than average samples, as a guide for future purchases. FDNB-available lysine and pepsin solubility tests are commonly used as indicators for this purpose.

However, for setting the "availability factors" for each amino acid in "average samples" of an ingredient, more elaborate information is required. This has usually been obtained by growth assays in which basal diets, deficient in only one amino acid, are supplemented with the test material at various levels and the responses compared with those to another series of treatments in which the same basal diet is supplemented with different levels of the limiting amino acid. This work is slow and imprecise, and still subject to ambiguities (cf. de Muelenaere *et al.*, 1967; Carpenter *et al.*, 1972).

II. DETERMINATIONS OF THE DIGESTIBILITY OF INDIVIDUAL AMINO ACIDS

In general, attempts to use ordinary digestibility values for the amino acids seem to have overestimated their availability in materials damaged by processing. There has been general agreement that this could be due to (a) fermentation of undigested amino acids in the large intestine (e.g. by deamination) so that they are not recovered in the faeces and (b) absorption of amino acids in the small intestine in complexed forms that are not nutritionally usable. The latter situation is certainly known to occur in heated milk powders and is described in Chapters 31 and 34. However, with other materials that do not contain reducing sugars there is less reason to think that this occurs to an important extent. It should then be possible to obtain a measure of the available amino acids by measuring their disappearance from the small intestine. This, in turn, might be measured as the difference between the amino acids in the test diet and the contents of the alimentary tract at the end of the small intestine (i.e. in the ileum), as originally suggested by Payne *et al.* (1968). A correction for the presence of endogenous amino acids could be made by feeding a nitrogen-free diet and measuring the amino acids present in the ileum after this. One also needs to know the amount of original food to which the residue in the ileum corresponds and this can be estimated by using an indigestible marker.

Soares and Kifer (1971) have reported the results of applying the technique to a number of materials. Differences in "digestibility" were found, but could not be related directly to the results of growth assays for individual amino acids. We have endeavoured to do this for four samples, with growth assays for lysine, methionine and tryptophan, and also to compare "ileal" and "faecal" digestibility values (Varnish, 1971; Varnish and Carpenter, 1971). The ileal procedure, with animals killed 3 h after a test meal, has proved to be actually more convenient and labour-saving than the determination of "faecal" digestibility, with chicks operated on to allow separate collection of faeces and urine. Our first pair of samples consisted of freeze-dried chicken muscle untreated or autoclaved at 14% moisture content for 27 h at 116°C. The second pair consisted of lactalbumen, untreated or subjected to a treatment that attached a propionyl group to 95% or more of its ϵ-NH_2 lysine groups (Bjarnason and Carpenter, 1969). The results of the study are summarized in Table I.

The methods used for the growth assays have been referred to previously (Varnish and Carpenter, 1970). As on previous occasions, good quality "control" proteins have given values corresponding to over 100% availability for tryptophan and lysine assays. For methionine, the same materials have given much lower values. It may be that this reflects systematic errors in the assay procedures or (less likely) in the analyses, rather than a true difference in the availability of methionine (as compared to the other amino acids) in such materials. In an attempt to correct for any such systematic errors, the data have been recalculated in Table II on

TABLE I. The methionine, tryptophan and lysine contents of the test materials together with estimates of their availability obtained in different ways

	Chick muscle		*Lactalbumen*	
	Untreated	*Autoclaved*	*Untreated*	*Propionylated*
METHIONINE				
(Total, g/16 g N)	(3·60)	(3·84)	(3·25)	(3·00)
% availability from:				
(i) growth assay[a]	86	55	79	85
(ii) ileal digestion[b]	99 ± 0·7	61 ± 8·6	95 ± 0·9	81 ± 2·3
(iii) faecal digestion[b]	98 ± 0·0	73 ± 3·7	94 ± 1·8	88 ± 0·5
TRYPTOPHAN				
(Total, g/16 g N)	(1·35)	(1·20)	(2·50)	(2·40)
% availability from:				
(i) growth assay	115	58	108	104
(ii) ileal digestion	97 ± 1·0	47 ± 6·5	96 ± 0·5	84 ± 2·5
(iii) faecal digestion	96 ± 0·6	56 ± 10·0	96 ± 0·3	92 ± 0·5
LYSINE				
(Total, g/16 g N)	(9·75)	(9·20)	(10·3)	(10·2)
% available from:				
(i) growth assay	114	67	121	59
(ii) ileal digestion	99 ± 0·3	52 ± 5·6	93 ± 0·5	72 ± 3·2
(iii) faecal digestion	98 ± 0·4	61 ± 5·9	93 ± 1·8	82 ± 3·4

[a] The growth assays are, in general, means from two assays. It is not possible to give a precise coefficient of variation for the values, but it is in the region of ±5–10%. The tryptophan assay gave particular trouble, and the values are from one assay only

[b] The figures for ileal digestibility are means of four independent values, those for faecal digestibility of three

TABLE II. Availability of amino acids in the processed material as a percentage of that in the corresponding unprocessed material, according to the method of assay

	Autoclaving			*Propionylation*		
	Met	*Try*	*Lys*	*Met*	*Try*	*Lys*
By growth assay	64	50	59	107	96	48
By ileal digestibility	62	48	53	85	88	77
By faecal digestibility	74	58	62	94	96	88

a relative basis. Given the inherent variability in all the determination, we can see that autoclaving has apparently caused a 40–50% reduction in the availability of all three amino acids as judged by growth response, and this has been detected equally by the ileal analysis technique. The "faecal" method has given values suggesting a somewhat smaller degree of damage, but it cannot, of course, be claimed that this one set of comparisons proves the superiority of the ileal procedure.

With the propionylation, it appears that the damage is, at any rate, mainly to the lysine, but that even ileal analysis has failed to measure the full extent of the damage. This was, of course, expected since it is believed that ϵ-N-propionyl lysine is absorbed to some extent and then only partially hydrolysed by the chick in its kidneys (cf. Varnish and Carpenter, 1970). Our conclusion, therefore, is that the "ileal" technique may well prove a useful one, but that it needs further refinement to increase its precision, and further testing with a variety of processed materials to determine which types of damage it can detect.

REFERENCES

Bjarnason, J. and Carpenter, K. J. (1969). *Br. J. Nutr.* **23**, 859–868.

Carpenter, K. J., McDonald, I. and Miller, W. S. (1972). *Br. J. Nutr.* **27**, 7–17.

de Muelenaere, H. J. H., Chen, M.-L. and Harper, A. E. (1967). *J. agric. Fd Chem.* **15**, 310–317.

Payne, W. L., Combs, G. F., Kifer, R. R. and Snyder, D. G. (1968). *Fedn Proc. Fedn Am. Socs exp. Biol.* **27**, 1199–1203.

Soares, J. H., Jr, and Kifer, R. R. (1971). *Poult. Sci.* **50**, 41–46.

Varnish, S. A. (1971). Ph.D. Thesis, University of Cambridge.

Varnish, S. A. and Carpenter, K. J. (1970). *Proc. Nutr. Soc.* **29**, 45A–46A.

Varnish, S. A. and Carpenter, K. J. (1971). *Proc. Nutr. Soc.* **30**, 70A–71A.

CHAPTER 23 (DISCUSSION)

What are the Problems in Evaluating Protein Quality?

A. E. HARPER
University of Wisconsin, Madison, Wisconsin, USA

J. A. CAMPBELL
Department of National Health and Welfare, Ottawa, Canada

D. M. HEGSTED
Harvard School of Public Health, Boston, Mass., USA

I. OBJECTIVES OF PROTEIN EVALUATION

There are two main reasons for developing methods of protein evaluation. The first is to provide a procedure for ranking proteins according to their efficiency of utilization under some set of standard conditions. The second is to predict the efficiency of utilization of proteins as sources of nitrogen and amino acids for meeting the amino acid requirements of man and animals. These are not different ways of saying the same thing, as is often thought, but are distinctly different objectives.

A. Procedures for Ranking Proteins

These are concerned with measurement of the maximum potential nutritive value of a protein. This may be achieved under conditions of limited protein intake, but is achieved rarely, if at all, under practical conditions where concern is with maximum performance such as a satisfactory rate of growth or maintenance of health. It is important to know the maximum potential nutritive value of a protein, protein supplement, food or feedstuff in order to devise diets or improve diets with the assurance that they are of high quality and can be highly efficiently utilized, whether this is actually achieved or not. The greater the potential for efficient utilization, the greater the degree of protection afforded if protein intake falls for any reason.

Moreover, methods that measure as closely as possible the maximum potential of a diet or protein are appropriate methods for assessing the potential effects of amino acid fortification, protein complementation, effects of processing or any other treatment or condition that may alter amino acid availability. Again, the objective of such methods is to measure the potential improvement or the potential deterioration. How closely this potential is attained in practice will depend upon a variety of other factors, so measurements of potential value may bear only a limited relationship to reality.

A source of considerable misunderstanding, of misdirection of effort and even of economic waste is the assumption that, because a procedure (such as lysine fortification of wheat) can increase the potential of a protein for satisfying human needs, this potential will be achieved in practice. Whether it is achieved depends upon how closely the amounts of amino acids in the quantity of unfortified protein being consumed correspond with the amino acid requirements. It is a relatively simple matter to demonstrate the potential for improvement. It is quite another to demonstrate that the potential is achieved.

All of the standard biological methods of estimating the nutritive value of proteins will assess the potential effect of amino acid fortification; they will assess the effect of heat processing on amino acid destruction and will rank both fortified and unfortified proteins in relation to other proteins. Values for the potential efficiency of utilization of a protein obtained with one standard procedure can be compared directly with those obtained with another and such comparisons yield highly significant correlation coefficients. Block and Mitchell (1946–7) demonstrated this for comparisons between net protein value and protein efficiency ratio.

This degree of correlation, even if it is not as high as one might desire, would not be observed if standard tests of protein quality did not regularly rank proteins in the same order. A similar relationship would be expected between results obtained with animal tests and those obtained with well standardized microbiological methods. Nevertheless, observations that the correlation between values obtained with two different methods is far from perfect and that the average value for a single protein measured several times by the same method has a high coefficient of variation, provide ample evidence that there is room for improvement in methods of evaluating the potential efficiency of utilization of proteins.

Moreover, methods for evaluating proteins are slow and expensive and, although refinements of existing methods are needed to improve their reproducibility, the major need is for a rapid and inexpensive procedure that is reliable. Progress with this is slow. The microbiological methods have given promise but have proved much less simple than was anticipated when they were introduced. It therefore remains important to continue to explore and develop new methods.

B. Predicting Efficiency of Protein Utilization

The second objective of protein evaluation, to predict efficiency of utilization of proteins as sources of nitrogen and amino acids to meet human and animal requirements, is much more difficult to achieve. Besides depending upon the amino acid composition of the protein, its digestibility and the availability of individual amino acids, efficiency of utilization is influenced by: the amount of protein consumed, particularly over the range approaching the requirement; energy intake; inadequacies in other components of the diet; and the stage of growth or maturity of the individual consuming the protein.

Changes in efficiency of utilization of proteins with changing protein intake have been long recognized. Protein intake is carefully controlled in methods of protein evaluation that depend upon measurement of the group of experimental animals. The standard methods require that proteins be evaluated under conditions in which performance is limited by protein intake in order to ensure high efficiency of utilization. Under such conditions the values obtained should be characteristic of the protein and should represent the maximum potential efficiency. However, a requirement must be set at a level of intake that does not limit performance. Hence, it represents an intake at which efficiency of utilization of the nutrient is not maximum. And not only that, for concern is not with average requirements but with allowances which must take into consideration individual variability. The allowance ensures that the requirements of almost all members of a population are exceeded and thus ensures that efficiency of utilization is below maximum.

Several groups of workers have used nitrogen balance studies to show that egg and milk proteins are utilized with an efficiency of 0·65–0·70 by human subjects at intakes that meet requirements. Therefore it cannot be assumed that proteins for which n.p.u. is 0·90–1·0 will be used with such high efficiency for meeting protein needs. Plots of growth as a function of protein intake for experimental animals also show this phenomenon at the requirement level of intake, indicating that evaluation of a protein at this level of intake will give a lower value for efficiency than is obtained under the standard conditions. Platt, Miller, Bender and Payne in recognizing these problems proposed that, although n.p.u. measured under standard conditions is satisfactory for comparing the potential value of proteins, n.p.u. measured under the conditions that would be encountered in practical situations (n.p.u. operative as they called it) would be a more meaningful value (cf. Campbell, 1969).

This subject is the crux of the protein evaluation problem. Many methods are available for ranking proteins according to their potential nutritive value. These methods will also detect improvements brought about by amino acid supplementation or through protein complementation; they will detect effects of processing and deterioration of protein quality but they will not provide a means of predicting quantitatively the efficiency of utilization of a protein for meeting requirements. Yet this is an equally important objective of protein evaluation.

This is relevant to the usefulness of chemical and microbiological methods. No doubt they can be developed and improved and can serve to rank proteins. Can they be standardized to provide a reliable assessment of the amount of protein needed to meet human requirements? If proteins can be ranked and differences in potential nutritive value can be measured by chemical and microbial assays, they can be standardized against measurements of n.p.u. in animals. But this is not enough; these methods provide comparisons of the efficiency of utilization of proteins under conditions in which protein is limiting. They must, in turn, be standardized against assays with human subjects that measure efficiency of utilization at levels of intake that meet requirements.

A major problem to be solved then is whether efficiency of utilization of proteins at levels of intake in the range of adequacy can be predicted from measurements made at low levels of intake. This problem has received little attention. A procedure for accomplishing this was proposed by Platt, Miller and Payne, the validity of which has been questioned by Morrison, Campbell and associates and Hegsted and associates. It is, however, appropriate to focus on this neglected aspect of protein evaluation, especially as it has long been known that high-quality proteins are not used with maximum efficiency for maintenance of adult man and that efficiency of protein utilization falls as intake approaches requirement level.

REFERENCES

Block, R. J. and Mitchell, H. H. (1946–7). *Nutr. Abstr. Rev.* **16**, 249–278.

McLaughlan, J. M. and Campbell, J. A. (1969). *In* "Mammalian Protein Metabolism" (H. N. Munro, ed.) Vol. 3, p. 411. Academic Press, New York.

II. BIOLOGICAL METHODS

Perhaps it would be most useful to direct our attention to the questions of the applicability to man of results with animal assays. Firstly, what method will best predict the value of protein in individual foods for human use? Secondly, does the evaluation of protein in individual foods have any meaning or use? There is, of course, no question that the value of a protein will vary according to the diet in which it is used. Furthermore, we must make a clear distinction between the assessment of diets as a whole and of foods individually. It does not follow, however, that the protein value of individual foods can be disregarded. There are at least two areas where such estimates are important i.e., in food processing and development, and in the framing of food regulations.

Human uses for protein include foods for the diets of infants, protein-deficient infants, growing children, adults, and the aged. Such foods are needed to satisfy requirements for growth, maintenance and other functions. I believe that a method that would predict the value of proteins for young children would be the most generally useful. This is probably the main need both in developed countries and in developing countries. The application of such a criterion might result in the production of foods of higher value than necessary for adults but the differences would not be serious. Supplements for severely protein-deficient infants must, of course, be looked at from a different point of view.

To focus our attention on the problem we might try to answer three questions: is there need for a bioassay; what is the most suitable method for routine evaluation of individual foods; and what level of protein should be used in such assays? Although we shall not obtain answers to the last two questions, they should form a framework in which to examine the results that have been presented.

A. Is There a Need for a Bioassay?

It has been suggested that if we had reliable amino acid data available we should not need the relatively crude bioassay with rats. On the other hand, I doubt that so many of us would be working with the rather tedious and costly methods we have, unless we were convinced that such were necessary. It was also evident that reliable amino acid data are not available in many cases, and there is a real need for bioassay results to establish the meaning and status of other simpler methods, such as microbiological assays and dye-binding methods. Furthermore, much more needs to be known about amino acid availability, interrelationships and requirements. Thus, there is no substitute for a reliable biological assay.

I cannot see a new protein source being accepted as a food constituent without very careful testing in a standardized rat assay.

B. What is the Most Suitable Method for Evaluating Individual Foods?

It is indicated in Chapter 15 that the determination of net protein utilization is a practical measure of protein quality. It includes both biological value and digestibility. It gives essentially the same results as the net protein ratio (NPR) determination which we prefer because it is simpler and the results seem more reproducible. It has been pointed out that there may be differences in body composition relating to the diet used and these differences may influence the results of n.p.u. (calculated from body water) or NPR determinations to a certain extent. Although such differences were not significant and therefore would not be expected to influence n.p.u. values, the possibility of their affecting NPR and PER assays cannot entirely be dismissed.

We in the Health Protection Branch have used the PER method for regulatory and other purposes for about 16 years. It has the advantage of simplicity but may be criticized from several points of view. Consideration is presently being given to the possibility of using another method, probably the NPR procedure, which is theoretically sounder than the PER determination. All methods appear to rank proteins in the same general order and it is our feeling that preference should be given to the simpler procedures. To overcome some of the problems in the PER assay, the use of the slope-ratio method, which requires the testing of protein at several levels and furnishes an estimate of the precision and validity of each assay, has been proposed (Chapter 18). It may be questioned, however, whether it is appropriate to assay a protein at both maintenance and growth levels and combine the results.

C. What Level of Protein Should be Used in Protein Evaluation Work?

It has been pointed out by several workers that the level of protein influences the results obtained by various methods. The model described in Chapter 16 would give constant results for biological value at all suboptimal protein levels. Whether or not it can deal with the problem encountered with foods limiting in lysine remains to be demonstrated.

Yáñez and McLaughlan (1970) demonstrated this effect in another way (Fig. 1). The relative value of two diets, one of which was limiting in lysine, was quite different when tested at maintenance and at growth levels. Undoubtedly this represented the ability of the food limiting in lysine to meet the varying requirements of the animal for these purposes. It is clear, however, that at maintenance the quality of the lysine-deficient protein is overestimated relative to that of the other protein. At the higher level, the protein limiting in lysine has a much lower relative value. This effect can be observed regardless of the method used.

The question then arises: what is the most appropriate level of protein for estimating protein value of foods for growing children or, more specifically, what requirements relate best to the growth requirements of a child? This question needs answering for whatever procedure is being used to assess protein value.

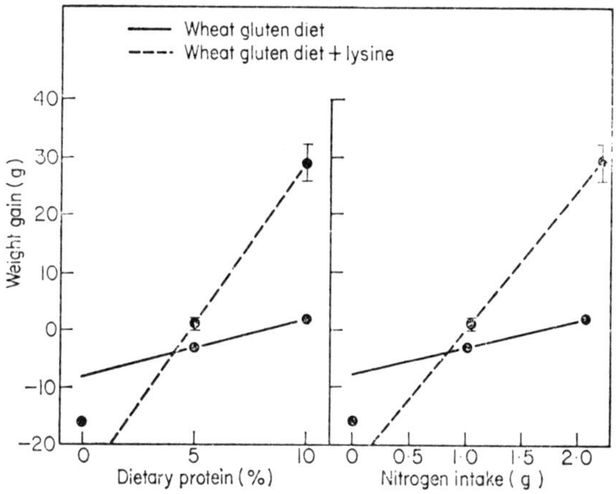

Fig. 1. Growth response curves of rats given wheat gluten and wheat gluten + lysine (Yáñez and McLaughlan, 1970)

After a review of the pertinent literature Campbell and McLaughlan (1970) concluded that the "relative lysine requirements for growth in the rat constitute a closer approximation of man's needs than do maintenance requirements of the rat. Although at this time the human requirement is not sufficiently well defined to establish the most appropriate protein level for rat assays, nevertheless, assays using the growing animal at the 8–10% protein level appear to give an accurate estimate of protein value for man". They also pointed out that "determinations at or below maintenance levels by the classical biological value method or by net protein utilization may give erroneously high estimates".

D. Conclusions

Finally, where should emphasis be placed in the future?

1. There is some difference of opinion as to the extent and magnitude of the protein problem. It has been suggested that it needs closer definition in terms of its extent, the need for protein foods and the actual use to which they will be put.

2. There is also controversy about the importance of the protein quality of individual foods. This aspect should be carefully considered for the benefit of those involved with plant breeding programmes and with the maintenance of quality in processed foods.

3. It is also evident that there is a real need for more quantitative results with human subjects to assess the value of foods and diets. Such information is necessary to standardize rat assay procedures so that they will produce results which are more directly applicable to the target animal, man. Particular attention should be paid to tests such as the analysis of body fluids that may be applied directly to man.

REFERENCES

CAMPBELL, J. A. and McLAUGHLAN, J. M. (1970). Symposium on Biological Evaluation of the Nutritive Value of Foods. *Int. Congr. Fd Sci. Technol. 3*, Washington, D. C.

YÁÑEZ, E. and McLAUGHLAN, J. M. (1970). *Can. J. Physiol. Pharmac.* **48**, 188–192.

III. CURRENT STATUS AND PROBLEMS IN ESTIMATING PROTEIN QUALITY AND PROTEIN REQUIREMENTS

A. Protein Quality

It is generally agreed that there is a real need for adequate measures of protein quality so that diets, foods, or protein sources which vary in protein quality as well as quantity can be compared. We need a measure of some factor, f, such that the amount of protein $\times$ f $=$ protein available to the animal.

It would seem self-evident that such a factor should vary from 0 to 1·0 and be *proportional* to the true quality. PER does not do this and is thus an unsatisfactory measure of protein quality. The fact that PER may show a high correlation with other measures of protein quality does not obviate this difficulty.

It would also seem that any diet which is completely lacking in an essential amino acid ought to yield a value of zero unless we propose that essential amino acids can be synthesized under some conditions. None of the methods which are generally assumed to be reasonably adequate, such as n.p.u., b.v. or NPR fulfils this condition. Net protein utilization standardized, the n.p.u. measured at approximately the maintenance level or below, is a very inaccurate measure of protein quality. Since the variance within a group of animals is largely relative to the difference in body protein content of the group given no protein and the group given the test diet, this inaccuracy is inevitable. For example, we find the n.p.u. of lactalbumin when given at these levels varies from 1·20 to 0·90.

The n.p.u. must obviously fall whenever the level of protein given is sufficient to allow the animal to achieve maximum or near maximum gain. Thus, to interpret such results one must make some correction such as that used in calculating n.d.-p : e. However, at these levels the calculated n.d.-p : e is *primarily* dependent upon the corrections applied rather than the performance of the animals. Hence, this is an unsatisfactory procedure for estimating protein quality.

These two problems are, in part, inherent in any type of biochemical or chemical assay, and application of correction factors is of little help when the basic results are unsatisfactory at very low or very high doses.

Another objection to the procedure for correcting the n.p.u. operative to n.d.-p : e is that it is based upon assumptions about the fall in n.p.u. with increasing levels of protein in the diet. This is a relatively ill-defined curve and depends primarily upon the performance observed at very high protein concentrations. These are of doubtful significance at crucial levels of protein intake.

Admittedly, one cannot determine whether a dose–response line is straight or has curvature. However, one can determine whether there is a statistically significant degree of curvature. All our results indicate that between maintenance intakes and those which allow near maximum growth, the intake–response line is *not* significantly curved. This part of the intake–response curve can be defined with reasonable accuracy as opposed to the % dietary protein–response curve.

A major difficulty in all of the work to date is the fact that with poor-quality proteins, particularly—but not exclusively—those low in lysine such as cereal proteins, all measures of protein quality appear to over-estimate the true protein quality.

The response in body protein is *not linear* with intake at *low levels* of intake. This appears to be due to the fact that certain amino acids are conserved when in short supply, especially lysine.

It is not possible to determine whether line A in Fig. 1 does in fact intersect the y axis at the expected point but it must come close. The linear portion of line B obviously does not. Thus, the n.p.u. of protein B falls substantially as the dose rises.

It should be emphasized that the "curvature" in line B at low intakes is a serious problem and that this "curvature" is not the kind that Miller and Payne assume. We believe that the slope of the line between points X_1 and

X_2 is the best measure of quality for *growth* of proteins since this is the increment in body protein per unit protein eaten.

The discrepancy at the low end of the curve should be of particular concern since protein quality is of primary importance with diets containing low-quality proteins. If n.p.u. measurements overestimate the true protein quality, this may be serious indeed.

For example, the n.p.u. of wheat gluten and of the protein of white flour is commonly stated to be about 0·40. We never find it to be this high. If the true quality of such proteins is indeed substantially lower, the estimates of the requirements with cereal diets would be raised markedly.

The true test of the adequacy of the assay methods ought to involve an assessment of the quality of the proteins being compared, the calculation of their equivalence, and then a retest giving them at presumably equal levels of available protein. None of the groups appears to have made

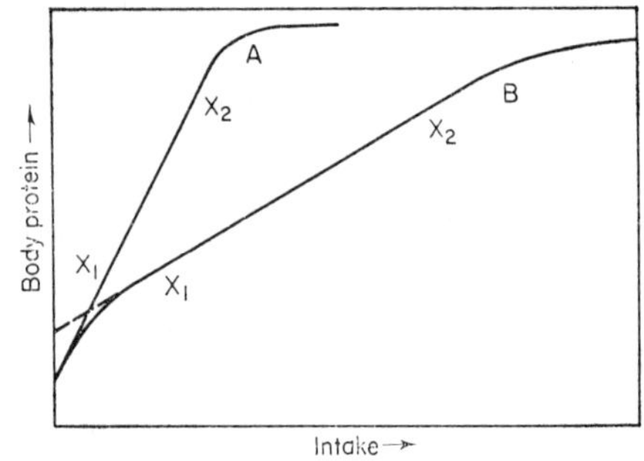

FIG. 1. The approximate shape of the dose–response curves for A, "good" and B, "poor" quality proteins

serious efforts to check their estimates in this way. However, when Hegsted and Chang (1965) tried to compare their estimates of the quality of lactalbumin, casein, soya-bean and gluten, the estimated relative value of gluten had to be reduced to only 0·14 that of lactalbumin in order to make the results "fit".

The slope–ratio method of Finney states that all dose–response lines have to have a common intercept. We have repeatedly pointed out that in our assays there were significant deviations from "blanks" and "intercepts" which we did not understand. We feel that the studies on response to various amino acids at low levels of intake (Said and Hegsted, 1970) make it clear what the problem is. Forcing all dose–response lines through a common intercept increases the slope somewhat for proteins like the one shown above as B and results in some overestimates of the quality of the protein. This will, however, be less of an overestimate than a simple measure of n.p.u. standardized.

B. Amino Acid and Protein Requirements

The fact that it takes a much longer time to produce a deficiency of lysine than of threonine, for example, does not indicate that lysine is any less "essential." It does, however, provide a warning that comparing proteins during a standardized test period, as is the practice in all measurements of protein quality, may lead to a considerable distortion of their true nutritional quality, tending to overestimate the quality.

Much of the available data can be interpreted to mean that the nutritional quality of proteins is different for maintenance and growth. Fortunately, it would appear that lysine and the sulphur amino acids are more critical for growth than for maintenance. This gives us some confidence that we shall not underestimate the nutritional quality for man in tests that are adequate to evaluate the quality for growth in young rats. However, we emphasize that since man is a slow-growing animal, the estimates of quality for maintenance are presumably most important and it is in this area that the rat tests are least adequate.

The estimates of the "maintenance requirement" by the use of n.p.u. or the slope–ratio assay with young rats have never been shown to be actually adequate for maintenance of animals in the long run. Such results as we have suggest that they are not. Adult rats given levels of lactalbumin that just allow maintenance of weight (nitrogen balance?) apparently develop fatty livers and certainly do not appear to be as "healthy" as those given higher levels. The maintenance of nitrogen balance or of body weight at low levels of intake does not tell us what is going on inside the animals. It is quite possible that modest changes in the protein content of a few organs, not detectable by these gross measures, may have long-term nutritional effects.

It is apparent that there is *similarity* in the amino acid pattern of requirements for various species as well as *similarity* in the nutritional value of proteins for various species with the methods now available. However, this does not mean that they are the *same*. Current work with baby monkeys (Hegsted, unpublished results) indicates that the maximum utilization of lactalbumin which is obtained when this protein is given at levels which limit the rate of growth is of the order of 0·70. Similar estimates for wheat gluten are about 0·15.

Furthermore, we also find that 0·10 of the energy supplied as protein from white bread (the diet being adequate in vitamins, minerals, etc.) is inadequate for the maintenance of adult monkeys although it takes months for such animals to become obviously depleted.

We cannot afford to be too confident of the applicability to man of results with rats.

Once we know how to measure protein quality, it will probably be desirable to express this as a proportion of the total energy in the diet. However, n.d.-p : e is *that number which is obtained by treating the results according to the ideas of Miller and Payne*. (See Chapter 6.) Since I believe that it is clear that several of their assumptions are seriously in error or only gross approximations, I believe that this nomenclature should not be used.

The available data on the protein requirements of man, the low protein content of breast milk, and so on, indicate that man is adapted to survive on relatively low-protein diets. However, since we are uncertain what the true nutritional quality of various diets is for children or adults, it is unjustifiable to conclude that cereal diets are adequate.

When we attempted to maintain dogs on diets which contained minimal levels of protein, we were unsuccessful in the long run.

Thus, when the diet is near requirement level the animals are unable to recover from their occasional failures to eat and even though they eat a full intake most of the time they gradually become depleted.

The same thing probably happens with children in ordinary circumstances. Thus, even though children in a controlled study situation might be shown to grow normally upon diets which are relatively low in protein quality and in protein content, this does not mean that they might not be better able to cope with the stresses of ordinary life if they had a somewhat better protein intake.

I agree that the "protein problem" has been overemphasized relative to the energy problem and have been making this point for about 15 years (cf. Hegsted, 1959). However, in spite of what we think happens, we do not know very much about what determines the protein and energy intakes of the children with whom we are concerned. If our estimates of the protein quality are wrong, it is possible that the low intakes may be due, in part, to the borderline protein intakes.

We do need to find some way to get food into the children. The easiest way might be with sugar or fat, if these were available, but this would in all likelihood really produce a diet too low in protein. The simple semantic problem of how this is stated is important. If energy can somehow be added, it should carry its share of protein (and might as well carry some excess).

We do not know enough to state that when energy is limiting the protein serves *only* as an energy supply. The inadequacies of short-term studies with either animals or man should be apparent. In studies with young rats the protein and energy needs change markedly within a few days—animals adapt to one or the other deficiency—and it is nearly impossible to devise an adequate long-term experiment. In human subjects temporary energy restriction shifts the energy metabolized from exogenous to endogenous sources but may not limit total energy metabolized. The relevance of short-term studies is open to debate.

Considering how little is actually known about protein–energy interrelationships, it is essential that we do not oversimplify. Miller (Chapter 6) goes too far in suggesting that protein quality makes no difference and that energy is the limiting factor in most situations.

The underestimation of protein needs is a more serious error than the overestimation. We should bear in mind that even adults want higher protein intakes than cereals supply or than our guess as to their needs. They may feel and perform better on such diets. We should not be anxious to discard all of the "conventional wisdom" of people everywhere. The major job is to get energy and protein into perspective without going overboard in either direction.

REFERENCES

HEGSTED, D. M. (1959). *Fedn Proc. Fedn Am. Socs exp. Biol.* **18**, 1130–1136.
HEGSTED, D. M. and CHANG, Y.-O. (1965). *J. Nutr.* **87**, 19–25.
SAID, A. K. and HEGSTED, D. M. (1970). *J. Nutr.* **100**, 1363–1375.

IV. GENERAL DISCUSSION

A. The Aims of Protein Quality Measurement

Dr G. D. Rosen considered that, on its own, the term "protein quality" was relatively meaningless. There was a need both for a better definition and one which related more closely to practical application. Moreover, one needed to know how to combine the figures and apply techniques to mixed feeds and complete dishes. He thought that what was missing from the literature was advice on how much more must be fed of a low-lysine batch of feed and how much less need be fed of a high-lysine batch. This was the sort of advice that a farmer or feed manufacturer needed. He also wished that more attention were paid to cereal proteins and the provision of proteins for ruminants.

Dr I. F. Duthie (Lord Rank Research Centre, High Wycombe) thought that the final use of the figures should be considered: were they for academic interest or to assess the requirements of human and animal populations and to attempt to fill them? There was also the question of quality control and the assessment of new protein sources. He thought that terminology should be agreed, especially when dealing with new protein sources such as single cell proteins. Protein was not necessarily the same as N $\times$ 6·25 and the availability of amino sugars, nucleic acids, etc. should be taken into account.

Dr P. L. Pellett asked if this presented a real problem; if nucleic acids had to be removed because they produced gout, measurements on the protein source should be made after their removal. Dr Duthie replied that development programmes had to be run well before nucleic acid removal was a practical possibility. Perhaps the value obtained should be called "nitrogen retention" rather than n.p.u.

Dr H. S. Bayley (University of Guelph, Ontario, Canada) said that amino acids were still required, and proteins differed in their capacity to provide these for human or animal use. Perhaps n.p.u. was an inadequate tool, and a better one should be found. Dr Hegsted added that everyone would be pleased by the advent of an improved method.

Dr D. S. Miller asked whether the aim was an academic desire to match chemical score and the measured n.p.u., or to evaluate the diets eaten by man in the field and to attempt to match them to human requirements. Professor A. E. Bender observed that the correlations made between two (or more) different methods of assay were often made with a group of proteins limited by the same amino acid, and the comparison was less independent than might at first appear.

B. The Difficulties of Protein Quality Measurement

Dr D. M. Hegsted thought that a major problem arose with low-quality proteins, and in particular with those deficient in lysine. The projection of response–intake plots for lysine-deficient proteins does not go through the origin, a result which is unaffected by the prevention of coprophagy. He thought that the curvature observed by Mr Dreyer and Professor Bender might be an important factor, although he disagreed with Mr Dreyer's assumption that different tissue stores were being filled. He suggested that obtaining an n.p.u. of 0·40 with a lysine-free diet implied that the body can conserve some amino acids but not others. Those whose absence produced the same effect as the giving of a non-protein diet were isoleucine, total sulphur amino acids and valine.

Dr D. S. Miller insisted that the value of the protein was n.p.u. standardized. Dr Hegsted, however, objected that a determination at a low protein level would give an equally false value, especially for poor proteins. He thought we really needed a complete response curve, as in a colorimeter standardization, and not a single determination at whatever level. Dr Miller thought that provided proteins could be distinguished, this was all that was necessary.

Dr K. J. Carpenter asked whether measurements carried out at high protein intakes were not tests of the adequacy of the diet rather than of protein quality. Dr Hegsted's criticism was that at such high protein levels all proteins were the same.

Dr P. L. Pellett objected that once a diet was diluted with starch it was not the same diet, so the estimate was not of the diet. However, as Dr Hegsted pointed out, the rat assay would remain valid. Dr Nicol thought that the experiment advocated by Dr Miller was to determine the adequacy of the diet. Professor Bender said that two separate questions were involved. Dr Miller was interested in the adequacy of the diet whereas Dr Hegsted's interest was in the quality of the protein utilized.

Dr J. A. Campbell said that it was to be regretted that so often n.p.u. values were quoted without any reference to the protein level and to whether the assay was standardized.

Dr J. Mauron suggested that, since Dr Miller wished to test the protein in the diet as it was eaten, then even if a vitamin deficiency reduced its utilization, this remained a result in this context, since a valid judgement had been made on the diet as a whole.

Professor A. E. Bender said that if energy supply did in fact control protein utilization, n.p.u. operative would be of no practical relevance, since enough food would solve any problem which existed. Dr Pellett said that his experience in the Middle East had shown that children could be malnourished even if there were adequate food within the household, since socio-economic factors were superimposed.

Professor H. Fisher said that some recent Indian work had shown that children eating wheat did not benefit from added lysine. Did this show that the child's requirement for lysine was low?

Professor A. E. Bender thought that children did benefit from added lysine and said that other work could be quoted to support this view. He considered that the use of low-protein diets tested the adaptability of the animal, rather than the protein: after Mr Dreyer's long adaptation period, for instance, the rats would no longer be the same animals. If the diet of rats in nitrogen balance were further restricted, then they would lose weight, but would establish a new balance at a lower body weight and a lower energy intake.

Mr P. R. Payne said that diets in excess of a child's requirement for growth would have a low n.p.u.; there was a need for work to be carried out under comparable physiological conditions. Many experiments which showed a response to lysine involved diets that were below requirement. Diets should be tested as they were eaten, not at artificially low levels.

Dr P. L. Pellett said that diet sheet calculations in the Middle East showed energy intakes of 7500–8400 kJ/day, levels at which no protein could be utilized efficiently.

Dr S. Buraczewski (Institute of Animal Nutrition and Physiology, Jabłonna, Poland) reported that in experiments at his Institute designed to evaluate proteins of low nutritive value it was found that the biological value (or n.p.u.$_{op}$) increased markedly during the 18 days of the experiment for such materials as yeast, horse bean, rye, alfalfa and dehydrated meals, although the digestibility did not vary. However, the values for casein, soya-bean meal and linseed meal, for example, remained constant. The level of nitrogen excretion in the protein-free group was found to depend on the preliminary feeding period, being markedly lower after 12 days. There was an additional factor, in that methionine added to the protein-free diet lowered nitrogen excretion immediately, regardless of the protein level in the preliminary diet.

Dr D. M. Hegsted had also observed that the addition of methionine reduced the urinary nitrogen of dogs in protein balance at maintenance levels of protein intake.

Mr J. J. Dreyer asked whether the water/nitrogen figures presented by Dr Hegsted would have differed if there had been a preliminary adaptation period of, say, 12 days on all diets. Dr D. M. Hegsted replied that all animals were given a preliminary lactalbumin diet and then put on the amino acid diets for 4–6 weeks. He did not know whether another preliminary period would have been an improvement, particularly in view of the long feeding period. It would not have affected the results with lysine and threonine, where the animals lost weight.

C. The Meaning of Protein Quality Measurements

Dr P. L. Pellett considered that these criticisms of the n.p.u. procedure were certainly valid when low levels of poor-quality protein were investigated, but he asked whether this was important in the contexts of real diets, where n.p.u.'s of 0·20, 0·30 and 0·40 never arose.

Professor A. E. Bender said that even in parts of Indonesia, where the protein–energy ratio was only 0·072, the n.p.u. never fell below 0·50. Dr D. M. Hegsted, however, said that diets were commonly limiting in either lysine or methionine, and such diets gave falsely high n.p.u.'s. Professor A. E. Bender replied that the correlation above n.p.u. 0·40 was in fact reasonably good, and all the diets under discussion were at least n.p.u. 0·50.

Dr D. M. Hegsted claimed to detect an inconsistency in Professor Bender's argument that biological methods for determination of nutritive value were inadequate—a point on which he agreed with him—and yet Bender accepted such data when discussing the difference between the poorest (n.p.u. 0·60) and best (n.p.u. 0·70) human diets. An n.p.u. of 0·40 for a lysine-free diet was certainly an overestimate. Why, in that case, should measured n.p.u.'s of *ca.* 0·50 measured on total diets not also be artificially high? A protein with no lysine had an n.p.u. of 0·40, yet animals given the diet died from lysine deficiency.

Dr M. Rakowska (Institute of Food and Nutrition, Warsaw, Poland) said that in her measurements of n.p.u. in children and in rats, it was found that n.p.u. measured in preschool children was about 40% lower than that determined by rat assay, e.g. 0·36–0·38 compared to 0·60–0·68.

Professor A. E. Bender drew attention to the differences between growth and maintenance. A protein devoid of lysine might have an n.p.u. of 0·40 but its PER would be zero, since there would be no growth. He would still stress the use of chemical score which was measured under standard conditions, rather than feeding tests carried out under widely differing conditions.

Dr B. M. Nicol thought that the figure for n.p.u. of 0·60 quoted for the poorest diets was, from the data published, too high. He agreed with Professor Bender's suggestion that too much emphasis was being placed on the careful definition of the biological value of proteins since this was not a very important factor, at maintenance levels, in determining protein utilization. He wished to stress the importance of the protein digestibility of human diets as it affects n.p.u. He and Phillips had found the following correlations between d., b.v. and n.p.u. (true) in adult Nigerian males given diets of traditional patterns based on sorghum or rice with cassava and beans, a little fish, vegetables and condiments at maintenance (N equilibrium) levels and energy intakes of 190 kJ/kg body weight: b.n./n.p.u., $r = 0{\cdot}60$; d./n.p.u., $r = 0{\cdot}86$. Home-pounded and winnowed sorghum had a higher true digestibility than did machine-milled sorghum. The inference for food processing and preparation was obvious.

Professor A. E. Bender said that d. was already implicit in n.p.u. figures. He added that the figures of 0·60 and 0·70 for the n.p.u. of diets were taken from FAO reports.

Dr B. M. Nicol said that the FAO report referred to by several speakers divided human diets into three groups: less than 0·60, 0·60–0·70, and over 0·70. There were some, although not many, below 0·50. These figures were based on direct measurements on human diets as eaten.

Dr R. G. Whitehead, referring to the comment that accurate determinations of nutritive quality were irrelevant because of the narrow range of total dietary n.p.u.s (0·60–0·70), thought that one would never know whether this was right until direct measurements had been made in man. In the case of animals, objectives were generally defined in terms of the cheapest way to produce eggs, or an acceptable carcass for meat, and this was very useful. For children the situation was vastly different. It was difficult to find any people with a diet inadequate in protein. What was needed was not more sophisticated assays but direct investigations in man, to determine the efficiency of human foods under the various physiological conditions which might apply.

Man must be the primary standard, and man varied considerably from farm and laboratory animals (as well as between individuals), particularly in such factors as the rate of growth and the proportion of protein used for growth and maintenance. Rat work was mainly applicable to the rate of growth. Man's requirements should be studied at different ages and under different environmental conditions. There was also a need to study the energy intake very closely, since without sufficient energy, the highest-quality protein would not prevent negative nitrogen balance. It should not be forgotten that n.d.–p : e varied with the activity of the individual. When judging diets intended for human beings, one should consider not only growth and maintenance but also function. For example, even the establishment of a positive nitrogen balance does not necessarily lead to rapid restoration of serum albumin. Thus functional tests are also needed.

Dr H. S. Bayley feared that in a reaction against the clinical viewpoint, there was a danger of giving the impression that the value of protein in the diet was underestimated.

Dr D. M. Hegsted thought that for nutritionists to underestimate this problem was worse than for them to overestimate it. The "protein problem" should not be written off as non-existent.

Dr B. M. Nicol said that protein production, considered at the world level, was sufficient for all, but since a proportion of this was used for animal feeds, fertilizers and so on, it was still true that there was a protein food problem.

D. Miscellaneous

1. *Claims for Commercial Products*

Mr J. J. Dreyer said that another problem was the evaluation of commercial products, and whether one could remain confident that the provision of additional protein was of value.

Dr P. L. Pellett said that in any case an n.p.u. figure measured in isolation gave no indication of its supplementary value.

Professor A. E. Bender thought that the question was whether the extra protein was of value to those people who needed it; if it was not, no claims should be made.

Dr J. A. Campbell thought that one of the questions was whether or not authority was available to forbid any specious claims about the protein value of foods.

Professor A. E. Bender said that since the [UK] Government refused to permit any specific advantages to be claimed for polyunsaturated fats, the same could be applied to protein.

2. *Dye-binding*

Dr T. C. A. McGann (The Agricultural Institute, Moorepark, Republic of Ireland) stressed the point that—apart from its theoretical interest—dye-binding techniques offered a rapid, precise and simple method for the analysis of milk products in process and production control.

Mr A. L. Lakin said that all one could expect from dye-binding was a measure of the total content of basic amino acids. A higher result could indicate more protein, more basic amino acids, or both. The advantages of the method were certainly known, and it was of great potential, but its development depended on a knowledge of what was being measured. For example, was the dye-binding loss found after heating milk due to a loss of lysine?

Dr K. J. Carpenter pointed out that measurements using dye-binding were affected by the total free amino acid content, thus the high value obtained with fish reflected largely the occurrence of autolysis (or gut contents) which had neutral biological effect.

Mr A. L. Lakin thought that this might explain why there was no lowering of the dye-binding value when milk was evaporated, although it was known that there was a loss of lysine availability.

3. *Free Amino Acid and Urea Studies*

Referring to Dr B. O. Eggum's statement that the measurement of blood amino acids gave no advantages over urea determinations, Dr H. Erbersdobler said that in the case of amino acid availability one could use amino acid digestibility in germ-free animals, ileal analysis or blood amino acid levels. It was possible to measure protein quality and to determine which amino acids were limiting by his own techniques of determining portal blood amino acids in high-protein adapted rats. Dr Eggum agreed that amino acid requirements and availabilities were usefully measured by blood amino acid techniques.

Dr O. P. Walz said that portal blood amino acids responded directly to the diet in the case of lysine but, as Dr R. Pion had remarked, methionine was entirely different. Each amino acid had to be tested. When zein was given to pigs there was no direct response of arterial blood to the diet. He thought that the urea method was less useful if the foodstuffs under test were of similar composition (e.g. cereals) and in any case needed to be confirmed by animal feeding trials.

Dr B. O. Eggum agreed with these comments on the amino acids and added that he was starting to test methods comparatively with rats and pigs. He conceded that the urea method might be insufficiently sensitive.

Dr O. P. Walz (Institute of Animal Nutrition, Giessen, GFR) added that wheat, oats and barley could not be distinguished by the urea method, but this was possible using rat bioassay.

Dr R. Pion said that measurement of the free amino acids in portal blood may be a good way of estimating the influx of amino acids from the gut. However, portal blood is formed by a mixture of gut amino acids and of arterial blood, which may differ from peripheral blood.

Mr M. A. Esnaola Lewis (NIRD) said that his work on methionine utilization in pigs had shown that measured plasma urea correlated very well with nitrogen retention. There was considerable work on plasma amino acids and he wondered what role the blood cell played in amino acid transport.

4. *Utilization of Methionine Sulphoxide*

To a suggestion that methionine sulphoxide might be utilized by rats in the presence of dietary cystine, Dr J. Mauron said that we should differentiate between free methionine sulphoxide, which could be used in some circumstances, and protein-bound material, which was not used.

Dr H. Erbersdobler said that from his own experiments with severely heated casein there was some evidence that methionine sulphoxide was used even in the bound form.

CHAPTER 24

New Uses for Fish Proteins

BO HALLGREN, LARS-BÖRJE SJÖBERG AND JAN STELLEMAN
Astra Research Laboratories, Fack, Sweden

The world catch of fish in 1970 was 69 million metric tons. There has been a great increase in world fishing which has more than tripled in volume from 20 million metric tons in 1948. More than 50 million tons of the catch is fish from the oceans and about half of this is not used for direct human consumption but is processed to fish meal. It is the oily pelagic species that can be caught most cheaply and in the greatest quantities. This favours their use for fish meal manufacture.

I. FISH PROTEIN FOR ANIMAL FEED

Fish meal has for a long time been used as a high-quality animal protein in various animal feeds. However, soya-bean meal and synthetic products such as lysine and methionine are increasingly applied in compounding animal feeds. It is therefore desirable to be able to use fish protein, which is a highly nutritious animal protein, as a replacer for other animal proteins, especially milk protein. The animal proteins are most needed in the feeding of young animals. As milk is an expensive ingredient in animal feeds cheaper substitutes have been sought, such as skim milk instead of whole milk. It was early found that skim milk and whole milk in equal parts gave acceptable growth in calves. About 25 years ago cheap non-milk fats began to be added to skim milk. This was the first step to a whole milk replacer. But it is, of course, of even greater interest to find substitutes for the milk proteins. It has been found that casein can be replaced by defatted fish meal in calf-milk replacers and that fish protein together with whey, which has been considered a waste product from the dairy industry, can form the basis of a new calf-milk replacer. This composition can also be justified from an economic standpoint, as the prices for skim milk protein, fish protein and casein are as follows:

	U.S. dollars/kg	U.S. dollars/kg protein
Skim milk	0·66	1·9
Fish protein	0·47	0·6
Casein	1·46	1·8

The amino acid compositions of fish protein concentrate, casein and the whey proteins, lactoglobulin and lactalbumin, are given in Table I. The whey proteins have a high biological value and are characterized by a very high content of lysine- and sulphur-containing amino acids. The sulphur-containing amino acids are limiting in casein. Fish protein is higher in sulphur amino acids than casein but lower than the whey proteins. The PER values in rats are *ca.* 3·0 for fish protein, *ca.* 2·5 for casein and *ca.* 3·1 for whey proteins. The proportions in cow's milk proteins are 80% casein and 20% whey proteins. During the first week after calving the whey

TABLE I. Amino acid composition (g/16 g N) of FPC, casein and whey proteins

	FPC	*Casein*	*Whey proteins*	
			Lacto-globulin	*Lactal-bumin*
Aspartic acid	10·7	7·1	11·4	18·7
Threonine	5·1	4·9	5·0	5·5
Serine	5·0	6·3	4·0	4·8
Glutamic acid	14·7	22·4	19·3	12·9
Proline	4·5	10·6	5·1	1·5
Glycine	5·4	2·0	1·4	3·2
Alanine	6·5	3·2	7·0	2·1
Valine	6·1	7·2	6·1	4·7
Methionine	3·7	2·8	3·2	0·95
Isoleucine	5·5	6·1	6·9	6·8
Leucine	8·5	9·2	15·5	11·5
Tyrosine	3·9	6·3	3·7	5·4
Phenylalanine	4·7	5·0	3·5	4·5
Lysine	9·0	8·2	11·8	11·5
Histidine	2·5	3·1	1·6	2·9
Arginine	6·4	4·1	2·8	1·2
Tryptophan	1·5	1·7	2·7	7·0
Cystine + cysteine	1·2	0·34	3·4	6·4

proteins are higher due to their content of immunoglobulins. In a milk replacer for calves based on fish protein and whey, the percentage of fish protein should be the same as for casein in milk proteins. The amino acid composition of such a mixture of fish protein and whey is not very different from the amino acid pattern of milk protein (Table II).

A calf-milk replacer, "Kalv-Manna", containing fish protein ("Prot-Animal") and whey, has been tested in many experiments on calves and compared with milk-based formulae. In 1969, two trials with a total of 216 calves were carried out at the Agricultural College of Sweden (Danell, 1970). Kalv-Manna and the skim milk preparation "Nötex" were compared. Both contained about 25% crude protein and 20% crude fat. Within each milk replacer group, the calves were weaned after either 5 or 7 weeks. The milk replacer was given twice a day and the amount of milk nutrient was the same during the whole period, calculated on an energy basis. Kalv-Manna had a slightly higher energy content than Nötex, and to correct for this the amounts given at each feed were 215 g of Kalv-Manna and 220 g of Nötex. The mean age of the calves at the start of the trial was 4 weeks in the first trial and 3 weeks in the second trial. Their average weight was 47 kg. During the milk feeding period, the calves had

TABLE II. Amino acid composition (g/16 g N) of cow's milk proteins and the milk replacer Kalv-Manna, based on fish protein and whey

	Cow's milk	*Kalv-Manna*
Aspartic acid	7·5	9·5
Threonine	4·4	4·9
Serine	5·7	5·0
Glutamic acid	21·8	19·2
Proline	9·0	7·1
Glycine	1·9	3·5
Alanine	3·4	4·7
Valine	5·7	6·2
Methionine	2·5	3·2
Isoleucine	4·6	5·2
Leucine	9·4	9·2
Tyrosine	4·7	3·9
Phenylalanine	5·3	4·6
Lysine	7·7	8·5
Histidine	2·6	2·5
Arginine	3·2	4·5

free access to a calf starter (20% protein) and hay. The calves were slaughtered when weighing about 230 kg. Growth and feed consumption can be seen from Table III. The growth was very good in trial I but quite

TABLE III. Comparison between milk replacers containing skim milk or fish protein concentrate (after Danell, 1970)

Milk feeding period		*5 weeks*		*7 weeks*	
Source of protein		*Skim milk*	*Kalv-Manna*	*Skim milk*	*Kalv-Manna*
Number of calves included		54	54	54	54
Culled		3	3	2	2
Growth, g/day					
0/5 weeks	I	592	614	617	549
	II	480	417	434	414
5/7 weeks	I	829	950	736	858
	II	643	529	614	643
0/7 weeks	I	661	710	651	637
	II	527	449	488	482
From 7 weeks	I	1202	1243	1248	1220
to slaughter	II	1106	1125	1125	1131
Feed consumption 0/7 weeks, kg					
Calf starter	I	42·4	45·8	36·8	34·1
	II	36·6	32·8	30·2	30·1
Hay	I	9·4	9·3	9·5	6·9
	II	8·9	8·6	9·3	8·5
MJ[a]/kg growth up to slaughter	I	41·4	40·6	41·0	40·6
	II	43·5	44·8	43·5	44·4

[a] metabolizable energy

satisfactory also in trial II. Small differences were found between the different milk replacers. In trial I, the calves receiving fish protein grew somewhat more rapidly than the others during the first 7 weeks, whereas in trial II, the reverse was found. Over the whole period up to slaughter no significant differences could be found either in the rate of growth or in feed utilization per kg of growth. At slaughter, the fleshiness and colour of the carcasses were judged in accordance with the usual Swedish standards and no differences were found between the different groups.

The successful incorporation of fish protein into calf-milk replacers marketed in Scandinavia and Western Europe has opened a new field of application for fish protein. It is expected that fish protein will find its use in other feeds for new-born animals.

II. FISH PROTEIN FOR HUMAN FOOD

A hygienic, safe and nutritious fish protein concentrate should increase the availability of fish protein for human consumption. There have been many scientific publications dealing with the production, safety, nutrition and use of various forms of fish protein in recent years. An extensive review on fish protein for human foods has been published by Finch (1970). As the fish protein concentrates have been used mainly in cereal-based foods the following discussion will be devoted to this field.

A. Enrichment of Flour for Bread and Bakery Products

The nutritional value of cereal proteins is limited by a deficiency of one or more essential amino acids. In wheat, lysine is the first limiting amino acid. In fish protein there is a surplus of lysine (Fig. 1). By adding increas-

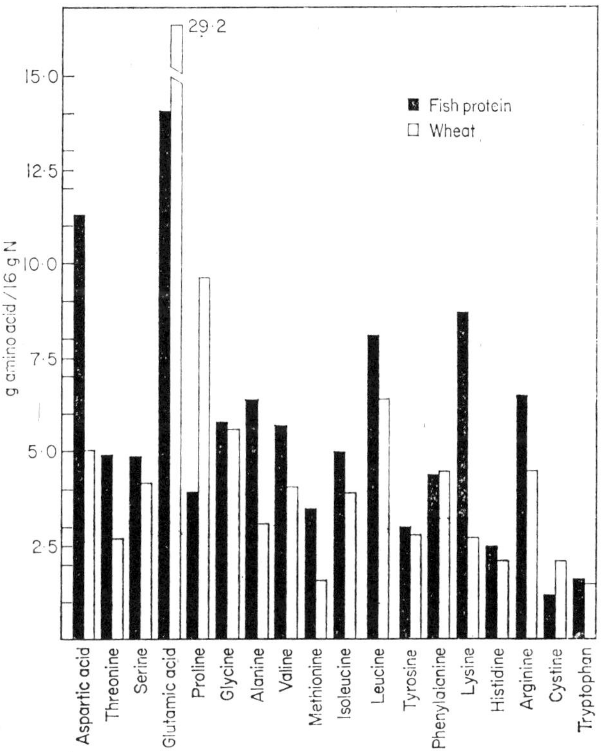

FIG. 1. The amino acid compositions of fish protein and wheat

ing amounts of fish protein to wheat flour its nutritional value is enhanced. Wheat flour contains about 10% protein. An enrichment with about 2% fish protein concentrate gives a protein mixture with a PER value of about 1·8. This PER value could also be achieved by adding 0·15% of lysine. When more fish protein is added to wheat flour the nutritional value of the protein mixture increases further but in this range it is an enrichment effect due to supplementation with other amino acids which are limiting in wheat protein, principally threonine (Fig. 2). Stillings *et al.* (1971) have studied the nutritional value of wheat flour and bread fortified with increasing percentages of fish protein from hake. Their results are

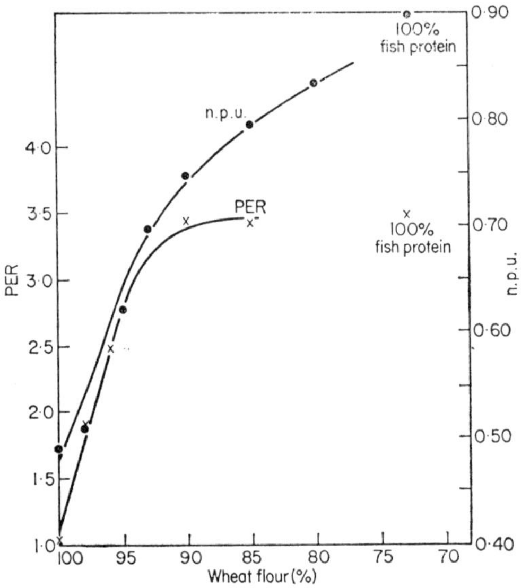

FIG. 2. The nutritional value of wheat flour enriched with fish protein (Herring EFP 90, 1753B)

similar to ours with fish protein from herring. Other studies also show the enriching effect of adding fish protein to wheat flour and bread (Ericson *et al.*, 1961; Jansen, 1969).

After adding 5% fish protein (corresponding to 6% FPC) from herring to wheat flour the protein mixture has a PER value of about 2·7. By this supplementation a flour is obtained which contains about 15% protein and has about the same biological value as casein. The supplementation of wheat flour with extracted soya-bean flour to the same protein level (corresponding to the addition of about 10% soya-bean flour) would increase the PER value to about 2·0, comparable with the supplementary effect of adding 2–3% fish protein concentrate.

Wheat flour enriched with 5–6% FPC has good baking properties and the fish protein does not affect the taste of the bread. The enriched flour can also be used in gruels and porridges and is thus a multipurpose food. It seems to us to be a very valuable product for distribution in developing countries, since the highly nutritious protein constitutes a needed supplement to the low-protein diet in these countries. A bread enriched with Astra fish protein was tested in a school in a village outside Teheran in 1970. The study was performed under the supervision of the Food and Nutrition Institute of Iran (Hedayat *et al.*, 1970). The bread was baked in the village and the acceptability, studied during 5 months, was very good.

The successful incorporation of fish protein into various cereal products such as bread, cookies and pasta has been reported in many studies (Autret and van Veen, 1955; Sidwell, 1967; Kwee *et al.*, 1969; Munro *et al.*, 1969; Yáñez *et al.*, 1969; Brinkman and Rose; 1970; Crisan, 1970; Moorjani and Lahiry, 1970; Woo and Erdman, 1971). Hofvander *et al.* (1972) have also studied its acceptability to school children in Uppsala, who were given a bun with or without Astra fish protein as a snack. The fish protein product was well accepted and it was very interesting to note that as many children preferred the somewhat greyish fish protein bun as preferred a white bun containing milk protein. Large-scale field tests with a premix of wheat flour and Astra's fish protein are under way in countries in South America, Africa and Asia under the supervision of the World Food Programme. Sidwell *et al.* (1971), have recently reported that a stable premix of wheat and fish protein can be made and transported.

A fish protein-enriched bread could also meet a need for nutritious food among people with bad dietary habits in the developed countries. A formula has been developed for a FPC-enriched bread intended for the Swedish market, and all the nutritional and food technology information required for a market introduction is available. Nabisco-Astra in the USA has developed many fish protein-enriched cereal products which are currently being evaluated.

B. Fish Protein in Weaning Foods and Baby Foods

Protein–energy malnutrition in developing countries is most prevalent in the age group ½–3 years. The Protein Advisory Group has laid down guide-lines for suitable weaning foods to be used in developing countries. The mixtures should contain approximately 20% protein having an n.p.u. value of at least 0·60. A weaning food consisting of maize, soya-bean and milk named CSM and meeting the PAG specifications has been developed in the USA and distributed through AID. Fish protein could be used with advantage in weaning foods in combination with different cereals. The weaning food "Faffa", developed at the Swedish Nutrition Institute in Addis Ababa normally contains 5% skim milk. In test trials the skim milk has been replaced by 5% fish protein with no adverse effect on acceptability. Two other weaning foods (Mx 52 and Mx 71) containing 5% fish protein have been tested and found acceptable in India and Ethiopia (WHO, 1970). In cases of lactose intolerance it could be an advantage that fish protein is free from lactose. There are, however, different opinions about the amounts of lactose that are tolerated by children with lactase deficiency.

The nutritional value and acceptability of the Astra fish protein have been studied by Hofvander (1972) in healthy Swedish children aged 4–6

TABLE IV. Composition of gruel powder

Ingredient	*Percentage*
Astra fish protein	16
Skim milk powder	8
Oat meal	24
Wheat flour	9·8
Sucrose	30·5
Cocoa oil	6·0
Soya-bean oil	4
Sodium chloride	1·2
Vitamins and minerals	0·5

100 g of powder give 1760 kJ
Proportion of energy from : protein 0·20
: carbohydrate 0·54
: fat 0·26
PER = 2·5 (Reference: casein, 2·5)
n.p.u. = 0·82

months given an infant food in which milk protein was replaced by FPC. The preparation was well accepted by all the children and there were no adverse intestinal reactions. The growth was fully comparable with that of a control group consuming a milk-based food. After these clinical studies a baby food was made up containing as much as 16% of fish protein concentrate (Tables IV and V). This baby food has been sold to the Swedish Red Cross for distribution to Bangladesh.

From studies in Chile, Yáñez *et al.* (1969) reported successful incorporation of fish protein into weaning food, as shown by the acceptability of the product and by their clinical findings. Similar results have been described from South Africa (Pretorius and Wehmeyer, 1964; Dreyer and Du Bruyn, 1968), from Peru (Graham *et al.*, 1965, 1966) and from Morocco

TABLE V. Amino acid analysis of gruel powder

	g/16 g N		*g/16 g N*
Aspartic acid	9·1	Isoleucine	4·5
Threonine	4·1	Leucine	8·3
Serine	4·4	Tyrosine	3·3
Glutamic acid	17·6	Phenylalanine	4·2
Proline	4·8	Lysine	7·4
Glycine	3·8	Histidine	2·4
Alanine	5·1	Arginine	5·4
Valine	5·5	Cystine	1·4
Methionine	2·8	Tryptophan	1·0

(Tavill and Gonik, 1969), although in the studies of Graham *et al.* (1965, 1966) low serum albumin levels were found in children suffering from kwashiorkor. However, the majority of clinical investigations have demonstrated the value of a good quality fish protein in treating malnourished children.

C. Fish Protein in Soups and Beverages

The Astra fish protein has been tested in a soup in Brazil and in a chocolate beverage distributed in Biafra. Available reports indicate that fish protein can be introduced even into these types of food. However, since FPC is insoluble in water some grittiness is often noted in drinks. Sidwell (1967) and Sidwell *et al.* (1970) have devised a formula for an FPC beverage similar to milk in its composition and without marked grittiness.

D. Future Market Developments of FPC

Protein supplements for human foods must be acceptable in the form and at the level used. They must contribute significantly to the total protein in the diet and they must be available at a reasonable price. Fish meal with a strong fishy odour and flavour may be acceptable in South-East and East Asia and in Equatorial Africa. There are peoples preferring fishy flavours who are reported to accept fish meal direct from a teaspoon. Both children and adults in these populations like fish meal added to rice or soup. However, the defatted and deodorized fish protein concentrates are more stable during storage and more generally accepted as they have a bland taste.

The market potential of a fish protein concentrate is determined by its nutritional and functional properties. FPC intended for use as a nutritive supplement must be cheap, since the need for an improved protein intake is greatest in the developing countries where income is very low. If FPC is to be added to traditional foods it should be neutral in odour and taste, and non-functional in properties in order not to modify the characteristics of the foods to which it is added. Addition of FPC to cereal flours requires central milling operations in which the supplement can be added.

Hegsted (1968) determined the relative nutritive value of wheat flour to which additions of amino acids and FPC were made. He calculated the total utilizable protein by dividing the cost of each fortified flour mix by the total utilizable protein in 100 lb, to obtain the cost per unit of utilizable protein. These costs were: wheat, 2·5; wheat flour + 0·2% lysine hydrochloride, 1·55; wheat flour + 5% FPC, 1·26; and wheat flour + 10% FPC, 0·91 dollars/lb. Lysine and FPC were taken as costing 1 dollar and 0·25 dollar/lb respectively, and wheat flour as 5·50 dollars/100 lb.

One of the conclusions which could be drawn from these calculations would be that it is an extravagance not to fortify wheat donated to developing countries. Supplementing with lysine alone would not increase the biological value sufficiently, *i.e.* to about 0·60. Threonine is still too expensive.

Hammonds and Call (1970) have investigated the US market for protein additives with special reference to various forms of FPC. They have shown that the amount of protein additives now used in the United States is large, and that there is a good probability that FPC products costing between 28·8 and 53·8 cents per pound of protein could compete in the US market as protein ingredients in beverages, breakfast foods, canned meat, processed meat and baked goods. Hammonds and Call (1970) consider the most likely area of competition to be in the soya-bean concentrate —soya-bean isolates markets for baby foods, baked goods and processed meats. Success in the higher-priced fields would depend upon a neutral flavour and suitable functional properties.

The currently available fish protein concentrates have a low functionality. They are greyish powders with no texture, low wettability and low fat absorption. Their use has therefore hitherto been limited to cereals, bread, biscuits and pasta products. As mentioned above, the lack of functional properties can even be an advantage in these types of foods as the FPC does not change the normal texture and appearance of the product. If functional properties could be developed along with acceptable taste, FPC could be used in many products where non-fat dried milk or other high-quality proteins are now used. This depends on further technical development as this technology is not yet available.

The success of FPC depends on many factors, *e.g.* fish supply, processing, marketing and economic development policy. A fish protein concentrate for human consumption must be processed from fresh edible fish. Astra Overseas Fishing has a factory ship, M/S *Astra*, accompanied by ten trawlers operating in the South Atlantic. Most of the catch of these trawlers is processed to ordinary fish meal on board the factory ship, but a part of the fish is used as raw material for FPC for human consumption. A preserved press-cake is solvent-extracted and deodorized in a land-based factory at the fishing village of Bua on the west coast of Sweden. There are great possibilities for producing a defatted and deodorized FPC in large amounts for enrichment of different cereals to be used in developing countries. This must be the most efficient use of a valuable protein supply. However, the future of the use of fish protein concentrates for their nutritional properties is very dependent on the decisions made by the government authorities involved in aid programmes.

Astra produces fish protein concentrates both from whole fish and from eviscerated fish. In both cases a deboning procedure is necessary to decrease the fluorine content to less than 100 mg/kg to fulfil the specifications laid down by FDA in the USA. When the fish is eviscerated the yield is lower than when whole fish is used. This means a more expensive product intended for markets with legal restrictions against using whole fish as raw material. In the USA fish protein concentrate from whole fish is a food additive, but eviscerated fish protein should be classified as a food ingredient. It seems probable that in the future the FPC intended for enrichment of foods will be manufactured from fresh, cleaned and deboned fish, and not from eviscerated fish. It is, however, uncertain whether the deboning procedure is really necessary for the production of a nutritious fish protein.

The main reason for the delay of the success of FPC as human food in the developed countries seems to be the common aversion to fish. The food companies have not dared to make use of an effective marketing campaign. The first step must be to convince the consumers that a deodorized fish protein does not impart a fishy taste to the enriched product.

Some negative reactions have been caused by the use of an inferior quality of FPC. One of the main obstacles to the large-scale production of a good-quality fish protein is the perishable nature of the raw material.

The most likely application of the currently available fish protein concentrates in the food market in the developed countries is in protein-supplemented foods in which nutritive value is the main selling point. Up to now nutrition has not played any decisive role in marketing.

III. CONCLUSIONS

Protein in fish is a highly nutritious animal protein. If it is to be used effectively it must be produced in a storable form with its biological value retained. Such fish protein concentrates are intended mainly to enrich products with a nutritional value limited by a relative deficiency of one or more amino acids. Fish meal has for a long time been used as a high-quality animal protein in various animal feeds. A defatted fish meal can be used as a protein source in milk replacers for calves. Fine grade, solvent-extracted steam-dried herring meal mixed with whey constitutes a useful base for a calf-milk replacer. Due to the generally low hygienic standard of the fish meal used as raw material, and also because of incomplete lipid extraction and deodorization of the product it is, however, not suitable for human consumption.

A fish protein concentrate for human consumption must be processed from fresh edible fish. The nutritional value, the price, the taste and the functional characteristics determine the market potential of the product. The amino acid composition of fish protein makes it an ideal protein for the enrichment of cereals low in lysine and other essential amino acids. Wheat flour supplemented with 5% fish protein has a high nutritional value and good baking properties. It is a much more valuable product than unsupplemented wheat for distribution in developing countries. From the nutritional point of view, fish protein is also suitable for enrichment of weaning foods, breakfast cereals, and bakery products. A very bland taste similar to that of non-fat dried milk is essential for a sizeable market potential.

The currently available fish protein concentrates have a low functionality. They are greyish powders with no texture, low wettability and low fat absorption. If functional properties can be developed along with acceptable taste, FPC can be used in many products in which non-fat dried milk or other high-quality proteins are now used.

REFERENCES

Autret, M. and van Veen, A. G. (1955). *Am. J. clin. Nutr.* **3**, 234–243.

Brinkman, G. L. and Rose, J. (1970). *Nutr. Rep. int.* **1**, 291–295.

Crisan, E. V. (1970). *Fd Technol., Champaign* **24**, 1132–1138.

Danell, B. (1970). Astra-Ewos AB, Feed Protein Symposium. 14 September.

Dreyer, J. J. and Du Bruyn, D. B. (1968). *S. Afr. med. J.* **42**, 600–604.

Ericson, L.-E., Larsson, S. and Lid, G. (1961). *Acta physiol. scand.* **53**, 366–375.

Finch, R. (1970). *CRC Critical Rev. Fd Technol.* **1**, 519–580.

Graham, G. G., Baertl, J. M. and Cordano, A. (1965). *Am. J. Dis. Child.* **110**, 248–257.

Graham, G. G., Baertl, J. M. and Cordano, A. (1966). *Am. J. clin. Nutr.* **18**, 16–19.

Hammonds, T. M. and Call, D. L. (1970). Utilization of protein ingredients in the U.S. food industry. Dept Agric. Economics, Parts 1 and 2 AE Res. 320 and 321 Cornell University, Ithaca, New York.

HEDAYAT, H., SHAHBAZY, H. and PAYAN, R. (1970). Personal Communication.
HEGSTED, D. M. (1968). *Am. J. clin. Nutr.* **21**, 688–692.
HOFVANDER, Y. (1972). *Am. J. clin. Nutr.* (In press.)
HOFVANDER, Y., MELLBIN, T. and KYHLBERG, E. (1972). Personal Communication.
JANSEN, G. R. (1969). *Am. J. clin. Nutr.* **22**, 38–43.
KWEE, W. H., SIDWELL, V. D., WILEY, R. C. and HAMMERLE, O. A. (1969). *Cereal Chem.* **46**, 78–84.
MOORJANI, M. N. and LAHIRY, N. H. (1970). *Fd Technol., Champaign* **24**, 56–59.
MUNRO, I. C., MORRISON, A. B. and MYER, M. (1969). *J. Am. diet. Ass.* **54**, 398–400.
PRETORIUS, P. J. and WEHMEYER, A. S. (1964). *Am. J. clin. Nutr.* **14**, 147–155.
SIDWELL, V. D. (1967). *Activities Report* **19**, 118–124.
SIDWELL, V. D., STILLINGS, B. R. and KNOBL, G. M. JR. (1970). *Fd Technol., Champaign* **24**, 876–882.
SIDWELL, V. D., STILLINGS, B. R. and KNOBL, G. M. JR. (1971). *Comml Fish. Rev.* **33**, 39–41.
STILLINGS, B. R., SIDWELL, V. D. and HAMMERLE, O. A. (1971). *Cereal Chem.* **48**, 292–302.
TAVILL, F. and GONIK, A. (1969). *Am. J. clin. Nutr.* **22**, 1571–1576.
WOO, H. C. and ERDMAN, A. M. (1971). *J. Home Econ.* **63**, 263–270.
WHO (1970). "Consultation on Human Testing of Protein-Rich Foods" WHO Headquarters, Geneva, 9–11 March.
YÁÑEZ, E., BALLESTER, D., MACCIONI, A., SPADA, R., BARJA, I., PAK, N., CHICHESTER, C. O., DONOSO, G. and MÖNCKEBERG, F. (1969). *Am. J. clin. Nutr.* **22**, 878–886.

CHAPTER 25

Factors Governing the Use of Soya-bean and Other Oilseed Proteins

G. D. ROSEN

Farnborough, Kent, England

I. THE IMPORTANCE OF ECONOMIC FACTORS

Protein research and development has for many years attracted liberal funds, firstly because the subject is basic to a better understanding of animal and human nutrition, medicine, health and longevity and, secondly, because there has been massive, world-wide propaganda on the present and potential significance of protein malnutrition and undernutrition. Setting aside for the present the vital role of scientific studies on the relation of virtually all cellular and tissue processes and mechanisms to the fundamental physical and chemical properties of protein molecules, it appears that progress in the development of new protein resources and the more efficient use of existing supplies has been hampered by a failure of many workers in this field to devote sufficient attention to economic aspects—a tendency underlined by the title of this symposium. Therefore, a major theme in this brief review of the position of soya-bean and other oilseed proteins is to underline some economic aspects and to see how they might usefully guide not only the use of existing resources for protein studies but also attract continued and perhaps expanded financial support from world agencies and charities and individual government and corporate bodies. There are signs of a certain disappointment among some financial sources that applied protein research and development has not generated or led to enough self-financing projects during the last two decades or so to justify even mild optimism concerning further efforts.

Some economic aspects are not, however, easy to relate to research and development programmes concerned with new protein use patterns because they are affected by many extraneous influences, including grain and animal fat commodity matters, oil and fat consumption patterns, national agricultural policies, and international trading and politics. In a 955-page book Anson and Altschul (1958) dismissed the topic by stating that "The problem of the costs of various plant processed foodstuffs for animals in relation to needs and financial resources and to the costs of alternative foodstuffs is so complex that it likewise cannot be even summarized here. . . . We must accordingly be content here to point out the crucial importance of the cost aspect of any protein feeding problem". This neglect can be illustrated further by my own contribution (Rosen, 1958) where, dealing with groundnuts and groundnut meal in a 49-page review with a 361-reference bibliography, only 2% of it was concerned with the economics of uses in foods and feeds of the then annual groundnut production of some 13 million tons. In this, the economic treatment was confined to a brief illustration of the influences of local and world supply conditions, of the availability and relative prices of other oils and fats, foods and protein concentrates and of guaranteed prices in some countries. This protein resource was in fact traded primarily on the basis of oil content.

The economic factors of importance in protein evaluation and utilization cover, of course, not only the variable costs of production and market values of protein materials (whether as protein sources or not) but also include at least (1) the influences of the proximity or otherwise of markets to production sites; (2) the cost of processing for progressive concentration or isolation of the protein; (3) the value of by-products and (4) the food appeal (and maybe the nutritional value) and hence the sales value of the original material or of its derivatives.

So far as direct use of oilseeds or their protein derivatives as food is concerned, there has been relatively little progress in the last hundred years compared, on the one hand, with their centuries-old consumption in classic raw, cooked or fermented forms and, on the other hand, with advances in the manufacture and consumption of fatty animal product substitutes such as margarine for butter.

The conversion of oilseed protein into the rich, appealing and relatively expensive forms of food, including milk, meat, fish and eggs has often been criticized and attacked as inefficient, in that several kilograms of dietary oilseed protein yield only 1 kg of animal food protein. But it must be realized at the outset that the animal process in fact is the most efficient known for endowment of real food appeal and consumer demand. Man has to date failed almost completely to approach, let alone equal, the detoxification and food-synthetic abilities of pigs, poultry, cattle and sheep in the transformation of oilseed fat, protein and carbohydrate into delectable foods with great palate appeal and high nutritive value. And in the transformation of leaf and microbial protein he is even further from any form of success.

It may be held by some that non-scientific forces or disciplines, including economics, are not the true province of protein evaluation. But the broader view is that protein evaluation is not merely a matter of nutrition and health, of improved understanding of the pathways of protein metabolism and of new product technology. Many other factors affect the size and shape of existing protein resources, their use patterns and their limiting factors. The strong influence of economics, marketing and education and the profitable and constructive use of finance to improve the quality and quantity of protein for mankind's individual and collective long-term benefit is especially evident in the field of oilseed proteins.

In my view it is only by greater study of and greater emphasis on these less scientific factors governing the use of proteins that we shall start to be able to stem the increasing gap, referred to by Mauron in Chapter 1, "between knowledge and its implementation, between a worthy intent and practical achievement".

Some of these factors will be stressed in surveying briefly the status of soya-bean and other oilseed proteins.

II. PRODUCTION INFLUENCES

Quantitatively the oilseeds do not produce as much protein as is available from cereals, which are reported to contribute about two-thirds of the total world protein production. Outline data are given in Table I on the main production characteristics for major oilseeds comparing, as an example only, 1956–7 with 1969–70. Table II contains the quantity of crude protein available from these resources in 1969–70, together with an illustrative financial value. The oilseeds included are those currently yielding more than 3 million tons per annum. Minor contributors, including castor, copra, palm kernel and sesame, totalled only 6·5 million tons in 1969–70 and are, therefore, omitted. From the mid 1950s to late 1960s output of the selected oilseeds increased by 45% with a most striking increment of some 20 million tons for soya-bean; the others combined increased by less than half this amount and linseed subsided slightly. In fact, in recent times soya-bean represents some 46% of the

TABLE I. Production of major oilseeds

Oilseed	1956-7 Production (million long tons)	1956-7 Area (million acres)	1956-7 Tons/acre	1969-70[a] Production (million long tons)	1969-70[a] Area (million acres)	1969-70[a] Tons/acre
Cottonseed (17)[b]	16·8	83·0	0·20	20·6	78·7	0·26
Groundnut (18)	12·6	32·8	0·38	15·7	41·3	0·38
Linseed (24)	4·1	23·9	0·17	3·4	17·5	0·19
Rapeseed (22)	3·3	15·6	0·21	5·6	20·0	0·28
Soya-bean (40)	23·7	55·4	0·43	44·0	82·6	0·53
Sunflower (12)	5·5	17·4	0·32	6·6	19·8	0·33
TOTALS	66·0			95·9		

[a] Except rapeseed and sunflower, 1968-9
[b] Figures in parentheses are % crude protein content

six materials surveyed. Its higher protein content of 40% compared with 12–24% for the others accounts for its outstanding position in protein value for money.

Soya-bean also tops the list in yield per acre and clearly the more so when protein content is taken into account. Yields per acre have been more or less static for groundnut, linseed and sunflower. Although yields per acre of cottonseed and rapeseed have risen by approximately one-third

TABLE II. Protein yields and financial values of major oilseeds in 1969–70

	Protein (million tons)	Value c.i.f. UK port (£/ton)
Cottonseed	3·5	38
Groundnut	2·8	92
Linseed	0·8	55
Rapeseed[a]	1·2	52
Soya-bean	17·6	48
Sunflower[a]	0·8	50
TOTAL	26·7	

[a] 1968-9

compared with one-quarter for soya-bean, it is noteworthy that the enhanced output of soya-bean material is primarily a function of the 49% expansion in acreage.

The dominant position of soya-bean in the oilseed production and utilization pattern is further stressed in that two-thirds of the protein output for the six oilseeds emanates from soya-bean. Its economic value as a source of protein is evident from the c.i.f. UK port valuations given for 1969–70 (Table II). In this connection oil content is of significance as is seen from the high price for groundnuts. After making allowance for oil yields of 16% from cottonseed, 32% from groundnut and 17% from soya-bean and for a rough comparison attributing the value of the residues to the protein content, it is found that groundnuts are five times as expensive as soya-bean and cottonseed almost twice as expensive as soya-bean as a source of protein.

From the viewpoint of protein quality, which is of considerable influence in animal feed applications, soya-bean is at least equal to and usually better than the other oilseed proteins. It might also be mentioned that the previous fertilizer "wastage" of many oilseed materials is now much diminished. Whether the move from fertilizer into animal feeds will be continued into human foods on a vast scale seems, from the evidence of the last two decades, to be questionable. Despite optimistic predictions that large quantities, notably of soya-bean, cottonseed and groundnut, will be used directly for human feeding, the scale will continue to be extremely restricted, until such time as the new derivatives can be classed as wholesome items of sufficient palate appeal to be attractive to a large populace.

Although soya-bean is not widely grown—taking into account those areas where cultivation is possible—it is clearly the primary protein source of choice from the point of view of supply, price and quality. Its move in the direction of becoming a more and more important protein resource can be illustrated by the changing relative values of soya-bean as a source of oil and oil meal in that in 1947 the oil/meal price ratio was 53/47, but this had declined to 33/67 by 1968. As will be discussed later, if yields per acre for soya-bean can be improved in the same manner as has occurred for cereals, then the outstanding position of soya-bean as a protein resource in the oilseed field can be expected to grow. It is concluded, therefore, that the basic criteria determining oilseed utilization are availability and price, influences which should be constantly borne in mind when contemplating new protein products or means of increasing the total protein supply on an economic basis.

III. PROTEIN-CONTAINING DERIVATIVES OF OILSEEDS

The fullest range of derivatives of oilseeds is known for soya-bean although analogous materials can in theory be prepared from other oil seeds and there has been some progress towards flours, concentrates and isolates with cottonseed and groundnut. Table III illustrates the many

TABLE III. Protein-containing derivatives of soya-bean

Derivative	*Process*
Full fat beans	(cooked), kibbled or ground
Full fat flours	de-hulled, (cooked), milled
Defatted meals	solvent extracted, (toasted)
Defatted flours	solvent extracted, milled, (heat-treated)
Partially defatted flours	expelled or solvent plus refatting
Oil-containing protein concentrates	water extraction of beans
Protein concentrates	water or solvent extraction of meal or flour
Protein–oil complex	aqueous extraction from beans and precipitation
Protein isolates	aqueous extraction and precipitation from meal or flour
Carbohydrate meals	insoluble residue from protein–oil complex or protein isolate production
Whey	non-precipitable solids from protein complex and protein isolation
Textured flours	flour compression, extrusion-cooking
Textured concentrates	concentrate compression, extrusion-cooking
Textured and spun protein isolates	isolate compression and/or extrusion
Whipping agents	enzymolysis of isolate
Gelling agents	aqueous extract of meal

ways in which soya-bean can be treated and refined progressively to obtain sixteen derivatives.

There is much versatility in the ways in which soya-bean is processed. The largest application is as meal for animal feeding which contains 44% or 50% protein according to whether or not hulls are removed: the latter meal finds specialist application mainly in poultry feeding. Interest has grown recently in the processing of full-fat beans on the farm with the development of a number of small machines, but it is still doubtful whether it is more economic for a farmer to process his beans in this way for feeding instead of selling his beans and purchasing soya-bean meal to supplement his grain. The process of grinding and cooking is fundamentally the same as that in the preparation of full-fat flour for various food uses, but without the need for the same standards of sanitation. For many food applications very careful control over the cleaning of the raw material and its handling in bulk production is essential to ensure high-quality baked goods, meat products, baby and diet foods, etc. The unheated enzyme-active flour is used mainly for bread improvement.

The main economic factors affecting the decision to process soya-bean in the various possible ways are:

(a) Scale of operation, i.e. in producing meal plus oil it is not uncommon to obtain great production economy by the active processing of $\frac{1}{2}$–1 million tons per annum in a plant. Solvent recovery is a key factor.
(b) Any aqueous extraction or concentration and isolation process is more expensive and this is reflected in the approximate sales values of flours, concentrates and isolates of 5–12 cents/lb, 18–26 cents/lb and 34–60 cents/lb respectively. The proportion of these sales values representing production costs is, of course, greatly affected by scale and it is only now, after 10–20 years, that isolates are becoming profitable.
(c) Texturing and spinning flours and isolates are also rather expensive processes and sales values are 25–80 cents/lb for the former and 45–175 cents/lb, including both wet and dry forms, for the latter.
(d) For whipping and gelling agents prices from 80–120 cents/lb are indicated.

Plant capital costs for the more complicated and sophisticated processes of isolation of protein are in the range \$1–5 million.

In addition to the relatively simple functions of water-binding and emulsification enjoyed by the use of simple soya-bean flours in foods, more highly specialized properties such as spinnability and coagulation call for protein concentration and isolation and the higher prices tend to place a limit on their use. With the removal of water-soluble material and insoluble carbohydrates there is a definite flavour and odour improvement but it cannot yet be stated that the protein derivatives are as bland as required for application in, for example, dairy products or substitutes. A troublesome problem that may be more costly to solve is that of the insolubility or feathering of oilseed proteins intended for application in drinks.

IV. NON-PROTEIN FACTORS AFFECTING UTILIZATION

Thus, the raw material price, the extent of processing needed and the scale of operation are extremely important factors affecting the utilization of soya-bean proteins. There are, in addition, a number of other compositional characteristics of oilseeds and oilseed meals which can be restrictive and difficult to eliminate.

Hydrocarbon and other solvents need to be removed from meals and flours not only for process economy but also for their acceptance by national and international authorities as free from health hazards. Recent work using dimethylformamide as extractant has shown much higher levels of residual solvent than hitherto known, in some cases ten times that expected: up to 1·5 g/kg. Residual solvent can be a bar to food use.

Aflatoxin primarily affects groundnuts but it is known to be present in other oilseed materials. It is an extremely difficult contaminant to remove and the tendency to date has been to set maximum levels controlling the use of groundnut materials as nuts or derivatives. In order not to condemn too much material compromise has been necessary. With the exception of badly contaminated material, the tendency is to divert from human to animal use and to restrict the level of inclusion in animal feeding or even to omit certain species. To date aflatoxin has had no real effect on the financial values of groundnut products but it may be a very serious bar to uses of groundnut flours and protein derivatives in foods. Avoidance of moulding at source is the answer.

Trypsin inhibitors have been studied most extensively in soya-bean. Heat processing to eliminate or minimize activity has to be carefully controlled to avoid damage to the protein that will affect its nutritional value. A recent development of considerable significance is the use of soya-bean materials to replace high-priced skim milk powders in calf and piglet feeding and to broaden the base of human food application of water-extracted soya-bean materials has been the discovery in France that there is, in addition to the free trypsin inhibitor normally detected and monitored, a bound form which is only revealed by prior pepsin digestion or treatment with hydrochloric acid. Processes for the complete elimination of the bound as well as the free trypsin inhibitor have led to the use of certain soya-bean materials in milk replacement at higher levels than before for both veal production and to lower the cost of rearing heifer replacement calves.

New techniques used in characterizing trypsin inhibitors in the nutritional context in which soya-bean or other oilseed is used will give a better characterization of the corresponding systems in groundnut. They have already shown that protein concentrates and isolates reputedly trypsin inhibitor-free are by no means so. The bound form has been undetected until recently.

A complex variety of molecules is generally responsible for the dark colours and unpleasant organoleptic properties of oilseed derivatives. Many originate in the hull and seed coat, and necessitate special raw material selection, special processing and chemical treatment of the products in order to eliminate or minimize their effects.

Gossypol is a well-known pigment and toxin of cottonseed materials which has restricted the use of cottonseed products, expecially for monogastric animals and in human foods. When it is removed, together with other bitter substances, cottonseed flour can be produced; this contains 69% protein and is claimed to be superior in colour and flavour to the corresponding soya-bean protein concentrates of the same crude protein content. The estimated selling price is 15–18 cents/lb. So far, neither the breeding of pigment-gland-free cottonseed nor the liquid cyclone process for the elimination of glands has proved to be of commercial significance despite many years of development and study.

Although it is relatively easy to remove soya-bean hulls and although the bean is relatively bland in colour, it is still necessary to bleach with oxidizing and/or reducing agents to achieve the requisite colour standards for use as a paper-coating agent or in certain food applications. Moreover, although a considerable degree of de-bittering is achieved through cooking and toasting and through extraction inherent in concentrate and isolate production, it cannot be claimed that soya-bean materials are yet as bland as many of the milk products they seek to displace. Recent work shows that aqueous treatment is costly but so far it is the only effective way of achieving a very high degree of odour and flavour improvement.

By contrast, the problems with colour are even more intractable for groundnuts, due to the virtual impossibility of removing all the red testa on a commercial scale. Treatment in aqueous or mildly alkaline media for the production of milk-like derivatives or isolated protein for fibre production has been responsible for serious product defects. The substances responsible—tannins, flavones and phlobaphenes—can also have undesirable effects on the physical properties of isolated proteins.

The tendency of highly unsaturated fat in free or phosphatide form to stick tightly to proteins is also a source of flavour reversion characteristics and common reports of fat contents of less than 1% in isolates should be discounted unless mixed (polar) solvents have been used in the estimation.

V. NEW SPECIALITY PRODUCTS

On a commercial scale new products containing oilseed proteins are primarily developed from soya-bean and have been largely the result of

TABLE IV. Use of some soya-bean speciality products in the USA in 1969-70

	Short tons	*Value* (million $)
Industrial isolates	26 000	12·5
Edible isolates	16 000	11·5
Whipping isolates	600	1·0
Protein concentrates	18 000	7·5
Soya-bean milk products	6000	—
Coffee whiteners[a]	35 000	63·0
Soya-bean isolate meat analogues	1500	3·2
Textured soya-bean flours	13 000	7·5
Soya-bean flours[b]		
Pet foods	100 000	
Calf-milk replacers	10 000	
Fermentation processes	6000	
Meat products	20 000	
Baked goods	40 000	
Food aid programmes	50 000	
Other food uses	18 000	
Industrial applications	70 000	

[a] Relatively little soya-bean material is used as yet in these materials due to inadequate functional and flavour properties

[b] Prices range widely between 6–19 cents/lb according to grade and quantity

work in the USA and Japan. "New" may be a misnomer since much of the work on the concentration and isolation of proteins commenced in 1935 in the USA and patents for textured proteins appeared in the 1950s. Some idea of the status of these products, including uses of soya-bean flours in the USA, is given in Table IV. There has, in fact, been a renewal of interest in the food applications of soya-bean flours due to the solution of certain raw material handling problems and sanitation procedures in manufacture giving better bacteriological qualities, and also due to the pressure for food ingredients at a lower price than the more refined concentrates and isolates.

Of the industrial protein isolate, most is used as a paper-coating adhesive, usually with casein, which it has to some extent displaced, or as starches and synthetics. The protein has to be considerably modified by chemical treatment in order to achieve suitable solubility and adhesive qualities. The meat industry has so far taken a considerable proportion of the edible products, some 9500 tons of isolate and 13 500 tons of concentrate. During the development of these products variation in the price of milk derivatives has at times assisted and at other times inhibited the progress of soya-bean.

Table IV refers to approximately 400 000 tons of soya-bean-based speciality products in the USA, and this should be compared with 17½ million tons of soya-bean cakes and meals used in animal feeding. Increases in these speciality products may be anticipated and there are those who predict a very rapid proliferation during this decade. The factors restraining development, however, are quite clear and much further research and development will be necessary to overcome (a) the high cost of concentration and isolation; (b) residual flavour and odour; (c) the present inability to equal the eating quality (flavour and texture) of the milk, meat and eggs some seek to replace; (d) inadequate functional properties and (e) legal restrictions on application.

With regard to (e), the American Food and Drug Administration, in co-operation with the Meat Inspection Division of the [US] Department of Agriculture has spent considerable time in agreeing nomenclature and specifications for some of the new derivatives, particularly textured products. Many proposals have been considered and abandoned, possibly because the soya-bean lobby wishes to set standards of nutritive value for textured vegetable proteins to exclude other oilseed derivatives. It seems to the author that the problem could be resolved by referring, for example, to textured soya-bean flours, spun soya-bean protein isolates: naming the oilseed and the derivative concerned instead of seeking a broad description to cover all.

VI. CURRENT AND FUTURE COMPETITION FOR OILSEED PROTEINS

Although oilseeds, in particular soya-bean, are relatively cheap protein resources, food development work has so far failed to provide us with a synthetic pig, bird or cow capable of competing in food appeal. So far the same may be said of other sources of proteins. Nevertheless, there is a number of competing materials holding a potentially threatening position and there are others that have already made an impact.

Urea used as one part together with six parts of maize is almost equivalent to seven parts of soya-bean meal in cattle feeding. Even if there is 10% superiority in production for soya-bean oil meal over the mixture, the 25–40% saving of ingredient costs using urea only up to safe levels without inhibiting production significantly, has led to the expansion of urea usage in this field in the USA from 314 000 tons in 1963 to 650 000 tons in 1970.

Although the increase in production of methionine or its hydroxy analogue has considerably assisted the application of soya-bean in animal feeds and will continue to do so as the price falls below 40p per kg, the increase in L-lysine production (now some 10 000 tons per annum—80% feed grade costing approximately 60p per kg) may have a tendency to reduce soya-bean inclusions. On the other hand it may well enhance the use of groundnut and cottonseed products. Similarly, high-lysine maize is a potential threat. Despite much publicity, it is by no means clear when this will make a real commercial impact and whether it can be produced sufficiently economically to compete with maize plus lysine.

Microbial protein has so far shown no real sign of being an economic competitor. The value of microbial protein for animal feeding is set by the availability and cost of other proteins including cereal, oilseed and animal derivatives. Feeding tests have shown microbial protein with or without methionine to be of good nutritive value, but published information on capital and raw material costs suggests that it may never compete economically with vegetable protein for feeds. It might make some impact on the use of very high-priced milk proteins but in this context soya-bean at least can almost certainly hold its own. Another unknown in this comparison is the high and increasing cost of water for fermentation production and the cost of solving the undoubted pollution problems of the waste waters.

Table I shows that compared with cereal grains there has been relatively little progress in increasing the output per acre of oilseeds by improved cultivation or by breeding new varieties. The success with cereals such as maize is not surprising because a great deal of money has been invested in research and development and there are over 400 breeders of corn varieties in the USA. By comparison, soya-bean has been relatively neglected despite a huge increase in output and utilization. Yields in bushels per acre have risen, but only from 23 to 28 between 1950 and 1970 and the breeding is in the hands of only about 40 interests. A recent grant for research into some of the difficult problems in soya-bean culture spread between six Universities amounted to only $185 000. If soya-bean interests wish to maintain their highly competitive position and be in a position to beat off competition by an ability to produce and sell soya-beans at a cost in the region of $2 per bushel, then much more attention than hitherto will need to be paid to enhancing output.

Inevitably this review has been incomplete. Topics such as use of oilseeds by the fermentation industries, development of village-type equipment for local use, production of soya-bean sauces and other traditional foods, success in breeding erucic acid-free rapeseed and destruction of myrosinase, use of oilseed materials in pet foods and hydrolysed vegetable protein, have been omitted or glossed over. The hydrolysed vegetable protein as a radical modification using hydrolysis with hydrochloric acid is a good instance of how much oilseed materials need to be modified in order to make them attractive, palatable and competitive. By comparison with the transformation in grain by baking and brewing processes to provide appealing foods, the simple and relatively cheap techniques of dry milling, wet cooking and fermentation will need to be more widely employed if real consumer demand for oilseed protein food is to be created and served and thereby made self-financing.

REFERENCES

Anson, M. L. and Altschul, A. M. (1958). *In* "Processed Plant Protein Foodstuffs" (A. M. Altschul, ed.), p. 9. Academic Press, New York.

Rosen, G. D. (1958). *In* "Processed Plant Protein Foodstuffs" (A. M. Altschul, ed.), pp. 419–468. Academic Press, New York.

CHAPTER 26

Quality Control in Industry

D. PEARSON

National College of Food Technology (University of Reading), Weybridge, Surrey, England

I. LEGAL ASPECTS OF QUALITY CONTROL

The basic sequences in quality control are as follows:

Agricultural control
Buying samples
Raw material (ingredient) control
Examination of trial batches
Process control
Product control
Storage control

In quality control we are aiming to standardize the product with respect to weight, composition and physical and organoleptic properties. This is attained in practice by attempting to standardize at each of these stages.

An example of agricultural control is the selection of the correct variety of wheat for bread. For canning, suitable varieties of fruit and vegetables are chosen, and we also take into account the best time to pick to give the best general quality. With pigs a consistent fat/protein ratio is sought for each animal purchased for manufacture. Buying samples are small representative samples taken from the bulk of raw material. The ingredients usually have to comply with specification requirements, which often include a statement that the material has to comply with all relevant legal standards. With trial batches and process control there is less control, perhaps, from the legal standpoint, but product examination is most important. Assuming that a figure is stated on the label, the Weights and Measures Act requires that all containers contain the correct weight, volume or number. Many foods can only be sold in multiple weights or volumes and the wrapper weight is sometimes restricted.

In Britain the composition of the product is controlled legally by Section 2 of the Food and Drugs Act, which states that it is an offence to sell any food which is not of the nature, substance or quality demanded by the purchaser.

Examples of the interpretation of these terms in the courts are as follows:

Foods not of the nature includes fish sold of a different species, and fruits of a different variety from that named.

Foods not of the substance, e.g. chicory in a food sold as coffee, margarine fats in butter and the presence of a piece of string in a loaf of bread.

Foods not of the quality are often products which fail to comply with compositional standards.

II. LABORATORY EVALUATION WITH SPECIAL REFERENCE TO PROTEINS

A. General

If we consider what actually occurs in the Quality Control Laboratories in the UK Food Industry, it is plain that over nine-tenths of the work done in connection with protein is the estimation of the total protein content (including polypeptides and amino acids) by means of the Kjeldahl procedure, or by some method which has been standardized against it.

In general the Kjeldahl method estimates the total nitrogen which is converted to total crude protein by means of an empirical factor, which depends on the proportions of the various nitrogenous compounds present in the particular food. The figure obtained therefore includes non-protein N, but nitrates, nitrites, nitroso- and nitro-compounds, for instance, are not estimated unless the procedure is modified in the early stages of the digestion.

The origins of the procedure go back to the last century. Kjeldahl (1883) was a Dane, who spent most of his working life investigating problems in the brewing industry at the Carlsberg Laboratory. The individual stages of the procedure have been studied and modified by various workers (Bradstreet, 1965), and important contributions were made by Gunning, Arnold, Wilfarth and Winkler. It should be noted that the large volume of literature on the subject includes much controversy.

The following represents the outline of the procedure most commonly used on the macro scale:

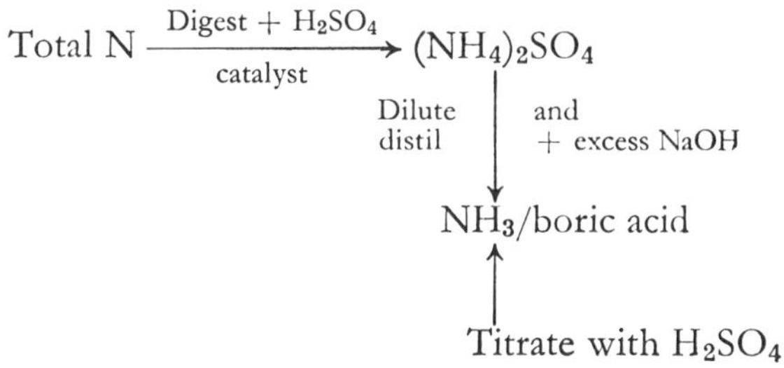

1. *Catalyst and digestion*

The term "catalyst" as used above is not perhaps scientifically accurate as it includes sodium or potassium sulphate whose action is to raise the boiling temperature. Of the genuine catalysts, copper is perhaps most frequently used, but it is considered to be inferior to mercury (Osborn and Krasnitz, 1933, 1934; Milbauer, 1938). Mercury, however, forms a complex which causes incomplete recovery of ammonia in the distillation with caustic alkali unless thiosulphate is also added to break down the complex. The conditions necessary for efficient digestion have been studied by Alcock (1946).

2. *Receiving acid*

We prefer boric acid for absorbing the distilled ammonia. It has the advantage that only one standard solution is required. Ammonium borate is formed, the boric acid is too weak to affect the titration and the ammonia is titrated directly with acid. The distillate must be kept cool, however, as ammonia is lost from boric acid above 50°C.

3. *Smaller scale modifications*

Modifications of the macro method using semi-micro distillation (Pearson, 1970b); or diffusion (Conway, 1933) possess certain advantages over the macro method but consideration must be given to the homogeneity of the sample.

4. *Non-distillation modifications*

It is possible to avoid the distillation step altogether. Alternative procedures include those using Nessler's reagent (Minari and Zilversmit, 1963), sodium hypobromite (Hashmi *et al.*, 1962) and a phenol–hypochlorite reaction (Mann, 1963).

B. Application of the Technicon Autoanalyser to the Kjeldahl Procedure

The Kjeldahl procedure has been applied to the Technicon Autoanalyser system, which can handle up to 20 samples per hour (Lento and Daugherty, 1971).

The digestion vessel consists of a Pyrex glass tube grooved helically along its length (Fig. 1). By continuous rotation, material introduced at one

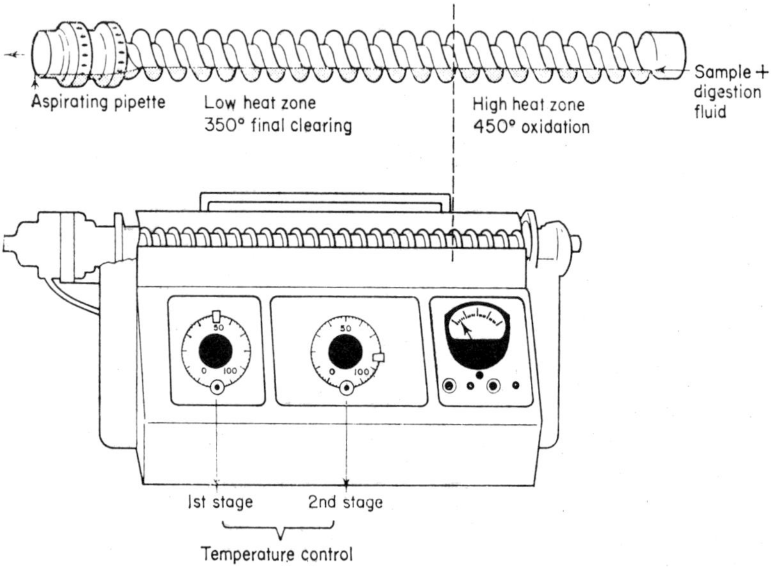

FIG. 1. The Kjeldahl digestion unit used in conjunction with the Technicon Autoanalyser. The upper part shows the glass digestion tube grooved helically along its length

end is spirally conveyed to exit at the other end. Between the individual samples the digestion fluid flows through the helix and cleans the system. The lower part of Fig. 1 shows the controls which regulate the heat in both stages. The colorimetric reaction used involves phenate, hypochlorite and alkali (Fig. 2) and the final measurement appears as a peak for each sample on the recorder.

The method has been applied to a fairly wide range of foods such as vegetables, soups, cereals and materials quite difficult to handle like meat products (Faint, 1970). With most foods, the material is wetted with water for 20 min and then concentrated sulphuric acid is slowly added, so that the heat generated helps to break down the tissue. The digestion is accelerated with the addition of perchloric acid or vanadium pentoxide.

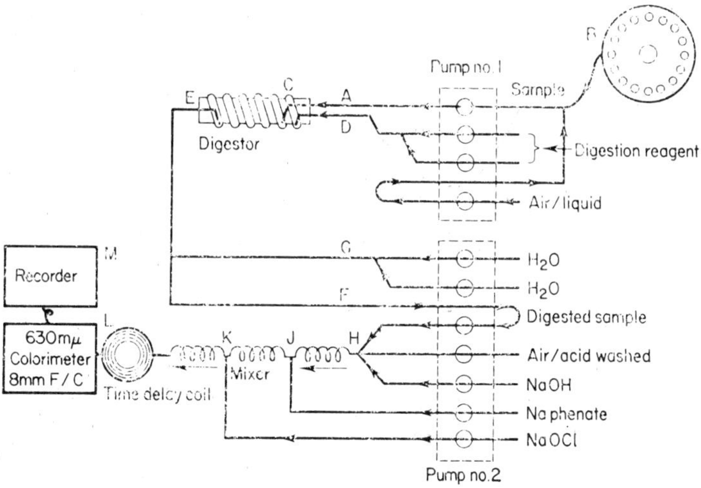

FIG. 2. Flow diagram for the estimation of protein using the Technicon Autoanalyser

With meat products more drastic treatment is necessary and the sample is allowed to stand initially for 30 min with 50% sulphuric acid at 60°. Recoveries are usually close to 100%, but special digestion conditions are required to attain this with some materials, including pure compounds such as creatine and arginine (Davidson *et al.*, 1970).

C. Non-Kjeldahl Procedures

Most of the other procedures for estimating protein are standardized against the results obtained using the Kjeldahl method. The simplest method is probably the formol titration, which depends on the ease of reaction of free amino groups on a protein with formaldehyde (Taylor, 1957). Using titrations in the presence of potassium oxalate to remove the effect of calcium salts, it has been shown that a definite reduction in the number of titratable amino acid groups occurs in dried milk protein compared to raw milk protein (Harrall, 1933). Formol titration is also of value for assessing the degree of proteolysis but its main applications are for estimating protein in liquids such as milk or food extracts. It represents a very useful routine control method for obtaining the milk solids-not-fat in ice-cream, for which there is a statutory minimum of 7·5%. The empirical factor employed depends on the actual analytical procedure adopted as well as the ratio of casein to whey proteins in the milk. Formol titration is also useful for differentiating a brewed vinegar from an artificial product prepared from synthetic acetic acid and caramel, and for detecting adulteration in fruit juices.

Of the other methods, the biuret reaction involves the formation of a coloured complex when peptides are treated with copper sulphate in alkaline solution, and has been applied to cereals (Pinckney, 1949; Williams, 1961).

Dye-binding methods are discussed in detail in Chapter 12 and may have useful applications for some foods, though we have worked with meat products using Amido Black and have found difficulties in standardizing the procedure so that it is applicable to unknown samples (Pearson and Parvaneh, 1971).

A turbidimetric method has been applied to cereals by Feinstein and Hart (1959). The turbidity is caused by the addition of sulphosalicylic acid to an alkaline extract of the cereal and the transmitted light is measured in conjunction with a 540 nm filter.

D. Interpretation of Results

1. *Identification of fruit and fish*
   (a) The following examples are not directly associated with the Kjeldahl method:
   The free amino acids in fruit juices have been separated by paper and thin-layer chromatography (Coussin and Samish, 1968) and this forms a possible method of identifying the fruit present in products.
   (b) The electrophoretic patterns of the proteins of fish have been employed to identify the species. Difficulties arise, however, if the fish has been heated in a product such as fish paste. Mackie (1969) at the Torry Research Station has, however, had some success with fish cooked to a lesser degree, but not pressure cooked. The water-extractable muscle myogens are extracted in 6 M urea. Using a single acrylamide gel, the method appears to be suitable for the identification of the fish present in fish cakes.

2. *General use of the protein figure in proximate analysis*

Together with the water, fat, carbohydrate and ash, the protein is one of the important estimations in the proximate analysis of many foods. The amount present should fall within normal ranges, and minimum percentages are quoted in commercial specifications. For example, flour for bread making should be a strong variety containing about 11·5% protein, and it has been established that the baking quality is positively correlated with the protein content. The baker is specially interested in the physical properties of the gluten. Further, the Bread and Flour Regulations 1963 prescribe that "Gluten Bread" should contain at least 16% protein in the dry matter and "High Protein Bread" at least 22%.

Other materials examined for total protein are barley intended for the manufacture of fermented liquids, dried egg and soya-bean flours. Good quality meat extracts should have a low content of gelatin and this is checked by the Kjeldahl procedure. Low protein levels in fruit juices suggest adulteration, and the determination of selected amino acids such as betaine (Lewis, 1966) and serine (Morgan, 1966) have been used as checks.

3. *The estimation of protein-rich materials in products*

The protein figure for a product can be used to estimate the content of a N-rich component in that product. Examples are: the rice and milk contents of canned rice pudding (Pim, 1964, 1967), almond in marzipan (Monk, 1963; Firth, 1969) for which there is a minimum (23·5% of dry almond) stated in a Local Authorities' Joint Advisory Committee Code of Practice, and the amount of gelatin in table jellies.

The most widely used application is, however, for meat products such as sausages, and examples of the types of calculation used are given below. The main problem is not the accuracy of the analytical data, but the selection of the figure for N content, since raw materials such as meat

TABLE I. Nitrogen factors for meats calculated on the fat-free material (SAC, 1961, 1963, 1965, 1967)

Type of Meat	*% N in fat-free material* Mean factor	Range of values
Pork	3·45	2·8–4·2
Beef	3·55	3·0–4·5
Veal	3·35	3·0–3·7
Tongue	3·0	2·2–3·6

TABLE II. Variation of the N factors for meats and wheat rusk filler since 1919

	Nitrogen factor used	*Stubbs and More* (1919)	*Jackson and Jones* (1932)	*SPA* (1940, 1952)	*SAC* (1961, 1963)
Pork	% N/FF	4·0	3·55	3·6	3·45
Beef	% N/FF	3·75	3·42	3·4	3·55
Wheat rusk filler	% N/carbohydrate	2·0	2·0	2·0	2·0 (1965a)[a]

[a] 2·3 for limited period

show considerable biological variation. This difficulty can be appreciated by considering that the fat/protein ratio may be as low as 0·13 for lean meat and as high as 100 for outside fat. Greater consistency can be obtained if figures are calculated on fat-free (FF) material, and even then the compromise N/FF factors proposed by the Meat Products Sub-Committee of the Analytical Methods Committee of the Society for Analytical Chemistry (1961, 1963, 1965a,b, 1967) are derived from wide ranges (Table I). Comparison of the factors proposed since 1919 shown in Table II indicate considerable variations. Thus whereas previous calculations indicated that the factor for pork was higher than that for beef, the modern view is that the positions should now be reversed. Apart from a short period in the early 1960s, the agreed percentage of N calculated on the carbohydrate for the wheat rusk filler has remained at 2·0 since 1919.

(a) *Example of the calculation of total meat content.* Supposing the analysis of a sample of beef sausage were as follows:

Water	50·2%
Extracted fat	24·9% $= F_E$
Protein (N × 6·25)	9·4% $= 1{\cdot}504\%\ N = N_T$
Ash	2·5%
Carbohydrate (by difference)	13·0% $= C$

$$\%\ \text{Total meat} = \%\ \text{Defatted meat} + \%\ \text{Extracted fat}$$

$$= \frac{\%\ \text{meat N}}{\text{mean N/FF for beef}} \times 100 + \%\ \text{Extracted fat}$$

$$= \frac{\%\ \text{Total N} - \%\ \text{Filler N}}{\text{Mean N/FF for beef}} \times 100 + \%\ \text{Extracted fat}$$

For wheat rusk filler, N/carbohydrate = 0·02 = 2·0%

$$\therefore\quad \%\ \text{Total meat} = \frac{1{\cdot}504 - 0{\cdot}02 \times 13{\cdot}0}{3{\cdot}55} \times 100 + 24{\cdot}9$$

$$= \frac{1{\cdot}504 - 0{\cdot}260}{3{\cdot}55} \times 100 + 24{\cdot}9$$

$$= 35{\cdot}0\ (\text{defatted meat}) + 24{\cdot}9\ (\text{extracted fat})$$

$$= 59{\cdot}9\%\ (\text{total meat})$$

The sample therefore complies with the statutory minimum for the total meat of 50%. The above assumes that the only sources of N in the sausage are meat and cereal filler. If protein-rich materials such as milk and soyabean were present the calculation would have to be modified accordingly (Pearson, 1970b).

(b) *Example of the calculation of the lean meat content.* Apart from the statutory minimum for the total meat content of beef sausage of 50%, there is a further minimum for the lean meat content of 25%, i.e. 50% of the minimum for the total meat. In practice various cuts of meat are used as raw material, containing varying proportions of lean and fatty tissue. For the purposes of The Sausage and Other Meat Product Regulations 1967, however, lean meat is defined as meat free of visible fat and the resultant material usually contains 4–11% fat (Pearson, 1968; Dalley, 1969).

For the calculation we decided to allow 10% fat in lean meat and assume that outside fat contains on the average 90% fat. The equations produced therefore allow for the intramuscular fat in the lean, and for the small amount of protein present in the outside fat. The general formula produced for beef sausage is as follows (Pearson, 1968; Pearson, 1970a; Pearson and Gardiner, 1971):

$$\%\ \text{Lean meat} = \frac{112{\cdot}5\ N_T - 0{\cdot}4437\ F_E - 2{\cdot}25\ C}{\text{Mean N/FF for beef}}$$

Using the analytical figures in the previous example:

$$\begin{aligned}\%\ \text{Lean meat} &= \frac{112{\cdot}5 \times 1{\cdot}504 - 0{\cdot}4437 \times 24{\cdot}9 - 2{\cdot}25 \times 13{\cdot}0}{3{\cdot}55}\\ &= \frac{169{\cdot}2 - 11{\cdot}0 - 29{\cdot}3}{3{\cdot}55}\\ &= 36{\cdot}3\%\ \text{(lean meat)}\end{aligned}$$

The sample therefore complies with the statutory minimum for the lean meat of 25%. Actually the defatted meat from the previous calculation is equal to the lean meat figure if the extracted fat exactly equals the defatted meat. If, however, the defatted meat exceeds the extracted fat, the calculated lean meat exceeds the calculated defatted meat. The difficulty here is in deciding how much fat to allow in lean meat. The problem is not that of attaining analytical accuracy, but rather what are reasonable averages for the N content of FF meat and for the amount of fat to allow for in lean meat.

REFERENCES

ALCOCK, R. S. (1946). *Analyst, Lond.* **71**, 233–234.

BRADSTREET, R. B. (1965). "The Kjeldahl Method for Organic Nitrogen." Academic Press, New York.

CONWAY, E. J. (1933). *Biochem. J.* **27**, 430–434.

COUSSIN, B. R. and SAMISH, Z. (1968). *J. Fd Sci.* **33**, 196–199.

DALLEY, R. A. (1969). *J. Ass. publ. Analysts* **7**, 33.

Davidson, J., Mathieson, J. and Boyne, A. W. (1970). *Analyst, Lond.* **95**, 181–193.

Faint, P. D. (1970). Paper presented at Technicon Colloquium On Automated Analyses for Foods, Beverages and Allied Industries, London (Technicon Instruments, Basingstoke).

Feinstein, L. and Hart, J. R. (1959). *Cereal Chem.* **36**, 191–193.

Firth, F. O. (1969). *J. Ass. publ. Analysts* **7**, 22–23.

Harral, J. C. (1933). *Analyst, Lond.* **58**, 605–606.

Hashmi, M. H., Ali, E. and Umar, M. (1962). *Analyt. Chem.* **34**, 988–990.

Jackson, F. W. and Jones, O. (1932). *Analyst, Lond.* **57**, 562–566.

Kjeldahl, J. (1883). *Z. analyt. Chem.* **22**, 366.

Lento, H. F. and Daugherty, C. E. (1971). *Fd Product Development* **5**, 86–92.

Lewis, W. M. (1966). *J. Sci. Fd Agric.* **17**, 316–320.

Mackie, J. M. (1969). *J. Ass. publ. Analysts* **7**, 83–87.

Mann, L. T. Jr. (1963). *Analyt. Chem.* **35**, 2179–2182.

Milbauer, J. (1938). *Z. analyt. Chem.* **111**, 397–407.

Minari, O. and Zilversmit, D. B. (1963). *Analyt. Biochem.* **6**, 320–327.

Monk, H. E. (1963). *J. Ass. publ. Analysts* **1**, 20–22.

Morgan, R. H. (1966). *J. Ass. publ. Analysts* **4**, 73–80.

Osborn, R. A. and Krasnitz, A. (1933, 1934). *J. Ass. off. agric. Chem.* **16**, 110–113; **17**, 339–342.

Pearson, D. (1968). *J. Ass. publ. Analysts* **6**, 129–134.

Pearson, D. (1970a). *J. Ass. publ. Analysts* **8**, 22–24.

Pearson, D. (1970b). "The Chemical Analysis of Foods." 6th edition. Churchill, London.

Pearson, D. and Gardiner, G. R. B. (1971). *J. Ass. publ. Analysts* **9**, 102.

Pearson, D. and Parvaneh, V. (1971). *J. Ass. publ. Analysts* **9**, 39.

Pim, F. B. (1964, 1967). *J. Ass. publ. Analysts* **2**, 62; **5**, 61–67.

Pinckney, A. J. (1949). *Cereal Chem.* **26**, 423–439.

Society for Analytical Chemistry (1961, 1963, 1965a,b, 1967). *Analyst, Lond.* **86**, 557–560; **88**, 422–423; **90**, 256–257, 579–580; **92**, 326–327.

Society of Public Analysts (1940, 1952). *Analyst, Lond.* **65**, 257; **77**, 543–544.

Stubbs, G. and More, A. (1919). *Analyst, Lond.* **44**, 125–127.

Taylor, W. H. (1957). *Analyst, Lond.* **82**, 488–498.

Williams, P. C. (1961). *J. Sci. Fd Agric.* **12**, 58–61.

CHAPTER 27

Determination of Functional Properties of Protein Foods

ANNE-MARIE HERMANSSON

Lund Institute of Technology, Sweden

I. INTRODUCTION

The development of protein products with high nutritional value is the subject of intensive research at various locations all over the world. The new products that should evolve from this work will be used mainly for incorporation into various types of existing foods. A suitable protein product must maintain or even enhance the quality and acceptability of the food. Thus apart from having intrinsically satisfactory properties such as nutritional value, flavour and colour, the protein products should possess certain functional properties which make them compatible with the various foods to which they are to be added. The market for new protein products will be determined to a large extent by their ability to meet these requirements. Therefore an important aspect of the development of processes for the production of new protein isolates or concentrates is to establish their functional physicochemical properties, which can be defined as those giving information on how the protein will behave in a food system. Hitherto very few results from systematic investigations of such properties have been published and basic research in this field seems to be badly needed.

The problem of functional characterization can be approached in different ways. The traditional method is to test the new products in a wide range of different types of foods. This trial-and-error technique is both time-consuming and expensive, and gives very limited information about the protein. An alternative approach is to study simple model systems from which information about the complex nature of the proteins can be obtained and then to test the performance of the proteins in a restricted number of foods. Properties of interest include emulsion stability, foaming, gel strength, solubility, sorption, swelling, viscosity and wettability. The behaviour of proteins in simple model systems can give valuable indications of their uses but the information should be used with caution when trying to predict how a protein will act in a food system containing lipids, carbohydrates, other proteins, salts etc.

As part of a programme aimed at determining whether results from model systems can be extrapolated to predict how proteins will behave in a food system, we have undertaken a systematic study of physical properties, especially those related to water–protein interactions. An understanding of the latter should be valuable since they have a fundamental bearing on most biophysical parameters.

Solubility, swelling, viscosity, gel strength and sorption will be discussed together with preliminary results on the effect of added proteins on the texture of meatballs.

The proteins chosen for this work have characteristically different properties. They are a commercially available soya-bean protein isolate Promine-D, a sodium caseinate and a whey protein concentrate (WPC). A fish protein concentrate (FPC) and a rapeseed protein isolate (RPI) have also been studied but to a lesser extent.

II. WATER SOLUBILITY

When extracting and precipitating proteins during production, information on changes in solubility is of prime importance. Solubility is therefore the first functional property to be studied.

Figure 1 shows the solubility as a function of pH in 0·2 M NaCl.

Solubility data give a clue as to the restrictions rather than the possible applications of a given protein. An insoluble protein such as FPC, for example, cannot be used in beverages but may be advantageous in products such as bread and snacks to which inert materials can be added (Hermansson *et al.*, 1971).

As can be seen in Fig. 1 the solubility behaviour of the four protein systems varies markedly. The differences are even more marked when solubility is studied as a function of ionic strength, as shown in Fig. 2 for Promine-D, caseinate and WPC at pH 7.

This variation is due not only to the degree of denaturation and the

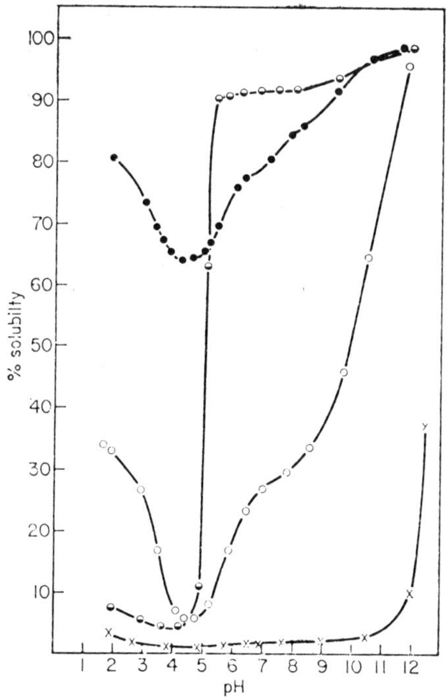

FIG. 1. Solubility as a function of pH in 0·2 M NaCl

- ○ Promine-D
- ◒ Caseinate
- ● WPC
- + FPC

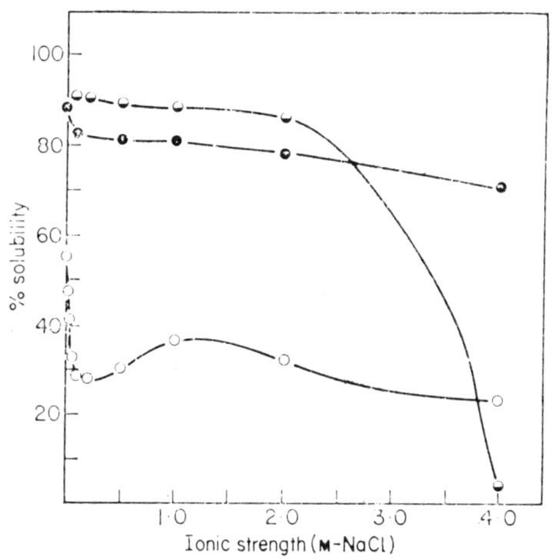

FIG. 2. Solubility as a function of ionic strength at pH 7

- ○ Promine-D
- ◒ Caseinate
- ● WPC

large number of proteins in the systems but also to changes in the interactions between the molecules, causing association and dissociation. Variations of pH and ionic strength cause such changes, which to some extent can explain the great differences in the solubility behaviour of complex protein systems.

Assuming that association leads to a decrease and dissociation to an increase in solubility, the characteristic behaviour of Promine-D (and other soya-bean protein isolates) can partly be explained by results from the ultracentrifugation studies of Wolf (1969) and Koshiyama (1968), who showed that at very low ionic strength the quarternary structure is unstable and dissociation occurs. This implies a relatively high solubility which is in agreement with the solubility data shown in Fig. 2. They also showed that the molecules associate at ionic strengths which correspond closely to our observed solubility minimum.

Caseinate has an even more complex quarternary structure than Promine-D. Therefore it is likely that the abrupt changes in solubility with pH and ionic strength are due to association–dissociation phenomena. Not only protein–protein interactions are of importance in determining solubility profiles but also association between protein molecules and other components with charged groups such as phytic acid.

Figure 2 also illustrates that caseinate and WPC possess similar solubility at moderate ionic strength, although WPC has a much simpler structure than does caseinate. They are also very different in many other respects and solubility alone cannot be used as a guide of functionality.

III. SWELLING

Since most foods are water-swollen systems, swelling should be a very important parameter but it is one that has been very little studied. This is due to the dearth of methods for investigating the swelling ability of partially soluble powders.

Swelling can be defined in terms of the spontaneous uptake of a solvent by a solid. It is a phenomenon frequently observed as the first step in the solvation of polymers, in which case swelling continues until the molecules are randomized within the system. In other cases solvation may be prevented by various intermolecular forces in the swollen sample, resulting in limited swelling and a definite volume increase.

As most proteins of interest as food additives are neither completely soluble nor insoluble in water, the concept of swelling cannot be defined rigorously and any description of their swelling behaviour must be empirical. In a typical semi-solid food product, an additive is supposed to bind a certain limited amount of water. This implies that, for proteins, swelling should be measured in terms of the ability to take up water in amounts smaller than those producing low viscosity dispersions.

A method has been developed for studying the relative swelling of proteins (Baumann, 1967; Hermansson, 1972). The spontaneous uptake of water is monitored in an apparatus, the basic design of which is shown in Fig. 3.

The glass equipment consists of a thermostated funnel connected with

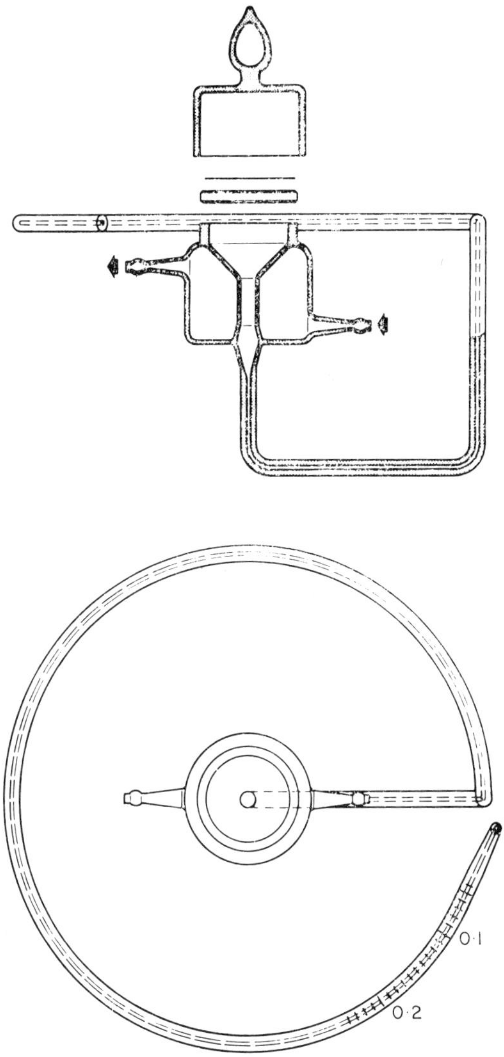

FIG. 3. The swelling apparatus

a horizontally located capillary. A sample is dusted on to a wetted filter paper fastened on a glass filter that is placed on top of the funnel filled with liquid. The uptake of fluid can be followed in the capillary. Loss of water vapour is prevented by the glass lid.

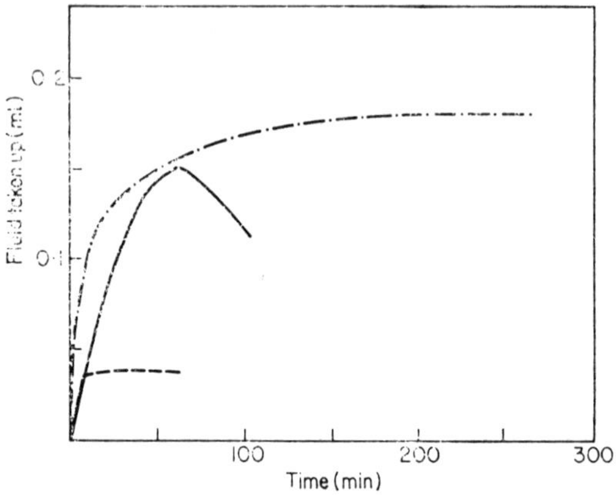

FIG. 4. Swelling as a function of time for 20 mg sample (Hermansson, 1972)

-·-·- Promine-D
—·— Caseinate
- - - - WPC

As can be seen from Fig. 4, Promine-D, caseinate and WPC have quite different swelling characteristics. The swelling of Promine-D reaches equilibrium after more than 3 h. The swelling of caseinate reaches a maximum after 1 h, then the protein loses its ability to hold water. Finally, WPC shows a low swelling ability. WPC swelling does not reach an equilibrium but a steady state. Thus, although both caseinate and WPC are highly soluble, their swelling abilities are markedly different. Further, the swelling behaviour of Promine-D is of a different character from that of caseinate and WPC, as is indicated by micrographs.

From Figs 5 and 6 it can be seen that the structure of both caseinate and WPC is rapidly destroyed by water uptake and swelling seems to be the first step in a solvation process. Promine-D, on the other hand, undergoes little structural change even after several hours, thus displaying a limited type of swelling (Fig. 7).

A. Swelling as Related to Viscosity

Whether or not swelling will reach a maximum and then decrease (as is the case for caseinate) depends on the ability of a soluble polymer to take up the amount of water necessary for solvation and for lowering the viscosity. When the molecules interact to a low degree and the viscosity is low, the solution will pass through the filter paper in the swelling apparatus. The WPC molecules are much smaller than those of caseinate and the viscosity of WPC dispersions are low. The degree of swelling is,

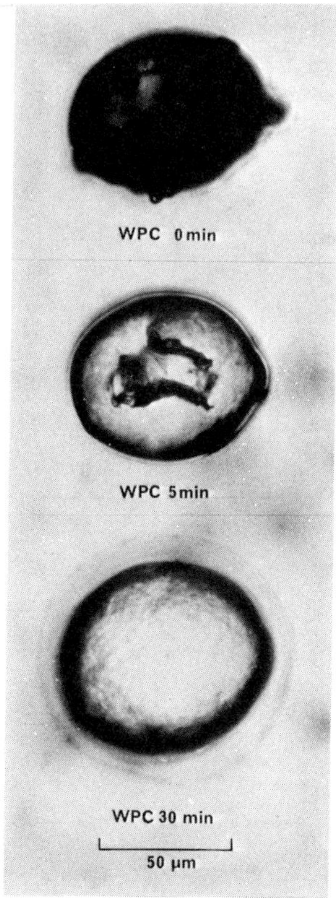

FIG. 5. Micrographs of WPC after swelling for 0, 5 and 30 min (Hermansson, 1972)

furthermore, dependent on osmotic pressure and Donnan effects. For small globular proteins such as those in WPC these effects are negligible and the degree of swelling before solvation is very low. Promine-D, which displays a limited swelling and has a high viscosity, will not pass through the filter paper.

B. Swelling as Related to Gel Strength

Gels are of importance for many types of foods as the gel structure can act as a matrix which holds moisture, lipids, polysaccharides and other ingredients. Brookfield viscosity is a measure of gel strength provided

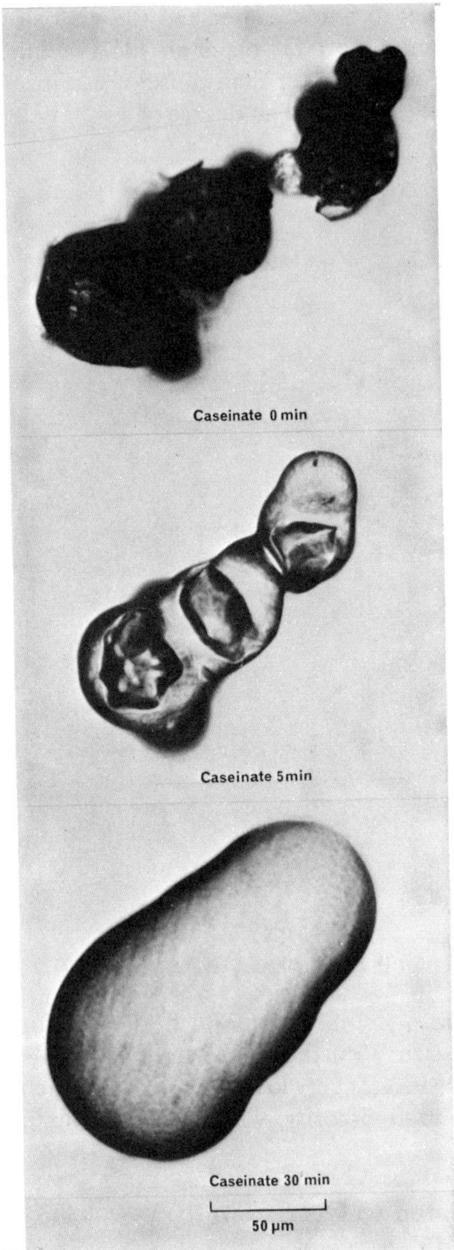

FIG. 6. Micrographs of caseinate after swelling for 0, 5 and 30 min (Hermansson, 1972)

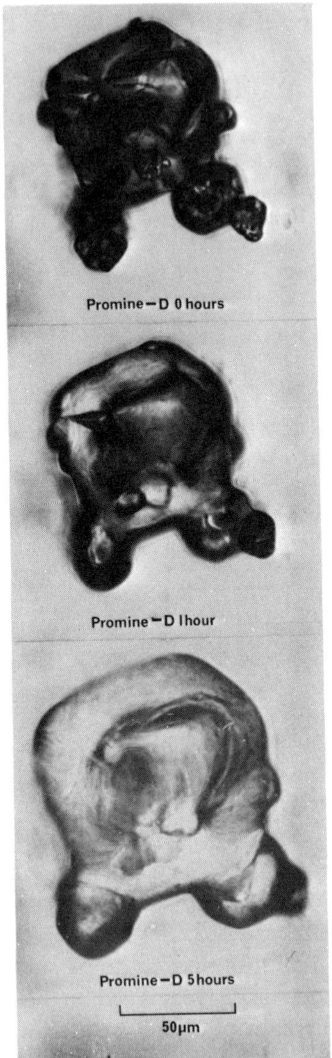

FIG. 7. Micrographs of Promine-D after swelling for 0, 1 and 5 h (Hermansson, 1972)

T-spindles and a Helipath stand are used. In this equipment the spindle moves down in a helical path through the material, always measuring undisturbed material. Gelation occurs for Promine-D and WPC but not for caseinate when dispersions of sufficient concentrations are being heated (Hermansson, 1972).

As can be seen from Fig. 8, the gel strength of WPC gels increases with heating temperature. The gel strength of Promine-D, on the other hand,

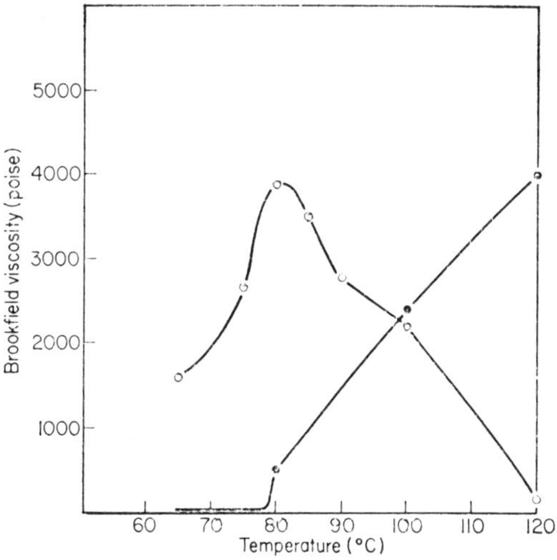

FIG. 8. Gel strength as a function of heating temperature. The TD-spindle at 2·5 rpm was used (Hermansson, 1972)

o Promine-D
• WPC

reaches a maximum and then decreases. According to work by Catsimpoolas and Meyer (1970) and Wolf (1970) the drop in gel strength for Promine-D is due to the disruption of the quarternary structure followed by dissociation, especially of the IIS-globulins.

It was considered of interest to see whether the formation of the gel structure had any influence on the swelling ability. The differently heated gels were accordingly freeze-dried, ground and the swelling ability rechecked.

From Fig. 9 it can be seen that gel formation increases the swelling ability of Promine-D and WPC, the former especially showing a very good correlation with gel strength.

Swelling, gel strength and high viscosity depend on the amount of free water associated with the macromolecules. (This constitutes the largest amount of water in fresh foods.) All these properties are highly influenced

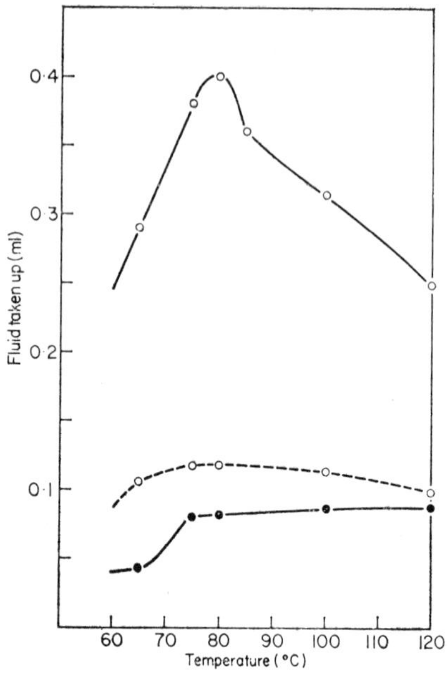

FIG. 9. Swelling as a function of heating temperature (Hermansson, 1972)

——o—— Promine-D in pure water
- - - -o- - - - Promine-D in 0·2 M NaCl
——•—— WPC in pure water

by changes in the electrostatic attractions between the molecules brought about by, for instance, pH and ionic strength changes.

C. Swelling as Related to Sorption

Sorption, unlike the properties mentioned above, gives a measure of the bound water that has physical properties different from those of free water. A sorption isotherm is shown in Fig. 10.

The isotherm can be divided into three regions.

(a) The first region of monolayer adsorption involves direct binding of water molecules to available polar groups on the protein with water–water interactions of relatively little significance.
(b) The addition of more water allows interactions among the water molecules and leads to the formation of a hydration shell, the structure of which is markedly different from that of free water.
(c) In the third region water–water interactions become more important and the water structure approaches that of free water.

Knowledge of sorption isotherms is of general importance for storage and drying conditions, as reactions responsible for deterioration in dehydrated foods are highly dependent on water activity.

It is of interest to determine whether sorption properties are related to the functional properties studied, especially swelling as sorption can be said to be the initial phase of swelling (Table I).

Table I shows the amount of water absorbed at three different water activities taken from region A, B and C and the swelling ability of the different protein systems. As well as protein systems already discussed, a non-heat-treated rapeseed isolate (RPI) is included in Table I. RPI is a protein product with poor swelling ability. It is seen that the sorption in

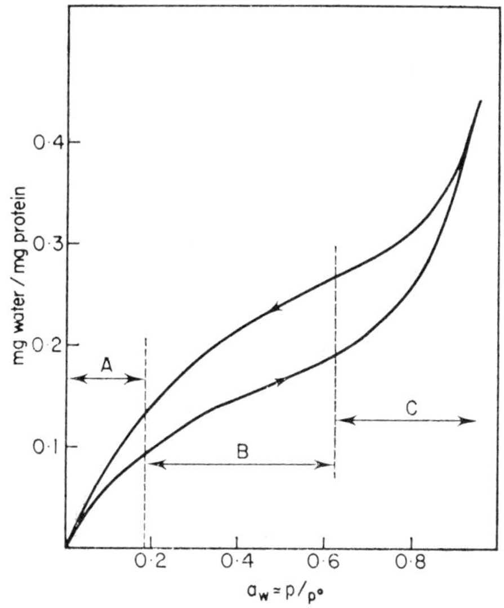

FIG. 10. General sorption isotherm

region B and to some extent in region C seems to increase with increasing swelling ability. The differences, however, are very small. It is, for example, not possible to distinguish between the differently heated Promine-D samples.

In the range of properties studied swelling is in an important intermediate position. Sorption seems to increase with swelling ability. Gel strength and swelling ability can be correlated. Swelling is also the first step in the solvation process. A highly soluble protein has poor water-binding properties, but a reverse relation between swelling and solubility is not observed. The results from studies in model systems on water–protein interactions indicate that swelling together with solubility data could be used as a guide to functionality.

TABLE I. Swelling and sorption

Protein system	*Swelling in pure water* (μl/mg)	*Sorption at three different* a_w (mg/mg)		
		0·10	0·40	0·70
RPI	1·6 max. value	0·038	0·080	0·149
WPC	1·8	0·042	0·087	0·172
WPC Heat-treated at 100°C	4·5	0·044	0·096	0·169
Caseinate	7·9 max. value	0·043	0·093	0·162
Promine-D	9·6	0·050	0·096	0·166
Promine-D Heat-treated at 120°C	12·5	0·047	0·101	0·170
Promine-D Heat-treated at 65°C	14·6	0·049	0·101	0·173
Promine-D Heat-treated at 100°C	15·8	0·049	0·101	0·175
Promine-D Heat-treated at 80°C	20·0	0·049	0·104	0·175

IV. DO PROPERTIES OF ADDED PROTEINS AFFECT FOOD TEXTURE?

Proteins to be incorporated into existing food products are usually added in relatively small amounts (*ca.* 5%). Therefore the most important questions are whether or not differences in the properties of added proteins really do cause differences in the texture of a processed food product and, if so, which of the properties are of importance for different types of textures. We feel that these questions have to be answered before the studied properties can be explained on a physical or chemical basis.

Recently a study was made on the influence of added proteins on the texture of meatballs, 50% of which was meat; 10% of the total mixture was replaced by 4% protein and 6% water. Table II shows some preliminary results when variously heat-treated Promine-D samples were incorporated. The same samples were used as in the swelling studies discussed above. The objective measurements were made in an Instron Universal Testing machine. The panel for sensory evaluation of firmness consisted of 10 experienced judges; 9-point scales were used.

It can be seen from Table II that heat treatment of the added soya-bean proteins caused some significant differences in both the objective and the subjective measurements. The addition of Promine-D, heat-treated at

Table II. Swelling and texture

Meat systems	*Swelling of added proteins in pure water* (μl/mg)	*Texture measurements on meatballs with 4% added protein*			
		Instrumental measurements		*Sensory measurements on firmness*	
		Extrusion force (Kp)	*Compression work* (g cm) (2nd cycle)	*Scoring*	*Ranking*
Reference Without added proteins		34·9	305·0	4·8	3·3
With Promine-D	9·6	38·1	236·6	3·7	2·4
With Promine-D Heat-treated at 65°C	14·6	38·5	282·6	5·2	3·7
With Promine-D Heat-treated at 80°C	20·0	48·5	305·0	5·3	3·9
With Promine-D Heat-treated at 100°C	15·8	39·2	228·0	3·2	1·7
Least significant Difference (5%)	$<$1·0	3·6	28·4	1·2	1·2

80°C, resulted in the highest values on firmness in the sensory evaluation and required the highest extrusion force and compression work. This protein sample also possessed the highest swelling ability and the highest gel strength before being freeze-dried. For this type of processed meat product it can be seen that changes in the properties of protein making up only 4% of the total mixture are of functional importance.

It seems that swelling is one property of importance for determining the texture of a semi-solid food product. In a complex food system, however, added proteins can interact with components such as other proteins, lipids and carbohydrates. Before any final conclusions can be drawn, these interactions have also to be thoroughly studied. It might then be possible to predict how a protein will behave in a food system and to choose a suitable application range for a new protein product by simple measurements in model systems.

ACKNOWLEDGEMENTS

Thanks are due to Mrs Margit Fjaervoll for her skilled and careful experimental assistance. Professors K. E. Thomé, B. Törnell and L. Å. Appelqvist are warmly thanked for their kind interest in this work and for valuable proposals and comments. The financial support of the Swedish Board for Technical Development is gratefully acknowledged.

REFERENCES

Baumann, H. (1967). *G-I-T* **6**, 540.
Catsimpoolas, N. and Meyer, E. W. (1970). *Cereal Chem.* **47**, 559–570.
Hermansson, A.-M. (1972). *Lebensm.-Wiss. u. Forsch.* **5**, 24–29.
Hermansson, A.-M., Sivik, B. and Skjöldebrand, C. (1971). *Lebensm.-Wiss. u. Forsch.* **4**, 201.
Koshiyama, I. (1968). *Agric. biol. Chem.* **32**, 879–899.
Wolf, W. J. (1969). *Baker's Dig.* **43**, 30.
Wolf, W. J. (1970). *J. agric. Fd Chem.* **18**, 969–976.

CHAPTER 28

Flavour Analysis of Protein Foods

E. VON SYDOW, T. PERSSON AND I. QVIST

Swedish Institute for Food Preservation Research, Göteborg 16, Sweden

I. INTRODUCTION

"Food has no nutritional value unless it is eaten", so the factors regulating consumption are indeed critical. Flavour is undoubtedly one of the more important factors involved. Thus, the understanding and analysis of flavour from the point of view of the consumer as well as from the point of view of food composition are important areas for research and development, particularly when it comes to developing new foods or introducing new raw materials such as unconventional proteins.

The sensory properties of foods are: appearance, texture, consistency and flavour, which is composed primarily of odour (aroma) and taste (von Sydow, 1971).

II. TECHNIQUES FOR MEASURING SUBSTANCES RESPONSIBLE FOR TASTE AND ODOUR

Taste and odour are physiologically and chemically different concepts which, however, interact at the psychological level in the human being, creating a combined sensation of flavour. A full understanding of flavour in foods demands, therefore, a psychophysical (sensory) study of the phenomena occurring in the human being, parallel to a physicochemical study and measurement of the chemical substances in the food which are acting as stimulants in the gustatory and olfactory systems.

What are the specific flavour problems involved when introducing new protein raw materials?

One of the main obstacles arises from the undesirable changes in flavour that frequently occur when using such proteins. In some cases it is a matter of the odour and taste of the protein raw material, which may differ from the conventional. In other cases, however, changes appear only after preparation and processing of the formulated food product. In this situation the proteins are acting as precursors for odour and taste compounds so that a change of protein also becomes a change in flavour.

In order to progress beyond trial-and-error testing, it was found essential to analyse the proteins—before and after heat treatment—with sensory and instrumental techniques in order to characterize the chemical changes which result in changes in flavour, i.e., in the taste and in odour.

The taste of these proteins originates mainly from salt, free amino acids, peptides and nucleotides. These compounds can be detected and their concentration determined by chromatographic techniques well known to the biochemist. Their contribution to flavour is more difficult to assess but various sensory techniques have been applied successfully by Japanese, American and Swiss scientists, enabling both qualitative and quantitative determinations to be made of their contribution to taste (cf. Solms, 1969; Kirimura *et al.*, 1969; Manley and Fagerson, 1971; Yamaguchi *et al.*, 1971). Heating mixtures containing proteins and carbohydrates often results in the formation of bitter-tasting compounds through Maillard-reactions (cf. Reynolds, 1970). These are difficult to determine either chemically or sensorially and more research is needed here.

Another source of substances contributing to taste is, of course, the presence of impurities derived from the manufacturing process.

This is also the case with odour. However, in many cases the protein raw materials can be made odour-free. As a result of heating, however, drastic changes in odour may occur.

In our experiments (von Sydow *et al.*, unpublished results) beef protein, soya-bean protein concentrate, sodium caseinate, fish protein concentrate and single cell protein concentrate are being analysed in model experiments with temperature, time of heating and formulation as the variable parameters. Beef protein is used as a reference material for the other proteins, but is also investigated from another point of view: the formation of "retort off-flavour" and the possibility of preventing the formation of this off-flavour during canning. The instrumental techniques being used are modifications of the head space gas chromatography and combined gas chromatography—mass spectrometry techniques described by von Sydow *et al.* (1970). About 100 volatile compounds can be traced, identified and measured quantitatively in each sample. The differences between the volatile compounds from the various proteins are mainly quantitative, although some qualitative differences are also found. It is believed that sulphur-containing volatile compounds are particularly important as sources of odours produced as a result of heating. A special photometric detector which is about 100 times more sensitive for sulphur-containing compounds than standard GC-detectors has proved to be particularly valuable (Brody and Chaney, 1966).

The sensory evaluation is carried out using an odour assessment technique previously applied in our laboratories (von Sydow, 1971; von Sydow *et al.*, 1970; von Sydow and Karlsson, 1971).

From a practical point of view it is crucial to be able to correlate sensory with instrumental data to permit the correct interpretation of the chemical results. Several mathematical and psychophysical models have been tested by us with varying degrees of success (von Sydow, 1971; Persson and von Sydow, 1972).

III. APPLICATIONS

The results so far show distinct possibilities of using the combined technique of instrumental and sensory methods for measuring food quality properties in quality control work. The combined technique may be used to evaluate such aspects as: deterioration during storage, over-heating during processing, and faulty raw materials. Many conventional processed foods suffer from certain undesirable properties such as retort flavour. The correlation technique described opens up new possibilities of relating the source of these properties to the chemical composition of the food, thus enabling new and improved food products to be developed.

An even more valuable application of this technique may be found in the development of food products from new, unconventional raw materials, such as protein preparations derived from fish, rapeseed and micro-organisms (single cell protein).

The results obtained so far support what was known from a practical, trial-and-error approach to the incorporation of proteins in foods and, more important, suggest a chemical basis for the undesirable and desirable changes. Thus they will enable recommendations to be made about product preparation and formulation and also about manufacturing procedures using the unconventional protein raw materials.

REFERENCES

Brody, S. S. and Chaney, J. E. (1966). *J. Gas Chromat.* **4**, 42–46.

Kirimura, J., Shimizu, A., Kimizuka, A., Ninomiya, T. and Katsuya, N. (1969). *J. agric. Fd Chem.* **17**, 689–695.

Manley, C. H. and Fagerson, I. S. (1971). *Flavour Ind.* **2**, 686–690.
Persson, T. and von Sydow, E. (1972). *J. Fd Sci.* **37**, 234–239.
Reynolds, T. M. (1970). *Fd Technol. Aust.* **22**, 610–611, 613, 615–619.
Solms, J. (1969). *J. agric. Fd Chem.* **17**, 686–688.
von Sydow, E. (1971). *Fd Technol., Champaign* **25**, 40–44.
von Sydow, E., Andersson, J., Anjou, K., Karlsson, G., Land, D. and Griffiths, N. (1970). *Lebensm.-Wiss. u. Technol.* **3**, 11–17.
von Sydow, E. and Karlsson, G. (1971). *Lebensm.-Wiss. u. Technol.* **4**, 152–157.
Yamaguchi, S., Yoshikawa, T., Ikeda, S. and Ninomiya, T. (1971). *J. Fd Sci.* **36**, 846–849.

CHAPTER 29

Evaluation of the Textural Properties of Protein Foods

P. SHERMAN

Queen Elizabeth College, London, England

I. INTRODUCTION

With the advent of proteins derived from hydrocarbon oils, microbiological sources and soya-beans the quantitative evaluation of the texture of food products into which these proteins are incorporated has developed into a problem of importance. The solution of this problem is not easy since the General Foods "texture profile" concept has clearly shown that the blanket term "texture" embraces a large number of properties which are sensorily identified in succession, but independently, by the consumer (Szczesniak, 1963; Szczesniak *et al.*, 1963; Brandt *et al.*, 1963). Consequently, instrumental techniques are required to quantify a wide range of textural properties rather than just "texture". For the purposes of the present discussion the term "texture" will be avoided; instead the phrase "textural properties" will be adopted.

Consumer studies involving controlled word-association tests (Szczesniak and Kleyn, 1963; Yoshikawa *et al.*, 1970a, 1970b, 1970c) have shown that although a large number of descriptive terms are used to indicate the textural properties of foods only a few terms have a high frequency of recurrence. These are: hard, soft, juicy, chewy, greasy, viscous, creamy, crisp, crunchy and brittle. Thus, in general terms the adjectives most frequently used denote different degrees of hardness, cohesiveness and moisture content (Szczesniak and Kahn, 1971). A recent study specifically related to hard and soft gels, and pastes, prepared from powdered soya-

TABLE I. Instrumental techniques utilized to evaluate the textural properties of foods

Technique	*Food on which employed*	*Reference*
1. Creep compliance-time studies		
(a) simple shear with parallel plate viscoelastometer	heat coagulated fish paste	Kishimoto and Makawa (1962)
	frozen ice cream	Shaw (1963); Shama and Sherman (1966)
	cake, margarine	Shama and Sherman (1968)
(b) compression between parallel plates	fruit, vegetables	Somers (1965); Mohsenin and Göhlich (1962) Mohsenin *et al.* (1963).
	bread	Cornford *et al.* (1964)
	margarine, butter	Sone (1961); Sone *et al.* (1962)
	natural cheese	Davis (1937)
	processed cheese	Szabó (1966)
(c) extension	noodles	Shimizu *et al.* (1958)
	meat	Bendall (1951); Bendall and Davey (1957)
	dough	Schofield and Scott Blair (1933a, 1933b); Glucklich and Shelef (1962a, 1962b); Shelef and Bousso (1964)
(d) coaxial cylinder viscometer	cream	Prentice (1968); Prentice and Chapman (1969)
2. Stress relaxation at constant strain	fruit, vegetables	Somers (1965); Mohsenin and Morrow (1968)
	noodles	Shimizu *et al.* (1958)
	milk gels	Scott Blair and Burnett (1959a; 1959b)
3. Chewing sounds recorded during mastication	rusks, crisp bread, crackers, potato chips, apples, beef, lettuce, peanuts, chewing gum	Drake (1963)
	apple, banana, peanuts, raw carrots, biscuits, rusks, crisp bread, wafers	Drake (1965)
4. Penetrometers	butter, margarine	Haighton (1959, 1965); De Man (1969a, 1969b)

Technique	*Food on which employed*	*Reference*
	margarine	Sambuc *et al.* (1969, 1970, 1971); Naudet *et al.* (1959)
	processed cheese, peanut butter	De Man (1969b)
	chocolate	Klienert (1969)
5. Instron Tensile Tester	(see Table III)	
6. General Foods Texturometer	large range of foods, cakes, dog food, bran flakes, strawberries, biscuits, apples, cheese, toffee, fish, banana, potato, turnip, chocolate	Szczesniak *et al.* (1963) Friedman *et al.* (1963) Szczesniak & Smith (1969) Brennan *et al.* (1970)
7. Kramer shear press	meat	Kramer *et al.* (1951)
	fruit gels	Kramer and Hawbecker (1966)
	apple, cheese	Brennan *et al.* (1970)
	peas	Angel and Kramer (1969)
	baked beans	Voisey and Larmond (1971)
8. Extrusion through fine orifice	hardened fats	Soltoft (1947)
	butter, margarine, shortenings	Prentice (1952, 1954, 1959); Naudet *et al.* (1959)

bean and wheat proteins (Toda *et al.*, 1971) using non-oral sensory evaluation in conjunction with instrumental evaluation suggests that the most important textural parameters are hardness, springiness and adhesiveness. Cohesiveness and gumminess were not considered to be very important properties of these gels.

II. INSTRUMENTAL METHODS FOR EVALUATING TEXTURAL PROTEINS

A. General

Procedures for the sensory evaluation of textural properties by texture profile panels and by consumer studies are now well documented, but much confusion still exists regarding instrumental evaluation of these textural properties. A large number of instruments has been used over the years and examples are quoted in Table I. With many of these one does not really know what is being measured because samples are subjected to complex mechanical actions which cannot be analysed easily. For example, the factors controlling the penetration of a punch into a food vary with the textural properties of the food. Penetration ". . . of cellular products

TABLE II. Test conditions employed with Instron tensile tester when evaluating the textural properties of foods

Food	*Crosshead speed*	*Data analysis*	*Reference*
Snap beans	10 cm/min	firmness evaluated as maximum force required to move 9·5 cm diameter piston to 0·635 cm from bottom of 10·3 cm diameter cylinder containing 250 g randomly orientated beans	Van Buren (1968)
Apple tissue	no speeds quoted	firmness evaluated as force necessary to compress a cylinder of 1 cm to 0·5 cm	Stirling (1968)
Meat	1 in./min		Pool (1967)
Wheat grain	0·02 in./min	based on uniaxial compression by parallel plates, indenter, punch etc.	Shelef and Mohsenin (1967)
Peas	20 cm/min	tenderness measured by puncture test with pin attachment	Casimir *et al.* (1967)
Meat	no speeds quoted	determined maximum force for puncture and also shearing force; penetration and shear measure tenderness	Kulwick *et al.* (1963)
Apples	punch speed or 5 cm/min; puncture test with Magness–Taylor pressure tips (1·11 or 0·79 cm diameter)	yield point force corresponds to "subjective thumb test" of firmness	Bourne (1965)

Food	*Crosshead speed*	*Data analysis*	*Reference*
Potato chips	2 cm/s needles, punches, and compression tests	crispness characterized by resistance to deformation under load up to point of sudden fracture; area under force-distance curve related to ease of mastication	Bourne *et al.* (1966)
Carrots	compression–0·05 in./min; shear (downwards) —2·0 in./min; compression and shear (upward) —2·0 in./min	evaluated compressibility; correlated with sensory evaluation, but no correlation between maximum shear force and sensory evaluation	Howard and Heinz (1970)
Peas	5 cm/min	calculated hardness, brittleness, elasticity, gumminess and chewiness	Bourne (1968)
Poultry meat	1 in./min	measured cohesiveness	Pool (1967)

such as fruits . . . may involve shear and compression factors. In products with strongly bound network structures, e.g. processed cheese, the main factors are shear and flow. In products with weakly bound network structures, such as plastic fats, flow is the only major factor involved" (De Man, 1969a). Furthermore, penetration may continue for a long time, albeit at a progressively slower rate, into very soft foods whereas it is complete in a few seconds with hard foods.

Another instrument showing variable behaviour is the Kramer Shear Press. It used to be assumed that shear and compression were the only forces involved in the extrusion of the food sample through the bars in the base of the sample cell, but recently it has been shown (Szczesniak, *et al.*, 1970) that extrusion forces play a major role, and that most foods are subjected to a combination of all three forces when they are evaluated with the Shear Press.

Proctor and his co-workers (Proctor *et al.*, 1955; Proctor *et al.*, 1956a, 1956b) designed a tenderometer utilizing artificial jaws with plastic dentures to simulate human chewing motions. However, little attempt appears to have been made to establish whether data obtained with this instrument correlated satisfactorily with sensorily evaluated textural properties. The dental literature suggests that wearers of complete dentures exert much smaller chewing forces, and consequently show lower chewing efficiencies, than subjects with natural dentition (Yurkstas and Emerson, 1964; Khang, 1966). Furthermore, teeth are displaced in their sockets during chewing, and consecutive chewing thrusts may be applied before teeth are able to return to their original positions. This means that each time opposing teeth come together in a series of chewing thrusts they tend to lie in different positions in their sockets relative to each other (Picton, 1962, 1964; Lewin, 1970). All these observations throw doubt on the validity of the assumption that data obtained with the Proctor tenderometer can be used to predict what occurs in normal masticatory processes.

B. Instron Tensile Tester

The instrument which has been used most widely to evaluate textural properties is undoubtedly the table model Instron Tensile Tester. Nevertheless, a perusal of published textural studies involving this instrument indicates quite clearly that there has been no uniformity in the test conditions which have been applied with respect to the load applied, the rate of load application, etc. In fact, it appears that test conditions have been selected quite arbitrarily with little consideration having been given to the conditions which prevail when the consumer evaluates textural properties. Table II quotes several examples of the test conditions which have been reported in published literature.

Since the results obtained with the Instron Tensile Tester depend on the way in which it is operated, i.e. the force–compression–crosshead speed interrelationship, it is imperative that the selected test conditions simulate as closely as possible the physical situation during sensory evaluation of textural properties by the consumer. Most foods exhibit viscoelasticity, which means that they can behave either as solids (elasticity) or as liquids (viscosity) depending on the test conditions to which they are subjected. Their behaviour will, therefore, be influenced by the rate of loading and the magnitude of the applied load. The rate at which force is applied to food during mastication depends on its textural characteristics, and the harder the food the slower the rate at which the teeth come together in a biting motion (Dahlberg, 1942).

A mathematical (Fourier) analysis of published chewing (force-time) curves shows that the "first bite" phase of mastication can be satisfactorily represented by a linear compression pattern up to the point of maximum force application (Shama and Sherman, 1972). Sensory evaluation studies with a "texture profile" panel have indicated that many textural properties, such as hardness, brittleness, crispness, are evaluated during the "first bite" phase using the front teeth or molars. Consequently, it is unlikely that saliva will have had much effect on the food at this stage,

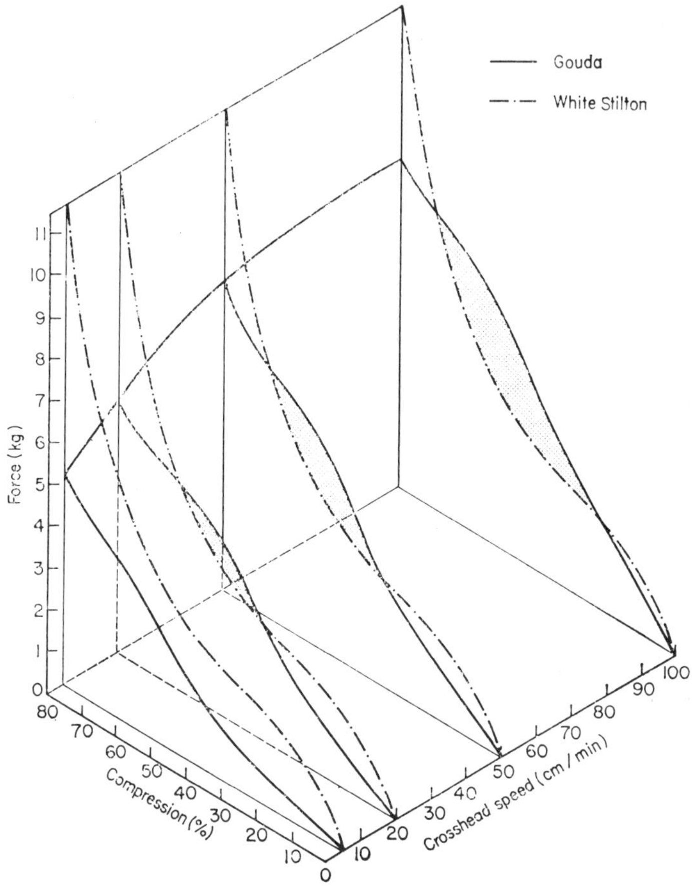

FIG. 1. Three-dimensional plot indicating the method for determining the judgment regions

and the evaluation of the aforementioned textural properties can be simulated by a compression test with the Instron Tensile Tester provided the correct loading conditions are employed.

The problem of correct test conditions can be exemplified by quoting a study on the relative hardness of the two cheeses, Gouda and White Stilton (Shama and Sherman, 1972). Figure 1 shows force–compression data obtained at several different rates of loading. At a crosshead speed of 5 cm/min the force–compression curve for White Stilton always lies above the curve for Gouda cheese, so that according to these instrumental test conditions White Stilton is harder than Gouda. Utilizing crosshead speeds of 20, 50 or 100 cm/min the curves for the two cheeses intersect and cross over at two points which, in terms of force or % compression, move further apart as the crosshead speed increases. Thus, at the three higher crosshead speeds instrumental evaluation of the relative hardness of the two cheeses depends on the operative conditions, with Gouda appearing to be the harder cheese under certain force–compression–crosshead speed conditions and White Stilton appearing to be the harder cheese under the other test conditions. In sensory evaluation tests with a "texture profile" panel Gouda cheese was always rated harder than White Stilton. The instrumental test condition regions which conform with this evaluation are indicated in Fig. 1 by the shaded regions. By combining these shaded regions a three-dimensional surface is obtained which delineates the instrumental test conditions which can be used when simulating the sensory evaluation of hardness of Gouda and White Stilton cheeses.

III. PROBLEMS OF TERMINOLOGY

A similar approach should be utilized to define permissible instrumental test conditions for evaluating other textural parameters. One serious drawback impedes progress at present in this, or any other, approach. This is the lack of generally accepted definitions for the various textural properties which need to be examined. Until these properties have been defined in clear and unambiguous terms we do not really know what it is that we require to identify and measure. Some idea of the confusion which exists at present over this problem can be obtained by referring to Table III, which summarizes various definitions for the textural properties stickiness, brittle and hardness. For example, in the case of hardness some of the definitions suggest that it is a bulk property of the food, whereas other definitions suggest that it is a surface property. It is interesting to compare these definitions with others which were derived from discussions with a "texture profile" panel. The definitions proposed by the panel members were as follows:

Hard—the force required to penetrate and/or compress the food with the teeth

Brittle—a sudden break of the sample following little or no penetration and characterized by the tendency to leave rough pieces with sharp edges when the sample is broken. Brittleness is often found in association with hardness.

Sticky—the work required to remove the food adhering to the teeth, gums, cheeks etc. during the process of mastication.

TABLE III. Published definitions for some textural properties of foods

1. ADHESIVENESS: STICKINESS

(a) The force that resists the separation of two bodies in contact (Reiner and Scott Blair, 1967).

(b) The force necessary to overcome the attractive force between the surface of the food and the surface of the other materials with which the food comes into contact (Szczesniak, 1963).

(c) Buccal sensation due to a pasty product, sticking to the teeth or palate (Centre National de Coordination des Études et Recherches sur la Nutrition et l'Alimentation).

(d) Sensed by the mouth while chewing foods with adhesive properties (Kramer and Twigg, 1959).

(e) Simple tactual perception which consists of a field of light contact or pressure points. It includes the deeper seated pull as well as the superficial light contact which are set up when the sticky stimulus separates from the skin. Stickiness is aroused by a moving stimulus only (Zigler, 1923).

2. BRITTLE

(a) Textural property characterized by breaking easily and leaving sharp edges (Amerine *et al.*, 1965).

(b) Force with which a material fractures. It is related to hardness and cohesiveness. In brittle materials cohesiveness is low and hardness can vary from low to high (Szczesniak, 1963).

(c) Disintegration of a food into small fragments due to the masticating process (Centre National de Coordination des Études et Recherches sur la Nutrition et l'Alimentation).

(d) Apt to break, fragile (Concise Oxford Dictionary).

(e) Behaviour of a solid which is not very deformable when it breaks without appreciable permanent deformation. Mode of rupture of a solid when the separation of the two parts is not preceded by slippage in the ruptured zone (*Fr. Soc. Rheol.*).

(f) Tending to break under the conditions of minimal previous plastic deformation (Reiner and Scott Blair, 1967).

3. HARDNESS

(a) Resistance of the surface of a body to penetration (Reiner and Scott Blair, 1967).

(b) Resistance of a solid to penetration i.e. to deformation of its surface (*Fr. Soc. Rheol.*).

(c) Capacity for resisting penetration (Mohsenin, 1970).

(d) That which offers resistance to mastication or deformation (Centre National de Coordination des Études et Recherches sur la Nutrition et l'Alimentation).

(e) Firm, unyielding to the touch (Concise Oxford Dictionary).

(f) Force necessary to attain a given deformation (Szczesniak, 1963).

(g) Hardness is not considered a fundamental property of solids but as a composite property dependent on the elastic moduli, the elastic limits, etc. (Matz, 1962).

It may also be mentioned that members of the "texture profile" panel did not use, nor did they understand, the term "elastic". It was confused with sticky and/or rubbery depending on the magnitude of other identifiable textural properties.

IV. A MODIFIED "TEXTURE PROFILE"

In this chapter the emphasis has been placed on sensory evaluation of the textural properties of a food while it is undergoing mastication in the mouth. This is in accord with the General Foods "texture profile" methodology, but it should be recognized that sensory evaluation of textural properties begins in some form as soon as the consumer sees or handles the food. Visual examination develops the initial impression, and this is modified when the food is handled. Further modification of the impression then follows when the food is inserted into the mouth and chewed. Therefore, a truly comprehensive "texture profile" of a food will incorporate the results of all possible modes of evaluating textural properties (Sherman, 1969, 1971). The force–deformation conditions appertaining to non-masticatory evaluation of textural properties will have to be identified, using principles similar to those adapted for simulating masticatory action, so that instrumental methods can be utilized on a broader basis.

REFERENCES

Amerine, M. A., Pangborn, R. M. and Roessler, E. B. (1965). "Principles of Sensory Evaluation of Food." Academic Press, New York.

Angel, S. and Kramer, A. (1969). *J. Texture Stud.* **1**, 90–108.

Bendall, J. R. (1951). *J. Physiol., Lond.* **114**, 71–88.

Bendall, J. R. and Davey, C. L. (1957). *Biochim. biophys. Acta* **26**, 93–103.

Bourne, M. C. (1965). *Fd Technol., Champaign* **19**, 413–415.

Bourne, M. C. (1968). *J. Fd Sci.* **33**, 223–226.

Bourne, M. C., Moyer, J. C. and Hand, D. B. (1966). *Fd Technol., Champaign* **20**, 522–526.

Brandt, M. A., Skinner, E. Z. and Coleman, J. A. (1963). *J. Fd Sci.* **28**, 404–409.

Brennan, J. G., Jowitt, R. and Mughsi, O. A. (1970). *J. Texture Stud.* **1**, 167–184.

Casimir, D. J., Mitchell, R. S., Lynch, L. J. and Moyer, J. C. (1967). *Fd Technol., Champaign* **21**, 427–432.

Cornford, S. J., Axford, D. W. E. and Elton, G. A. H. (1964). *Cereal Chem.* **41**, 216.

Dahlberg, B. (1942). *Acta med. scand.* Suppl. no. 139.

Davis, J. G. (1937). *J. Dairy Res.* **8**, 245–264.

De Man, J. M. (1969a). *J. Texture Stud.* **1**, 109–113.
De Man, J. M. (1969b). *J. Texture Stud.* **1**, 114–119.
Drake, B. K. (1963). *J. Fd Sci.* **28**, 233-241.
Drake, B. (1965). *Biorheology* **3**, 21.
Friedman, H. H., Whitney, J. E. and Szczesniak, A. S. (1963). *J. Fd Sci.* **28**, 390–396.
Glucklich, J. and Shelef, L. (1962a). *Cereal Chem.* **39**, 242.
Glucklich, J. and Shelef, L. (1962b). *Kolloid-Z. u. Z. Polymere* **181**, 29–33.
Haighton, A. J. (1959). *J. Am. Oil Chem. Soc.* **36**, 345–348.
Haighton, A. J. (1965). *J. Am. Oil Chem. Soc.* **42**, 27–30.
Howard, P. L. and Heinz, D. E. (1970). *J. Texture Stud.* **1**, 185-195.
Khang, L. (1966). *Malaysian dent. J.* **6**, 18.
Kishimoto, A. and Makawa, E. (1962). *Bull. Jap. Soc. scient. Fish.* **28**, 803.
Kleinert, J. (1969). *Int. Choc. Rev.* **24**, 406–412.
Kramer, A. and Hawbecker, J. V. (1966). *Fd Technol., Champaign* **20**, 209-213.
Kramer, A. and Twigg, B. A. (1959). *Adv. Fd Res.* **9**, 153–220.
Kramer, A., Burckhardt, G. J. and Rogers, H. P. (1951). *Canner* **112**, 34.
Kulwich, R., Decker, R. W. and Alsmeyer, R. H. (1963). *Fd Technol., Champaign* **17**, 201–203.
Lewin, A. (1970). *J. dent. Res.* **49**, 699.
Matz, S. A. (1962). "Food Texture." Avi Publishing Co., Westport, Conn.
Mohsenin, N. N. (1970). "Physical Properties of Plant and Animal Materials", Vol. I. Gordon and Breach, New York.
Mohsenin, N. N. and Gohlich, H. (1962). *J. agric. Engng Res.* **7**, 300.
Mohsenin, N. N. and Morrow, C. T. (1968). *In* "Rheology and Texture of Foodstuffs" p. 50. *S.C.I. Monogr.* no. 27.
Mohsenin, N. N., Cooper, H. E. and Tukey, L. B. (1963). *Trans. ASAE* **6**, 85.
Naudet, M., Sambuc, E. and Desnuelle, P. (1959). *Revue fr. Cps gras* **6**, 4–9.
Picton, D. C. A. (1962). *Archs oral Biol.* **7**, 151.
Picton, D. C. A. (1964). *Archs oral Biol.* **9**, 565.
Pool, M. F. (1967). *J. Fd Sci.* **32**, 550–553.
Prentice, J. H. (1952). *B.F.M.I.R.A. Res. Rep.* no. 37.
Prentice, J. H. (1954). *Lab. Pract.* **3**, 186–189.
Prentice, J. H. (1959). *B.F.M.I.R.A. Res. Rep.* no. 94.
Prentice, J. H. (1968). *In* "Rheology and Texture of Foodstuffs", p. 265. *S.C.I. Monogr.* no. 27.
Prentice, J. H. and Chapman, H. R. (1969). *J. Dairy Res.* **36**, 269–278.
Proctor, B. E., Davison, S. and Brody, A. L. (1956a). *Fd Technol., Champaign* **10**, 327–331.
Proctor, B. E., Davison, S. and Brody, A. L. (1956b). *Fd Technol., Champaign* **10**, 344–346.
Proctor, B. E., Davison, S., Malecki, G. J. and Welch, M. (1955). *Fd Technol., Champaign* **9**, 471–477.
Reiner, M. and Scott Blair, G. W. (1967). *In* "Rheology: Theory and Applications", Vol. 4 (F. Eirich, ed.). Academic Press, New York.

SAMBUC, E. and NAUDET, M. (1969). *Revue fr. Cps gras* **16**, 701–712.
SAMBUC, E. and NAUDET, M. (1970). *Revue fr. Cps gras* **17**, 221–233.
SAMBUC, E., REYMOND, G. and NAUDET, M. (1971). *Revue fr. Cps gras* **18**, 215–225.
SCHOFIELD, R. K. and SCOTT BLAIR, G. W. (1933a). *Proc. R. Soc.* A**139**, 557–566.
SCHOFIELD, R. K. and SCOTT BLAIR, G. W. (1933b). *Proc. R. Soc.* A**141**, 72–85.
SCOTT BLAIR, G. W. and BURNETT, J. (1959a). *Br. J. appl. Phys.* **10**, 15–20.
SCOTT BLAIR, G. W. and BURNETT, J. (1959b). *Br. J. appl. Phys.* **10**, 97–99.
SHAMA, F. and SHERMAN, P. (1966). *J. Fd Sci.* **31**, 699–706.
SHAMA, F. and SHERMAN, P. (1968). *In* "Rheology and Texture of Foodstuffs", p. 77. *S.C.I. Monogr.* no. 27.
SHAMA, F. and SHERMAN, P. (1972). Paper to be presented at 5th Int. Congr. Rheology, Lyons, France, September.
SHAW, D. J. (1963). *In* "Rheology of Emulsions": proc. symp. 1962 (P. Sherman, ed.) pp. 125–131. Pergamon Press, Oxford.
SHELEF, L. and BOUSSO, D. (1964). *Rheol. Acta* **3**, 168–172.
SHELEF, L. and MOHSENIN, N. N. (1967). *Cereal Chem.* **44**, 392.
SHERMAN, P. (1969). *J. Fd Sci.* **34**, 458–462.
SHERMAN, P. (1971). *Rheol. Acta.* **10**, 121–126.
SHIMIZU, T., FUKAWA, H. and ICHIBA, A. (1958). *Cereal Chem.* **35**, 34.
SOLTOFT, P. (1947). Doctoral Dissertation, Copenhagen.
SOMERS, G. F. (1965). *J. Fd Sci.* **30**, 922–929.
SONE, T. (1961). *J. phys. Soc. Japan* **16**, 961.
SONE, T., FUKUSHIMA, M. and FUKADA, E. (1962). *Int. Dairy Congr. 16, Copenhagen* **B**, 165–174.
STIRLING, C. (1968). *J. Fd Sci.* **33**, 577.
SZABÓ, G. (1966). *Int. Dairy Congr. 17, München* **D**, 257–262.
SZCZESNIAK, A. S. (1963). *J. Fd Sci.* **28**, 385–389.
SZCZESNIAK, A. S., BRANDT, M. A. and FRIEDMAN, H. H. (1963). *J. Fd Sci.* **28**, 397–403.
SZCZESNIAK, A. S., HUMBAUGH, P. R. and BLOCK, H. W. (1970). *J. Texture Stud.* **1**, 356–378.
SZCZESNIAK, A. S. and KAHN, E. L. (1971). *J. Texture Stud.* **2**, 280-295.
SZCZESNIAK, A. S. and KLEYN, D. H. (1963). *Fd Technol., Champaign* **17**, 74–77.
SZCZESNIAK, A. S. and SMITH, B. J. (1969). *J. Texture Stud.* **1**, 65–89.
TODA, J., WADA, T., YASUMATSU, K. and ISHII, K. (1971). *J. Texture Stud.* **2**, 207–219.
VAN BUREN, J. P. (1968). *Fd Technol., Champaign* **22**, 790–793.
VOISEY, P. W. and LARMOND, E. (1971). *J. Texture Stud.* **2**, 96–109.
YOSHIKAWA, S., NISHIMARU, S., TASHIRO, T. and YOSHIDA, M. (1970a). *J. Texture Stud.* **1**, 437–442.
YOSHIKAWA, S., NISHIMARU, S., TASHIRO, T. and YOSHIDA, M. (1970b). *J. Texture Stud.* **1**, 443–451.

Yoshikawa, S., Nishimaru, S., Tashiro, T. and Yoshida, M. (1970c). *J. Texture Stud.* **1**, 452–463.
Yurkstas, A. A. and Emerson, W. H. (1964). *J. prosth. Dent.* **14**, 931.
Zigler, M. J. (1923). *Am. J. Psychol.* **34**, 73.

CHAPTER 30 (DISCUSSION)

What is the Role of Food Science and Technology?

E. J. ROLFE

National College of Food Technology (University of Reading), Weybridge, Surrey, England

I. SOME PRACTICAL PROBLEMS IN FOOD TECHNOLOGY

Perhaps the most difficult aspect of the food problem is the conversion of proteins into articles of diet acceptable in terms of both palatability and price. Present effort in terms of protein production is designed to fulfil one of the following three main areas of consumer need:

1. Feed for animals (which are in turn used for food or to produce food for human consumption).
2. Food for affluent communities.
3. Food for poorer communities, which must be cheap but also palatable and nutritious.

Our attention has been directed to the conversion of dietetically unattractive proteins into forms more palatable in terms of flavour, appearance and texture. At present this is largely accomplished by route (1). Those in the affluent community prefer, and are able to choose, to eat one fresh egg rather than the 2–3 oz of cereal, soya-bean or single cell protein that the hen must consume in order to produce the egg.

Food conversion by means of animals is an inefficient and wasteful process, and this has stimulated the attempts being made to use science and technology to convert new or unconventional proteins directly into acceptable foods.

It is becoming apparent, however, that developing the new protein food is the easiest hurdle to overcome: the really difficult problems arise from a complex interplay of many economic factors, not least of which is to persuade people to eat a novel food. The problems are no less difficult in the developing countries. A food, no matter how cheap, still costs money to buy, and can be purchased only where employment is provided. The economic situation is complex and the solution elusive and difficult. Apparently cheap novel protein foods turn out to be too expensive for the people for whom they were developed and one is still faced with the resistance to change in food habits.

In many parts of the world the real income of the bulk of the population is rising as a result of increasing industrialization, and consequently the structure of demand is changing with a move towards luxury and leisure. This is apparent not only from the increased sales of television sets and cars but from its influence on the demand for food, in two aspects in particular: convenience foods that reduce the drudgery of food preparation in the kitchen and greater pressure on the limited supplies of the more attractive foods such as dairy products and meat. The latter is costly to produce, and in addition prices tend to be enhanced by scarcity.

The question many are attempting to answer is to what extent such considerations justify an increase in the stimulus of the search for novel foods such as meat analogues based on vegetable and other cheap protein sources. The quality of such products will improve with the development of the synthesizing ability of the technologist and manufacturer.

At present attempts are being made—with considerable success—to produce more cheaply foods of animal origin such as barley beef and broiler chickens. However, the "synthetic" substitutes should still be less costly, and they have what could be a very significant advantage: the manufacturer could control precisely the important quality aspects of texture, flavour and composition to meet the preference of the consumer.

The health aspects of diet are a matter of concern, for instance sugar and animal fats are both suspect as factors causing the increased incidence of atherosclerosis. By allowing precise control of composition, "synthetic" foods can be used to provide balanced nutrition and remove or reduce the level of undesirable components of the diet. A "synthetic" steak can be made completely free of animal fat.

To what extent is reasoning of this kind likely to influence the consumer? The expansion in the demand for so-called "health" foods indicates some concern, but represents only a small section of the public. Margarine is eaten more as a cheap substitute for butter than as a means of avoiding the ingestion of animal fats. Publicity about the adverse effects on health of smoking appears to have had little effect on tobacco consumption. It could be concluded that considerations of health play little part in influencing the consumer's choice of diet, but this could be an overpessimistic view. The widespread problem of obesity has given rise to an interest in nutrition and food requirements in a large section of the public, and one can expect the teaching of health and nutrition to increase in schools.

At the moment, however, whether or not the production of a new food is a successful operation will depend on cost and quality relative to competitive alternative foods.

But should force of circumstance—such as war or economics—cut off a food supply, there may be no alternative to the "synthetic" food, and effort would be directed to producing the substitute. Such conditions led to the preparation of what was probably the first protein food analogue. Wiking Eiweiss, an egg-white substitute, was produced from fish in Germany in World War II. The fish was solvent-extracted, hydrolysed with alkali, neutralized and spray dried to give a pure, white, water-soluble powder. This clearly indicates that new functional properties can be built into readily available protein foods and thus extend their consumption.

In some areas of development progress is disappointingly slow. At the First International Conference on Fish in Nutrition organized by the FAO in Washington in 1961 it was reported that Astra had built a factory to produce fish flour (fish protein concentrate). Yet even now, eleven years later, FPC is consumed only in small amounts and one still reads adverse reports on its quality. Why is progress so slow?

In developing countries the problems of nutrition become really difficult. Lack of foreign currency necessitates the development of indigenous food supplies. As mentioned before, the cheapest food costs money and adequate nutrition depends on employment for the population. In these circumstances, mechanization on the farm or elsewhere becomes undesirable as it contracts the size of the required labour force. The use of Incaparina as a food has been frustrated by its cost, although it may appear cheap to those in affluent societies.

The human animal shows great adaptability, and the adult appears able to survive on a surprisingly small amount of energy and with a limited protein intake. Thus the problem is essentially in the "vulnerable" groups, particularly children. As has been pointed out elsewhere (8th Report of the Joint FAO/WHO Expert Committee on Nutrition) the prevalence of protein deficiency is imperfectly defined. The high death rate among children under five in developing countries and often ascribed to infectious disease is now known to be a sign of malnutrition: malnutrition has made the child susceptible to infection. Measles has already been mentioned in this context (Chapter 7).

Protein deficiency in the diet of very young children has been given a new and sinister connotation through the possibility of irreversible adverse effects on mental health. Developing countries therefore need to develop protective schemes for young children based on a health care scheme linked with some form of controlled food supply to ensure that adequate supplies of essential foods are provided at the critical times in the course of their development.

This spells out the need for adequate supplies of cheap protein supplements and the development of institutional feeding and welfare schemes. Consideration must be given to evaluating the potential contribution from novel proteins such as algal and single cell protein as well as from fish and vegetable proteins, together with ways and means to convert them into cheap and palatable foods for children.

To be economically viable, production must be carried out in the developing country, and this will almost certainly introduce special difficulties through such factors as lack of uniformity in raw material for conversion and limited or non-existent public utilities.

II. GENERAL DISCUSSION

A. Production

1. *Fish Protein Production*

Professor A. E. Bender commented that fish protein seemed to be frozen in a permanent state of being a promising material, although it was used by the Romans and incorporated into biscuits in the last century. If scientists do not know how to market foods, neither do professional marketers. To catch fish, produce fish flour and disguise it in bread seems little removed from the ultimate illogicality of texturing it into synthetic fish. Furthermore the price was exorbitant: at a time when the local supermarket offered a high-protein baby food at 50 cents/kg with all the manufacturers', wholesalers' and retailers' profits, fish protein concentrate was still selling at 80 cents/kg. Would it therefore not be better to encourage the consumption of fish?

Professor F. X. Aylward thought that Professor Bender's criticisms of fish protein concentrate could be applied to any protein concentrate. From the trading viewpoint, the more people who worked on a product the better, but developing countries were not helped by the export of foods from advanced countries other than in disaster situations. He felt that there was no reason why fish flours should not be produced on the spot by simple methods and that the role of advanced countries was to provide the basic information to make this possible. As an example he quoted the fish meal made by an amateur in Africa, which would not have passed any tests since it contained 15% fat. However, it lasted for six months in Northern Ghana in a simple wrapping. Incidentally, the fish was not eaten as such: the local dietary custom was to drop it into soup in small pieces. When a sample was sent for analysis it was found that although it contained 15% fat the correct amount of antioxidant had been included quite fortuitously. He felt that more should be done to encourage such enterprises with modern sciences, simple methods and local labour, and that the training of such people was an important function of food science departments such as his own.

Dr K. J. Carpenter said that Professor Bender had asked why the FAO and other organizations should have tried to convert fish into characterless powders when fish as such might be developed as an attractive food in its own right for underdeveloped countries. This sounded a convincing argument, but he believed that it oversimplified the situation and was unrealistic. It conjured up in one's mind the idea of an attractive fillet of sole being taken away from a poor man and turned into something inferior. Most of the fish eaten in Britain had, of course, been caught in the far north off Iceland and Greenland, and had then been filleted immediately and frozen. The types of fish that could be found in large shoals near the coasts of South America, South Africa and, to a lesser extent, India, were mostly of the anchovy type, with small, sharp bones that were difficult to separate by filleting, and they were consequently unattractive even to local people. Moreover, in the tropics the "life" of fresh fish was short and, where the only practical transport was by boys on bicycles, the effective distance inland to which it could be transported was about 20 miles. If the costs of refrigerated transport and storage were taken into account, fish ceased to be an economic food for the people of average or below-average income.

The Icelanders had a traditional way of drying cod to produce the stockfish that they exported to West Africa, but this was possible only under cold, dry conditions with prevailing winds. One could not expect the same thing to happen if one hung up a round-fish, of much higher fat content, in the humid tropics. There was, therefore, a real problem in some areas of people in need of more, cheap food while there were large numbers of fish off their coasts, at present unusable except as fish meal which made only an indirect contribution to the human diet through animal production. So far, attempts to produce *and* market a comparable, but upgraded fish flour had not been successful, and he agreed that the reason for this needed careful consideration, but it would be wrong to think that the work was not worth attempting because there were simpler alternatives that the organizations concerned had chosen to ignore. For these reasons he thought that more sympathy should be shown to attempts to develop new products.

Dr L. R. Njaa said that it was quite obvious that fish which could be presented as such was sold as such. The raw material for fish flour was small shoal fish that only the Japanese were prepared to eat as such. Part of the reason for trying to make human food from this material was political, in that this fish was available and potentially useful in human diets.

Professor A. E. Bender replied that he was still puzzled by the lack of success of such ventures. He had no objection to the treatment of fish, but failed to see why it should be overtreated, defatted, deodorized and disguised as different foods. Scrap meat, for example, was made into meat products and he saw no reason why the same should not be attempted with these fish.

Dr G. D. Rosen suggested that the thing wrong with fish flour was that it was not a food. He asked whether the manufacture of fish protein concentrate was a profitable enterprise. Professor E. J. Rolfe said he thought that fish protein concentrate could be described as a food in the sense of its composition.

Dr B. Hallgren said that the whole question of the commercial viability of fish protein was complex. Soya-bean products, for example, used not to be accepted as human food, and the popularity of groundnut flour has declined since the aflatoxin trouble. Although a maize–soya-bean–milk product is made in the USA for distribution to developing countries there was a long time-lag before production started, largely due to political factors. Thus, there was a surplus of maize and soya-bean which it was intended to combine, and then the milk lobby insisted on the inclusion of milk. In Sweden, where the lobbies were much less powerful than those in the USA, fish protein was added to wheat flour for developing countries. Other reasons for the lengthy development of fish protein were the difficult technical problems and the large investment costs in the processing plant.

In reply to questions from Dr J. Abraham, Dr Hallgren said that fish protein concentrate contained 85% protein, very low levels of fat (*ca.* 0·1% lipids) and 8·0 g/100 g lysine by Carpenter's method. The bacterial content was very low, less than 1000/g. The best raw material was herring, but less attractive South Atlantic fish were now being used.

Dr N. R. Jones (Tropical Products Institute, London) asked whether the microbiological aspect of foods was considered important; most paediatricians would certainly think it was. He added that fish protein concentrate would not seem to be a viable proposition for low-income groups, and the economic opening for such material should be assessed. It was often possible to control flavour in fish by reducing those substances which would produce undesirable flavour factors, and this could be done in developing countries by washing. It did, however, seem pointless to remove a good texture. In high-temperature regions it was better to work with high-temperature species of fish, which kept longer under normal refrigeration than did temperate-zone species. This was often not realized, and wasteful deep-freezing equipment was installed, which was unnecessary provided that the reasons for flavour or odour deterioration could be determined and simple preventative techniques applied.

Dr D. M. Hegsted thought it ironic that fish should be caught, but not eaten, in Peru.

Mr J. J. Dreyer said that there seemed to be a tendency to reduce the bone content (and fluoride content) of fish flours, even though this was an excellent mineral mixture. There was also a stripping of vitamin content, and he felt that adding products low in vitamin E to cereals could be potentially harmful. He thought that a combination of animal proteins with the less palatable plant proteins might make the latter more acceptable.

Dr B. Hallgren agreed that the fluoride content should not be lowered too greatly, and added that if the American Food and Drug Authority could be persuaded to accept a level of 150 mg/kg this would obviate the need for deboning and the removal of valuable minerals.

Dr Hallgren thought that the adverse reactions to fish protein concentrate during a trial in Morocco which were mentioned by Dr J. Abraham (CNRS, Meudon-Bellevue, France) might be due to poor extraction techniques.

Dr H. Erbersdobler asked whether fish protein was suitable for veal calf feeding. Dr Hallgren replied that fish protein contained appreciable levels of iron, so that the veal calves did not remain anaemic and produce light flesh.

2. *Production of Other Protein Foods*

Taking up Professor Rolfe's point about the wasteful conversion of cereal to animal products, Dr G. D. Rosen argued that this was not entirely wasteful since it produced desirable foods. He also urged that the development of new foods should be self-financing within a reasonable period.

Professor E. von Sydow agreed that self-financing was important for new products, but asked how this should be defined. Commercial barriers were artificial from the viewpoint of a food technologist, but government restrictions could ruin the success of a good product. Furthermore, aid was often needed initially, even if manufacture became self-financing once a certain production volume was achieved.

Dr G. D. Rosen said that higher sales sometimes meant nothing more than higher losses. The writing-off of investment was often a political question, but he would say that a new product should be self-financing within 5 years. Of the costs of a new product, the basic research formed a very small part. He gave as an example of another form of tariff the EEC control of soya-beans.

Professor H. Haenel asked whether textured vegetable proteins had proved failures and should be abandoned. Dr G. D. Rosen replied that the raw material question was rather difficult. Fish was already a food, and in his opinion should be left as such, but soya-bean was not, and needed processing before it became food. He thought that soya-bean flour, rather than the more expensive protein isolate, should be the raw material for textured analogues. Certainly investment was a major problem in the manufacture of textured soya-bean products.

Referring to Mr Dreyer's earlier point about protein mixtures, he said that soya-bean products were frequently mixed with such animal products as meat and egg, and in this instance no attempt was being made to create a food in its own right.

Mr J. J. Dreyer said that a product containing egg, milk and soya-bean had proved quite acceptable, but that he still had doubts about adding protein isolates to cereal products.

3. *Production of Practical Complete Diets*

Dr R. G. Whitehead remarked that one of the complete diets intended for distribution to countries at times of disaster had a protein–energy ratio of 0·20. This was very high for a complete meal, and a reduction to—say—0·15 would presumably reduce the cost. This would be quite justifiable as normal children needed a ratio of 0·05 and even malnourished children required only 0·08 – 0·09.

Dr B. Hallgren thought that the reason was probably that Swedish baby foods had a protein–energy ratio of 0·20, whereupon Dr Whitehead pointed out that the most famous of all baby foods, human breast milk, had a ratio of only 0·06.

Dr B. M. Nicol asked about the cost of the gruel supplied to Bangladesh and Dr Hallgren said that this was sold to the Red Cross for about 80 cents/kg.

4. *Problems of Marketing New Products*

Mr J. C. McKenzie (Food and Drink Research Ltd, London) drew attention to the almost total failure of well-intentioned international organizations in promoting nutritionally desirable food products in developing countries, a record of failure that would not be tolerated in any commercial enterprise.

He thought that this could be partly attributed to the climate in international agencies, cushioned as they were from commercial pressures or insistence on success. Moreover, products were too frequently handled not by professional food manufacturers but by the scientist playing at marketing. Demonstration of a food's superior nutritive value was not enough, especially if—as was too often the case—it was expensive and unpalatable. However, it must be realized that to change the food habits of people was a considerable task. Food was an integral part of our culture, subject to emotional and socio-psychological influences; rarely was it chosen for its nutritive value. Even some businessmen, faced with marketing nutrient supplements, became convinced, perhaps for the first time, that their products were really good and that they need make less effort to promote them.

He thought that the answer was to introduce protein supplements in staple foods—as, say, margarine was fortified—or to imitate an existing attractive food as closely as possible while making the new product cheaper.

Professor A. E. Bender thought that Mr McKenzie must meet only those firms that studied their marketing problems adequately. Only last year, for instance, a large firm brought out a new product for the elderly and found only afterwards that it was quite unacceptable. If market analysis provided a foolproof or even valid method there should be very few failures. The problems in developing countries were well known; they had no food and no money, but how could this be explained to the appropriate authorities? On the credit side, one group of companies was beginning to study the acceptability of textured foods.

Dr B. M. Nicol said that it was true that international agencies used not to make use of market research and he himself had urged that they do so. In the past five years, however, when they had been doing so, there had been no greater degree of success.

Dr A. Uzel (Hacettepe University, Ankara, Turkey) pointed out that developing countries were usually agricultural countries, and they had no desire to import food. If the aim were to improve the nutritional status in developing countries, then why not help them to improve their own food industries? Food aid would certainly not help, for even in emergencies the food provided was not eaten by those people who really needed it.

Mr H. Turgut (Turkey; present address, National College of Food Technology) thought that there was a tendency to overlook the problem of education in developing countries. It was not the whole story to say that they had no money or food; often they lacked the knowledge for preservation and preparation of available foods.

Dr R. A. M. Delaney (The Agricultural Institute, Moorepark, Republic of Ireland) asked whether the nutritional value of a food were ever of any importance in selling it.

Mr J. C. McKenzie replied that there were foods in which this was a factor. Negatively, in that the promotion of milk-drinking was inhibited by the idea that it was a cold, clinical food that did one good; and positively in that eggs were often bought for their food value.

He thought that Professor Bender's expectation of a 100% success rate was unrealistic. For any commercial product there were many equally heavily advertised products in competition and—in that there was a limit to the amount that one could eat—all products were essentially competitive. Failures were a result of this competition: after all, someone else may have an inherently better product. Of those products introduced by the food industry, those accepted—i.e. continuously purchased—by the public were a relatively small proportion. Yet, having admitted this, it must be said that the successes in promoting products in the developing countries were far fewer.

He thought that market research organizations had to be given the right tasks: how to improve a product rather than the study of the food habits of a particular indigenous population. It was true that money was scarce in developing countries, but every individual had a list of priorities for expenditure. The problem was to persuade people to re-allocate their money so that they bought less carbonated soft drinks of negligible nutritive value and more high-protein food.

B. Laboratory Evaluation

Opening a general discussion on laboratory methods, Dr B. Drake (Swedish Institute for Food Preservation Research, Göteborg, Sweden) said that some of the nutritionists present might feel that the topics were irrelevant to their field. This, however, was a short-sighted attitude, as was that of the food technologist who ignored the nutritional aspects. Both approaches were needed.

He emphasized once more that there was no point in producing a nutritionally perfect food if people did not eat it. In order to promote the consumption of foods of high nutritive value collaboration between nutritionists and food scientists and technologists was essential. He felt that this was important both at the laboratory level and in the higher echelons of organizations such as the FAO. The question was, how could such collaboration be encouraged and made fruitful.

1. *Functionality of Fish Protein Concentrate*

Dr R. A. M. Delaney asked whether the limited use of fish protein concentrate might be due to its low functionality. Could this be enhanced, perhaps, by the introduction of whipping or foaming capacity? Dr A.-M. Hermansson said that fish protein concentrate had good foaming properties despite its low solubility; a surprising finding, as one would expect foaming capacity and solubility to be related. Probably there was a small soluble fraction responsible for the foaming.

Dr J. T. Worgan pointed out that fish has functional properties, although fish protein concentrate does not, and he wondered whether it was possible to restore them. Dr A.-M. Hermansson said that this was not possible as the changes were irreversible; one had to treat further to introduce new functional properties.

In reply to a question from Dr L. R. Njaa, Dr B. Hallgren said that the water-binding properties were lost at the defatting stage.

2. *The Implications of Textural Studies*

Dr E. W. Evans (NIRD, Reading) asked to what extent texture properties were those of the continuum or of its defects, since many physical properties were limited by the interfaces in a material. Dr P. Sherman said that a rheologist treated the material as a continuum, and in any case the properties could result from the basic linkages rather than from flaws.

Mr A. Ossai (Nigeria; present address, National College of Food Technology, Reading, England) said that although no one instrument measured all the factors involved, a human subject did so at once. Was there any correlation? Dr P. Sherman replied that there was no general correlation between the instrument and a human panel, but only on each textural factor, such as fragility or stickiness. It was difficult to reach definite conclusions about comparisons of different instrumental techniques. Dr B. Drake said that there were electronic methods for studying chewing habits, but they had not been used extensively.

Dr R. Harper (University of Reading, England) asked to what extent one could calculate from instrumental techniques common physical properties other than those such as viscosity. It seemed to him a difficult problem: for example springiness could involve not simply elasticity but also rate of recovery.

Dr P. Sherman said that no advance had been made with solid foods beyond hardness testing. Further progress may involve complex stress–strain calculations. Liquids could be defined in terms of simple physical properties. Elasticity was easily measured, but did not correspond with anything tested by taste panels.

Dr V. C. Mason asked whether any work had been done which related functional properties to the material's digestibility or utilization. Dr A.-M. Hermansson said there was a lack of such studies.

Mr A. Ossai asked whether there were ways of inferring the structure of a food by rapid textural measurements. Dr P. Sherman replied that this was already done in some cases, for instance the ripeness of fruit could be tested by a very simple technique and the picking time thus determined. This could certainly be extended to other factors such as soil conditions.

Mr A. Ossai then asked whether—if there were a single dominant textural factor in a specific food that corresponded exactly with a panel test—the panel would be replaced by the instrument. Dr P. Sherman thought this quite possible, provided that it was borne in mind that the machine was testing the factor and not any sort of acceptability. In any event, one would first have to determine whether the sensory test, be it panel or instrumental, was itself related to consumer preference.

3. *The Implications of Odour Studies*

Professor H. Haenel asked whether there was any relationship between the structure of chemicals and their type of odour; whether such chemicals were of toxicological interest; whether it was true that the combination of odours produced new sensations and whether it was possible to make simulated foods such as "orange juice" containing no oranges.

Professor E. von Sydow replied that there was some general classification possible: thus, mercaptans and certain aldehydes had similar odours, but many chemically related substances had quite different odours. He thought that it seemed likely that all foods would be found to contain at least one factor that would not be permitted as an additive. This was merely a fact that had to be accepted and was partly a question of how carefully analysis was performed; it did not apply only to new foods. When different odours were combined it was sometimes possible to preserve the distinction, but there were cases where new odours arose that the components did not possess. He said that for most food odours the synthetic material was more expensive than the natural product.

Mr J. J. Dreyer asked whether the results depended on the specific palates of the particular tasting panel. Professor E. von Sydow thought that this could be argued, but he felt almost certain that his panel would be representative. They were, after all, detecting specific odours, not passing judgement on their pleasantness or palatability.

4. *Quality Control and Analysis*

Dr R. Harper said that quality control seemed to be oriented towards the developed countries. Professor E. von Sydow said that food technologies differed in the developed and developing countries. His own Institute's work was performed on behalf of the Swedish food industry, and they had to keep their aims in mind.

Dr L. R. Njaa asked whether international conventions had any local applications. Dr D. Pearson replied that the Codex Alimentarius was set up in ten parts: at stage 9 the Codex itself accepted it and at stage 10 governments adopted it. Many of the provisions may be accepted in stages, and some developing countries may never apply them, but it is hoped that most countries will do so. There might well be regional variations: for instance colours acceptable in one country may be considered unattractive elsewhere.

He went on to say that from the time of the first [UK] Food and Drug Act until 1940 firms analysed solely to comply with the legal requirements. Nowadays the question of quality in a broader sense was considered; indeed the term now used was "quality assurance", that is, assurance of the process at each stage.

He described some work that had been done at the National College of Food Technology on damage in proteins. Spoilage in meat and fish, for example, followed protein changes. One useful method for testing such damage was distillation from magnesium oxide. Extensive deamination was produced by boiling meat and fish in water.

Professor I. E. Liener asked whether the presence of nitrate and nitrite in meat affected the protein analysis. Dr D. Pearson said that fresh meat contained no such additives, and even in cured meat the sources of error tended to cancel out.

Dr C. Sørensen (State Laboratory for Soil and Crop Research, Lyngby, Denmark) pointed out that the nitrite and nitrate content varied in different products and wondered whether the methods excluded them or whether the total nitrogen result varied with the product. Dr D. Pearson said that the Kjeldahl method could be modified to include all the nitrogen, by the use of phenol or sulphosalicylic acid, for instance, but he preferred to estimate nitrite and nitrate separately.

Dr J. Abraham asked how frequently sampling would be carried out commercially. Dr D. Pearson said that this was a statistical question which would involve several considerations.

CHAPTER 31

The Normal Course of Digestion of Food Proteins

H. ERBERSDOBLER

Institut für Tierphysiologie der Universität München, GFR

I. INTRODUCTION

The main limitations on the availability of amino acids in proteins result from retardation of digestion and, possibly, from a delay of amino acid absorption. Digestibility is largely dependent on the type and sequence of the amino acids in the peptide chain, their spatial configuration and the presence of various cross-linkages between functional groups.

II. THE ROLE OF THE STOMACH

The digestion of proteins starts in the stomach with the disorganization of the "bulky" protein molecule through denaturation with hydrochloric acid. The other functions of the stomach are to mix, moisten and store the food, and to initiate enzymic hydrolysis. Moreover, the stomach plays an important part in regulating the rate of digestion by feed-back mechanism which may include hormonal controls. One such regulatory control is of the rate of release of the food proteins from the stomach. The influence of the protein on the rate of stomach emptying has been reviewed, e.g. by Rogers and Harper (1964) and recently by Porter and Rolls (1971). The rate of passage of food proteins from the stomach depends on the amount and type of the protein in the diet, and generally does not seem to be related to protein quality (Rogers and Harper, 1966; Zebrowska, 1968; Porter and Rolls, 1971).

However, there was a decrease in the stomach contents when heat-treated rather than unheated soya-bean protein or casein was given (Erbersdobler *et al.*, 1968; Weber, 1972). After test meals of severely heat-treated proteins the amino acid concentrations in the portal blood of rats adapted to a high-protein diet were much lower than after meals of the unheated or mildly heat-treated samples (Fig. 1). The heat-treated proteins, which showed a lowered digestibility (Erbersdobler *et al.*, 1972b) passed more rapidly from the stomach than did the unheated or mildly-heated

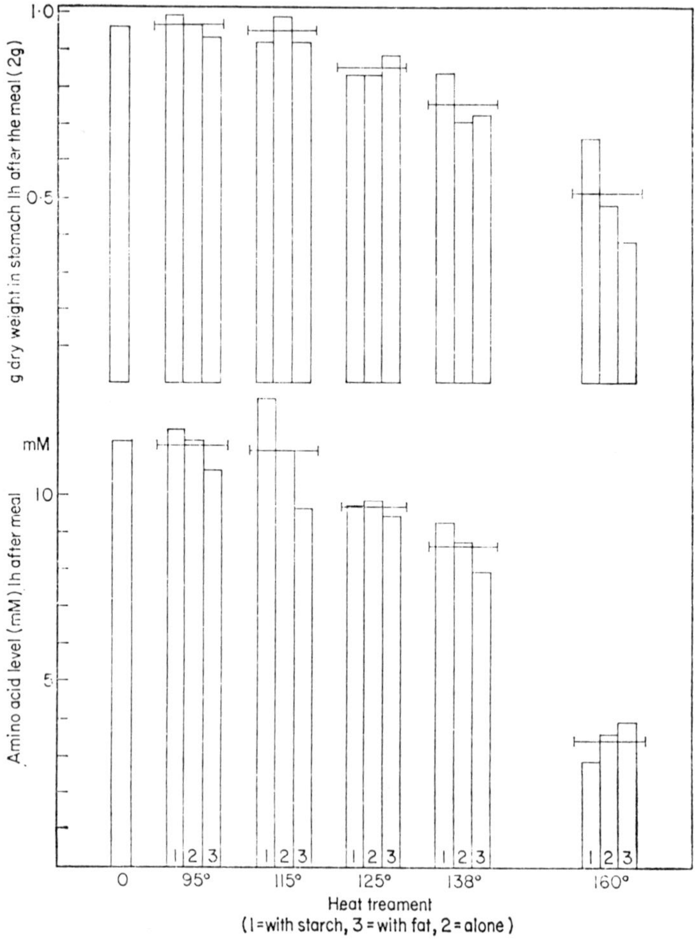

FIG. 1. The dry matter content of the stomach and the concentration of free amino acids (excluding cystine and tryptophan) in the portal plasma 1 h after giving a single meal of 2 g of heat-treated soya-bean proteins (75% protein) to rats adapted to a high-protein diet

samples. These findings agree with the observations that the rate of emptying of proteins from the stomach was most rapid when low protein diets were given (Gitler, 1964) and that this rate decreased as the level of protein (casein) increased up to 30% (Peraino *et al.*, 1959). Furthermore, there was a high correlation between the rate of stomach emptying and the amino acid concentrations in portal blood (Fig. 2). However, these findings are not in accord with those of Buraczewski (1966) and Buraczewski *et al.* (1966, 1967), who reported no change in the rate of stomach

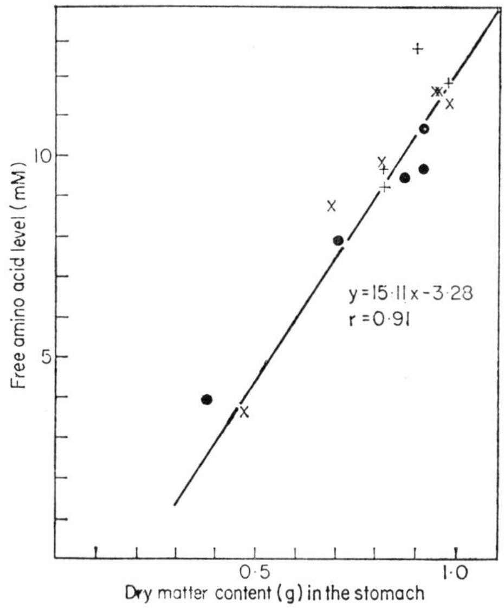

FIG. 2. Correlation between the concentrations of free amino acids in the portal plasma and the dry matter content of the stomach of rats 1 h after a meal of 2 g of heat-treated proteins. (×, alone; ●, with fat; +, with starch)

emptying after a meal of heat-treated proteins. The different pretreatment of the animals may be the reason for this discrepancy. We used rats that had been adapted to the test diets for two weeks. In the last week the animals were trained to consume their daily food in two meals within 30 min (morning) or 45 min (evening), at exactly the same time. Then after a fasting period of 24 h they consumed their test meals of 2–3 g in the morning within 15 min. According to Chen *et al.* (1962) it is important that the rat has been adapted to a diet of the same composition as that of the test meal actually used.

The mechanisms controlling stomach emptying require further elucidation. We may assume the presence of some feed-back mechanism dependent on the concentrations of free amino acids in the blood or in the duodenum, but we cannot completely exclude the possibility that heat-damaged proteins do not elicit the secretion of the same amounts of endogenous N as do the more digestible proteins (Valle-Riestra and Barnes, 1970).

III. THE ACTION OF PROTEASES

Initially in the stomach, and even more after the passage of the pre-digested protein into the duodenum, the combined action of the proteases and peptidases results in a rapid splitting of the protein molecule to smaller fragments and finally to free amino acids. Some of the peptidases, e.g. trypsin, show a high substrate specificity depending on the structure of the substrate binding site (Hartley, 1970; Shotton and Hartley, 1970; Steitz *et al.*, 1969). Trypsin is only able to split the peptide chain close to lysine or arginine if their reactive amino groups in the side chain are free. For this reason it is possible to inhibit the action of trypsin by blocking the ε-amino group of lysine. The action of the other less specific proteases is, however, only partially inhibited when the ε-amino group of lysine is blocked (Bjarnason and Carpenter, 1969; Tazawa, 1943).

Alterations in the side chains of some other amino acids do not hinder the action of the less specific proteases. Experiments in our laboratory (Erbersdobler, 1969; Weber, 1972) have shown that methionine sulphoxides are liberated very easily from the peptide chain. The concentrations of methionine and methionine sulphoxides in portal plasma after single meals of casein treated under different conditions are shown in Fig. 3.

When casein that had previously been heated with oil or with oxidized oil in the open air was given, there was a rapid influx of large amounts of methionine sulphoxides into the portal vein. These high concentrations indicated that there must have been an enzymic hydrolysis of the peptide chain containing the methione sulphoxide. It seems, therefore, that the oxidation of the peptide-bound methionine to the sulphoxide is a less important factor in methionine availability than Ellinger and Palmer (1969) suggested.

The animal is able to adapt itself to alterations in protein digestion, as Pavlov (1913) suggested. When foods containing protease inhibitors are given, the animal responds by an enlargement of the pancreas (e.g. Chernik *et al.*, 1948; Corring and Aumaitre, 1970). Desnuelle *et al.* (1962), Ben Abdeljlil *et al.* (1963), Snook and Meyer (1964), Zucker *et al.* (1968) and Aumaitre (1971) have shown that there was an increase in trypsin and/or chymotrypsin activity in the intestine when the protein content of the diet was increased. There was a further increase in trypsin activity when heat-damaged proteins were given (Erbersdobler, 1967).

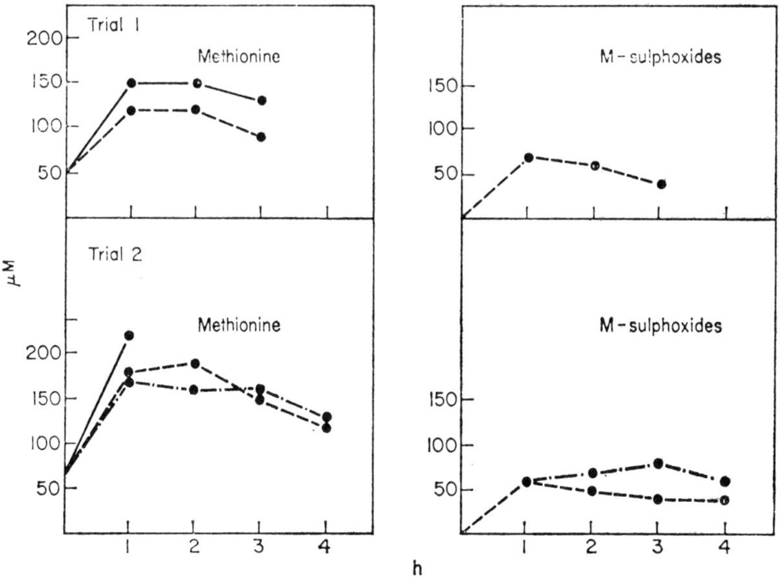

FIG. 3. The concentrations of methionine and methionine sulphoxides in the portal plasma 1–4 h after a single meal of heat-treated (110° for 24 h) samples of:
———— casein
- - - - - - - casein + oil
—•—•— casein + oxidized oil

IV. AMINO ACID ABSORPTION

The main part of the digested protein is absorbed as free amino acids. There are at least three separate mechanisms of intestinal amino acid transport: one for the acidic and neutral amino acids, one for lysine and arginine and one for the imino acids. Glutamic and aspartic acids are not actively transported (Wiseman, 1968). The differences between the transport rates of the different amino acids are attributed to the concentrations and to their individual affinities toward the transport systems. Figure 4 shows the range of the transport rates of eleven amino acids present in the incubation medium in equimolar concentrations (1 mM) (Scharrer and Brüggemann, 1971). For these experiments the everted sac technique was used (Wilson and Wiseman, 1954). There was a high transport rate for lysine since lysine and arginine are transported by a special system and arginine was omitted from the medium. Among the neutral amino acids, isoleucine, methionine, valine and leucine were preferentially transported, whereas low values were found for the transport of histidine, serine, threonine, glycine and alanine.

When rats were adapted to diets with a high protein content of 75%

for 2 weeks, significantly higher transport rates were obtained (clear columns in Fig. 4). This indicates that the transport systems are able to adapt to dietary changes to some extent. In similar experiments with chicks Scharrer (1971) found the same range of rates of amino acid transport with the exception that threonine and serine were absorbed at a higher rate.

If amino acids have different affinities for the same transport system, competitive inhibition can easily occur (cf. Gitler, 1964). This inhibition depends on the nature and the concentration of the inhibiting amino acid. We have recently started to investigate the inhibition of amino acid

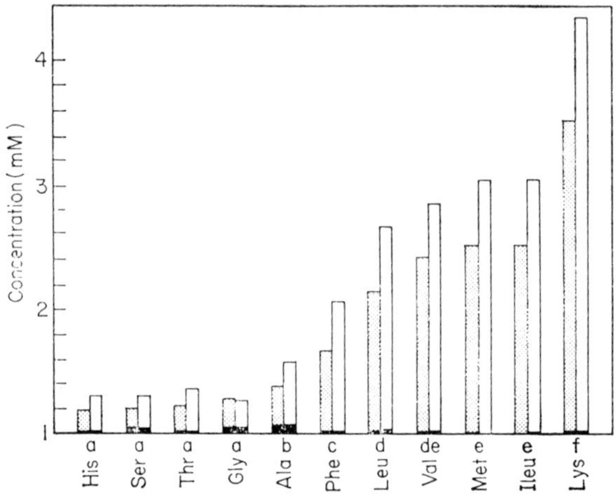

FIG. 4. Mean increases after incubation in the concentrations of amino acids in the serosal fluid of everted sacs from seven rats

□ Rats adapted to a high-protein (75%) diet

::: Rats adapted to a low-protein (11%) diet

■ No amino acids added to the mucosal fluid

Initial mucosal concentration of each amino acid, 1 mM. Differences between columns with different letters are significant in one or both groups

transport caused by some amino acid derivatives in order to follow up some of the results and suggestions of Buraczewski (1966), Buraczewski *et al.* (1967, 1971) and Ford and Shorrock (1971). These authors postulated that some peptides or peptide-like compounds may interfere with amino acid absorption. Our preliminary results show that lysine does not interfere with the transport of a neutral amino acid such as threonine. However, ε-*N*-acetyl-lysine, which is only poorly utilized by the rat (Bjarnason and Carpenter, 1969), also had no effect on threonine transport. Furthermore, the transport of lysine can be inhibited in the presence of acetyl-lysine, indicating that acetylation had not fully eliminated the basic character of the blocked ε-amino group.

Preliminary results indicate that there was some inhibition of threonine absorption by fructoselysine (ε-*N*-deoxy-fructosyl-lysine). Fructoselysine or lactuloselysine (ε-*N*-deoxy-lactulosyl-lysine) are formed by heating proteins in the presence of glucose or lactose during the initial stages of the so-called Maillard reaction. As can be seen in Fig. 5 this lysine–sugar complex is itself absorbed at a slow rate (Erbersdobler, 1971b). These and recent results obtained with the everted sac technique, using ^{14}C-labelled fructoselysine, make it likely that there is no active transport of fructoselysine but that it is absorbed by diffusion. These findings do not contradict

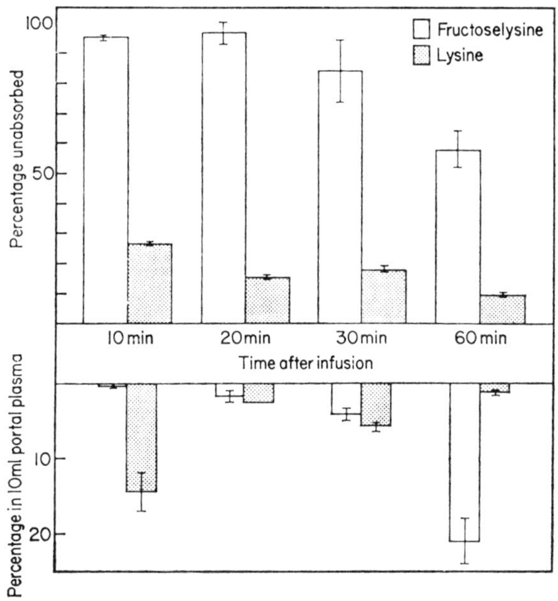

FIG. 5. Absorption of ^{14}C-labelled fructoselysine and lysine from the jejunal segments of rats

the results of Mauron (1970) and Finot (Chapter 34) who found large amounts of fructoselysine in the urine of rats that had been given pure fructoselysine. Although relying on passive diffusion, an appreciable uptake of fructoselysine is possible, since the concentration differences between the intestinal contents and the blood are large. We assume that no active reabsorption takes place in the renal tubules, so that excretion in the urine would occur rapidly. During incubation of everted sacs for up to 2 h (two trials) the labelled fructoselysine present in the incubation medium remained stable.

These model experiments are also relevant to peptide absorption, which is of some clinical and physiological interest (Fisher, 1967; Porter and Rolls, 1971). Recently Bjarnason and Carpenter (1969, 1970) and Ford and Shorrock (1971) have found that rats given proteins that have been heated alone can absorb some undigested peptide-like molecules which are excreted in the urine.

On the other hand the intestinal transport of a single amino acid may be stimulated by the presence of another amino acid. We supplemented protein poor in methionine (isolated soya-bean protein) with DL-methionine and found, compared with the unsupplemented control, not only the expected increased concentration of methionine in the portal and aortic plasma, but also an increase in lysine and arginine (Erbersdobler *et al.*, 1972a). These *in vivo* results confirm the *in vitro* findings of Robinson (1968) and Reiser and Christensen (1971) that methionine stimulated the uptake of L-arginine and L-lysine.

A significant portion of the amino acids liberated in the intestinal lumen is used for synthesis of the proteins of the mucosal cell (Dawson and Holdsworth, 1962) or is metabolized or transaminated (Neame and Wiseman, 1957).

V. AMINO ACID INFLUX INTO THE PORTAL VEIN

The size and duration of the amino acid influx into the portal blood depends on the amount, nature and digestibility of the protein meal. Figure 6 shows the lysine concentrations after single meals with a high

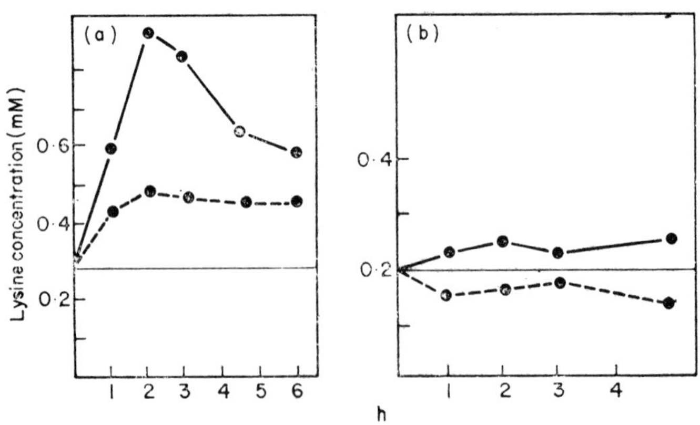

FIG. 6. Lysine concentrations in portal plasma of adapted rats after a single meal of unheated (————) or heat-damaged (– – – – –) proteins.

A, rats given 3 g of food containing 2·2 g protein from casein

B, rats given 3 g of food containing 0·96 g protein from dried skim milk

(75%) or medium (32%) content of unheated or heat-damaged protein. For several years we have used the technique of estimating the concentrations of free amino acids in the portal plasma of rats that have previously been adapted to high-protein diets. This treatment results in high concentrations of free amino acids in the plasma (Scharrer *et al.*, 1967; Erbersdobler, 1967) and increases the differences between the fasting value and those found after the influx of amino acids from the dietary protein. In this way a low amino acid availability, such as that resulting from heat-damage, can be evaluated (Fig. 7). It must be emphasized, however, that

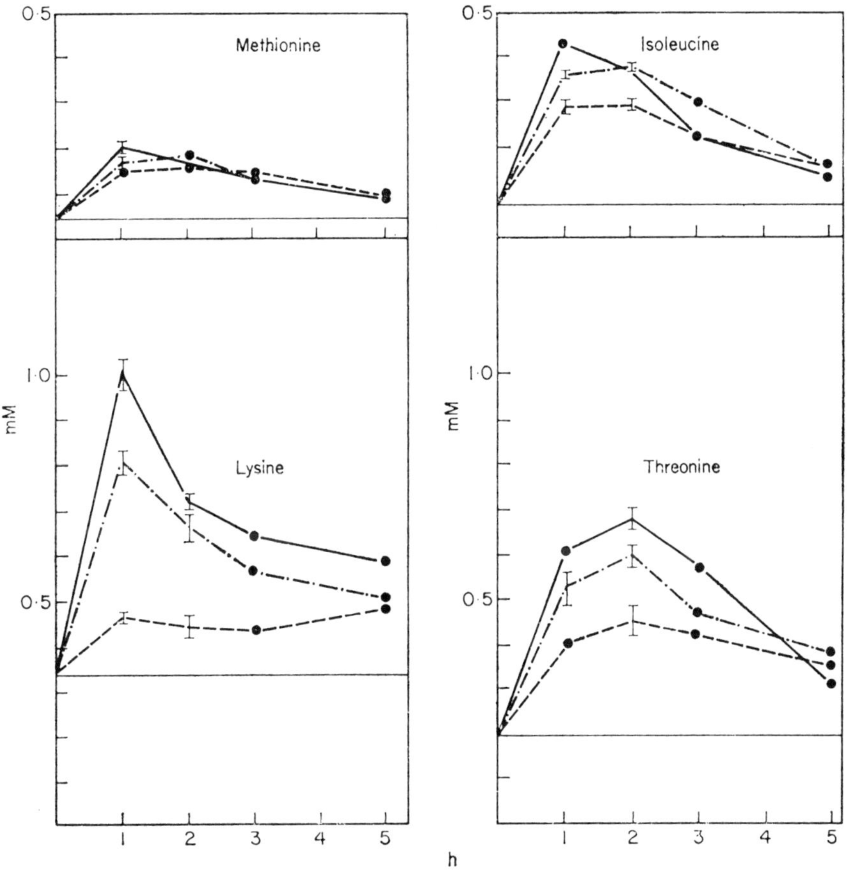

FIG. 7. Concentrations of some amino acids in the portal plasma of rats 1–5 h after a single meal of:

———— unheated casein
— • — • — casein heated at 138° for 30 min
- - - - - - casein heated with 10% w/w glucose at 138° for 30 min

the experimental procedures must be strictly observed to obtain reliable results (cf. Erbersdobler *et al.*, 1968, 1972b).

Since in most cases enzymic hydrolysis and not amino acid absorption is the limiting factor in protein digestion, free amino acids in the diet appear earlier in the portal vein than do peptide-bound amino acids (cf. Zimmermann-Nielsen and Schønheyder, 1962; Scharrer and Zucker, 1968). This more rapid influx into the blood and—what is even more important—the much earlier decrease may hinder the efficiency of protein utilization in diets supplemented with the limiting amino acid.

These problems are only likely to arise with animals that are fed only once or twice a day, such as dogs and pigs (Walz, 1972).

VI. PROTEIN DEGRADATION BY THE INTESTINAL FLORA

For several years many authors have recommended the use of balance techniques for the measurement of amino acid availability (e.g. Kuiken and Lyman, 1948; Dammers, 1964; Eggum, 1966; Kristen, 1968; Poppe *et al*, 1969, 1971a,b).

Rapid developments in analytical techniques have allowed the determination by balance methods of so-called amino acid digestibilities or amino acid absorbances. It was soon realized, however, that the protein and amino acid digestibility did not usually decrease to the extent to be expected from the reduced nutritional value (e.g. Ford *et al.*, 1967; Nesheim and Carpenter, 1967; Erbersdobler, 1967; Varnish and Carpenter, 1971; Valle-Riestra and Barnes, 1970; Erbersdobler *et al.*, 1972b). It was suggested that the microflora of the large intestine destroyed some absorbed amino acids and hence they did not appear in the faeces.

Figure 8 shows the results of some *in vitro* experiments with a protein rich in the lysine–sugar complex lactuloselysine. This protein, which was isolated from a heat-damaged dried skim milk, was incubated together with the contents of the large intestine of rats under nitrogen for up to 48 h (Erbersdobler *et al.*, 1970).

During this incubation aliquot samples were removed for the determination of total N, lysine and the frustoselysine group (and in some cases ammonia). Fructoselysine and lactuloselysine, which are very unstable during acid hydrolysis, were estimated by measuring the product formed during hydrolysis with 7·75 M hydrochloric acid. We discovered this useful indicator some years ago (Erbersdobler and Zucker, 1966; Erbersdobler, 1967; Erbersdobler and Bock, 1967; Brüggemann and Erbersdobler, 1968). Heyns *et al.* (1968) and Finot *et al.* (1968) have determined the structure of the compound and named it furosine (*ε*-*N*-

(2-furosyl methyl)-L-lysine). The result of these experiments (Fig. 8) and the results of other trials with pigs (Erbersdobler, 1971a) demonstrate that the gut micro-organisms are able to destroy fructoselysine. These findings confirm with a well-defined unavailable product the results and suggestions of Nesheim and Carpenter (1967), Ford *et al.* (1967), Salter and Coates (1971) and Valle-Riestra and Barnes (1970).

In these cases the unavailable and undigested peptides or peptide-like

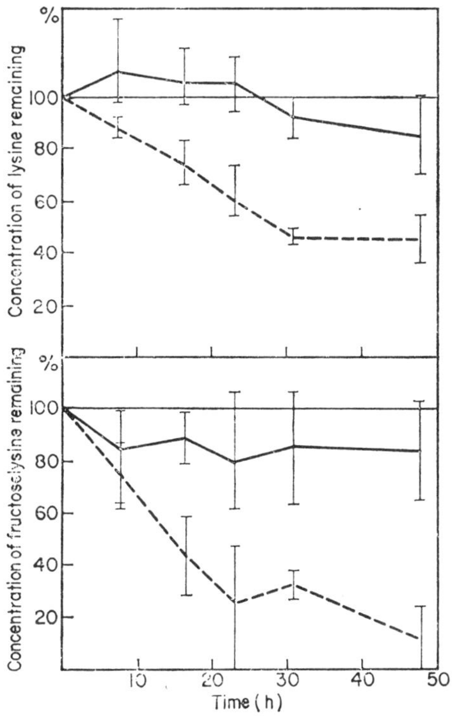

FIG. 8. Degradation of fructoselysine by the intestinal flora. Incubation of a heat-damaged protein with gut contents (- - - - -) or with gut contents that had been inactivated by the addition of mercuric chloride (————). (Concentrations before incubation, 100)

complexes were transformed to ammonia and fatty acids or were even completely destroyed. Since some of these compounds, such as ammonia, may be absorbed, the intestinal microflora may be said to have increased the digestibility of heat-damaged proteins.

Sometimes microbial activity may result in the release of substances from derivatives in which they are unavailable. Recent experiments with DL-acetyl-methionine led to the conclusion that rats can utilize part of the D-isomer if it reaches sites in the intestine where it is hydrolysed by microbial activity. The regenerated methionine may be absorbed directly or after coprophagy (Erbersdobler *et al.*, 1972a). Proteins subjected to severe heat treatment cannot be degraded by gut micro-organisms, as we have shown in digestibility trials with germ-free and conventional chicks (see Table I), and with rats (Table II) (Erbersdobler *et al.*, 1972b). The

TABLE I. Effect of heat treatment of isolated soya-bean protein on apparent digestibility of amino acids in germ-free, monoinfected (*B. subtilis*), polyinfected and conventional chicks. The diets contained 38% protein (A, unheated; B, heated at 140° for 24 h)

		Chick				
Amino acid		*Germ-free*	*Mono-infected*	*Poly-infected*	*Conventional 1*	*Conventional 2*
Mean of	A	90	90	91	88	—
all[a]	B	32	33	32	33	34
Lysine	A	92	92	92	89	—
	B	31	30	31	32	31
Cystine	A	74	80	82	76	—
	B	19	19	15	16	21
Threonine	A	86	87	88	86	—
	B	31	32	33	33	34
Leucine	A	92	91	92	88	—
	B	30	29	31	29	31

[a] Except Met and Gly (supplemented), Try

TABLE II. Effect of heat treatment of soya-bean protein on results of protein quality measurements

	Heat treatment		
	95°	138° + 146° (mixture)	160°
FDNB-available lysine	100	73	34
Lysine level in portal plasma	100	60[a]	33[b]
Digestible protein	100	91	18
Digestible lysine	100	81/83	20/5
Weight gain of rats	100	60	*ca.* −15

[a] Only the protein heated at 138°

[b] Fasting level also 33

results when severely heated protein was given showed good agreement among the methods, but when the mildly-heated proteins were given they agreed less well, and in particular the results of the digestibility trials with rats appeared to be too high.

REFERENCES

AUMAITRE, A. (1971). *Annls Zootech.* **20**, 551–575.

BEN ABDELJLIL, A., VISANI, A. M. and DESNUELLE, P. (1963). *Biochem. biophys. Res. Commun.* **10**, 112–116.

BJARNASON, J. and CARPENTER, K. J. (1969). *Br. J. Nutr.* **23**, 859–868.

BJARNASON, J. and CARPENTER, K. J. (1970). *Br. J. Nutr.* **24**, 313–329.

BRÜGGEMANN, J. and ERBERSDOBLER, H. (1968). *Z. Lebensmittelunters. u.-Forsch.* **137**, 137–143.

BURACZEWSKI, S. (1966). Ph.D. Thesis, University of Reading, England.

BURACZEWSKI, S., BURACZEWSKA, L. and FORD, J. E. (1967). *Acta biochim. pol.* **14**, 121–133.

BURACZEWSKI, S., PORTER, J. W. G., ROLLS, B. A. and ZEBROWSKA, T. (1971). *Br. J. Nutr.* **25**, 299–306.

BURACZEWSKI, S., PORTER, J. W. G. and WILLIAMS, A. P. (1966). *Int. Congr. Nutr.* 7, Hamburg **5**, 95–100.

CHEN, M.-L., ROGERS, Q. R. and HARPER, A. E. (1962). *J. Nutr.* **76**, 235–241.

CHERNICK, S. S., LEPKOVSKY, S. and CHAIKOFF, I. L. (1948). *Am. J. Physiol.* **155**, 33–41.

CORRING, T. and AUMAITRE, A. (1970). *Annls. Biol. anim. Biochim. Biothys.* **10**, 443–457.

DAMMERS, J. (1964). Ph.D. Thesis, University of Leuven.

DAWSON, R. and HOLDSWORTH, E. S. (1962). *Br. J. Nutr.* **16**, 13–25.

DESNUELLE, P., REBOUD, J. P. and BEN ABDELJLIL, A. (1962). *In* Ciba Foundation Symposium on the exocrine pancreas. pp. 90–114. Churchill, London.

EGGUM, B. O. (1966). *Z. Tierphysiol. Tierernähr. Futtermittelk.* **22**, 32–38.

ELLINGER, G. M. and PALMER, R. (1969). *Proc. Nutr. Soc.* **28**, 42A.

ERBERSDOBLER, H. (1967). *Habilitationsschrift*, Munich.

ERBERSDOBLER, H. (1969). *Wiss. Z. Univ. Rostock* **18**, M 1/2, 211.

ERBERSDOBLER, H. (1971a). *Z. Tierphysiol. Tierernähr. Futtermittelk.* **27**, 217–218.

ERBERSDOBLER, H. (1971b). *Z. Tierphysiol. Tierernähr. Futtermittelk.* **28**, 171–173.

ERBERSDOBLER, H. and BOCK, G. (1967). *Naturwissenschaften* **54**, 648.

ERBERSDOBLER, H., DÜMMER, H. and ZUCKER, H. (1968). *Z. Tierphysiol. Tierernähr. Futtermittelk.* **24**, 136–152.

ERBERSDOBLER, H., GROPP, J. and SCHARRER, E. (1972a). *Z. Tierphysiol. Tierernähr. Futtermittelk.* **30**, 142–143.

ERBERSDOBLER, H., GUNSSER, I. and WEBER, G. (1970). *Zentbl. VetMed. A* **17**, 573–575.

ERBERSDOBLER, H., WEBER, G. and GUNSSER, I. (1972b). *Z. Tierphysiol. Tierernähr. Futtermittelk.* **29**, 325–334.

ERBERSDOBLER, H. and ZUCKER, H. (1966). *Milchwissenschaft* **21**, 564–568.

Finot, P. A., Bricout, J., Viani, R. and Mauron, J. (1968). *Experientia* **24**, 1097–1099.

Fisher, R. B. (1967). *Proc. Nutr. Soc.* **26**, 23–27.

Ford, J. E., Henry, K. M. and Porter, J. W. G. (1967). *Proc. Nutr. Soc.* **26**, ix.

Ford, J. E. and Shorrock, C. (1971). *Br. J. Nutr.* **26**, 311–322.

Gitler, C. (1964). *In* "Mammalian Protein Metabolism" Vol. 1, pp. 35–69. (H. N. Munro and J. B. Allison, eds) Academic Press, New York.

Hartley, B. S. (1970). *Phil. Trans. R. Soc.* B **257**, 77.

Heyns, K., Heukeshoven, J. and Brose, K.-H. (1968). *Angew. Chem.* **80**, 627.

Kristen, H. (1968). *Habilitationsschrift*, Rostock.

Kuiken, K. A. and Lyman, C. M. (1948). *J. Nutr.* **36**, 359–368.

Mauron, J. (1970). *Int. Z. VitamForsch.* **40**, 209–227.

Neame, K. D. and Wiseman, G. (1957). *J. Physiol., Lond.* **135**, 442–450.

Nesheim, M. C. and Carpenter, K. J. (1967). *Br. J. Nutr.* **21**, 399–411.

Pavlov, I. P. (1913). "The Work of Digestive Glands." Charles Griffin, London.

Peraino, C., Rogers, Q. R., Yoshida, M., Chen, M.-L. and Harper, A. E. (1959). *Can. J. Biochem. Physiol.* **37**, 1475–1491.

Poppe, S., Kristen, H., Meier, H., Uhlemann, H. and Wiesemüller, W. (1969). *Wiss. Z. Univ. Rostock* **18**, M1/2, 67–79.

Poppe, S. and Meier, H. (1971a). *Arch. Tierernähr.* **21**, 447–455; 515–529.

Poppe, S. and Meier, H. (1971b). *Arch. Tierernähr.* **21**, 531–542.

Porter, J. W. G. and Rolls, B. A. (1971). *Proc. Nutr. Soc.* **30**, 17–25.

Reiser, S. and Christiansen, P. A. (1971). *Biochim. biophys. Acta* **241**, 102–113.

Robinson, J. W. L. (1968). *Eur. J. Biochem.* **7**, 78–89.

Rogers, Q. R. and Harper, A. E. (1964). *In* "The Role of the Gastrointestinal Tract in Protein Metabolism" (H. N. Munro, ed.) pp. 3–24. Blackwell Scientific Publications, Oxford.

Rogers, Q. R. and Harper, A. E. (1966). *Wld Rev. Nutr. Diet.* **6**, 250–291.

Salter, D. N. and Coates, M. E. (1971). *Br. J. Nutr.* **26**, 55–69.

Scharrer, E. (1971). *Arch. Geflügelk.* **25**, 21–25.

Scharrer, E. and Brüggemann, J. (1971). *Z. Tierphysiol. Tierernähr. Futtermittelk.* **27**, 327–337.

Scharrer, E., Erbersdobler, H. and Zucker, H. (1967). *Z. Tierphysiol. Tierernähr. Futtermittelk.* **22**, 265–275.

Scharrer, E. and Zucker, H. (1968). *Z. Tierphysiol. Tierernähr. Futtermittelk.* **23**, 321-330.

Shotton, D. M. and Hartley, B. S. (1970). *Nature, Lond.* **225**, 802–806.

Snook, J. T. and Meyer, J. H. (1964). *J. Nutr.* **82**, 409–414.

Steitz, T. A., Henderson, R. and Blow, D. M. (1969). *J. molec. Biol.* **46**, 337–348.

Tazawa, Y. (1943). *Acta phytochim., Tokyo* **13**, 177.

Valle-Riestra, J. and Barnes, R. H. (1970). *J. Nutr.* **100**, 873–882.

Varnish, S. A. and Carpenter, K. J. (1971). *Proc. Nutr. Soc.* **30**, 70A–71A.

Walz, O. P. (1972). Ph.D. Thesis, University of Giessen.

WEBER, G. (1972). Ph.D. Thesis, University of Munich.

WILSON, T. H. and WISEMAN, G. (1954). *J. Physiol., Lond.* **123**, 116–125.

WISEMAN, G. (1968). *In* "Handbook of Physiology, Section 6: "Alimentary Canal", Vol. III. "Intestinal Absorption" (C. F. Code ed.) p. 1277. Am. Physiol. Soc., Washington, D.C.

ZEBROWSKA, T. (1968). *Br. J. Nutr.* **22**, 483–491.

ZIMMERMANN-NIELSEN, C. and SCHØNHEYDER, F. (1962). *Biochim. biophys. Acta* **63**, 201–203.

ZUCKER, H., HABEDANK, W.-D., KORNDÖRFER, L. and SCHARRER, E. (1968). *Z. Tierphysiol. Tierernähr. Futtermittelk.* **23**, 205–211.

ACKNOWLEDGEMENT

Figures 4 and 8 are reproduced by permission of Paul Parey, Hamburg and Berlin.

CHAPTER 32

The Value of Amino Acid Supplementation

H. ZUCKER

Sandoz Research Institute, Vienna, Austria

Amino acid supplementation of diets for animal and man as a means of improving protein nutrition depends mainly on (a) knowledge of (available) amino acid concentration in dietary protein sources, (b) definition of amino acid requirements and requirement interrelationships, (c) economical availability of the respective amino acids and (d) feasibility of convenient incorporation of amino acids into diets at levels which meet the requirements.

It is widely agreed that free amino acids supplied in a meal are utilized to the same extent as amino acids which are supplied "the natural way", that is in a peptide chain. The extensive secretion of proteins into the gut lumen by the intestinal mucosa and by the pancreas, providing a relatively constant milieu for the various hydrolytic and absorptive mechanisms, may be a partial explanation. At least for the supplementation of protein-containing diets with small amounts of limiting amino acids, the assumption of equal utilization can be taken as generally valid. This assumption allows us to look at supplementary free amino acids in the same way as we do at amino acids in dietary proteins.

Disregarding questions such as palatability, reactions with other food ingredients, imbalances due to large excesses of a single amino acid, utilization of D-isomers and other potentially complicating factors, we are left with the question of the amino acid content of foods and feeds and with requirements.

I. ANALYSIS

Ion exchange chromatography after acid hydrolysis has become the most commonly used method for the determination of the amino acid composition of foods and feedstuffs. Kwolek and Cavins (1971) have recently estimated coefficients of variation for individual amino acids from 18 references, taking into account variation between independent hydrolysates and independent samples. Although the mean coefficients of variation for most amino acids were 6–7% of the mean, the values calculated for lysine, tryptophan, methionine and cysteine were 8·4, 10·6, 11·1 and 14·1 respectively. With the variations evenly distributed, one could be confident that such errors would have relatively little effect on mean values based on a large number of independent analyses and presented in widely-used tables. On the other hand, much of our information on requirements is based on experiments in which basal diets or their components are analysed once and graded levels of the amino acid in question are added. This yields fairly good agreement of results within a series of experiments within one laboratory, but the results may easily differ by 10–15% from those another laboratory would find from an identical experimental design.

Unfortunately, the most important candidates for supplementation, methionine, lysine and perhaps tryptophan, are associated with circumstances which complicate easy assessment. The sulphur-containing amino acids are subject to extensive oxidation depending on the procedure employed. The use of lysine values is complicated by the availability problem, and tryptophan, besides being present and required in particularly low concentrations, is quite frequently omitted from routine analyses since it requires a special procedure.

II. REQUIREMENT

Specification of requirement remains a confusing issue. Stated as "per cent of diet", the requirement may easily vary by $\pm$ 20%, if the range of possible energy densities and protein levels is taken into consideration. If expressed as level or amount per unit of energy, a certain ratio of energy to protein has to be assumed. It seems preferable to define amino acid requirements in g/16 g N at the minimum protein intake which fulfils the desired performance, relating protein intake at the same time to energy intake. Expressing amino acid needs in per cent of protein would also facilitate comparison between ages, levels of performance and species more satisfactorily than do other systems.

Criteria for measuring requirements seem simple in the case of chickens, where rate of growth, feathering, rate of lay, egg size and feed conversion are usually employed. In swine, carcass quality is highly dependent on protein nutrition, and response to its improvement may be confined in some cases largely to a change in the ratio of fat to lean tissue. Interactions between breed and feeding technique—restricted or *ad lib.*—may also occur. Desired and achieved growth rates at various ages vary much more with pigs than with poultry, and so do staple feedstuffs and environmental conditions. These factors may account for the particularly poor reproducibility of results of amino acid supplementation with swine. Carpenter (1971) has recently given examples and pointed to possible sources of errors.

Variation in amino acid content of natural protein sources, errors in assays, variation in protein and energy content (which governs feed intake), variation in requirement and errors in its estimate: all these independent factors combine to give a rather broad range of uncertainty about the effectiveness of amino acid supplementation under practical conditions.

III. SUPPLEMENTATION

So far, there has been only one notable exception of widely-recognized importance. The growing chicken, with its need for extensive feather production on a comparatively large body surface at a time of fast body growth, has a requirement of at least 3·5 g of sulphur amino acids/16 g of dietary N. A mineral- and vitamin-supplemented maize–soya-bean meal diet meets its needs for all nutrients most economically in many parts of the world. About 0·5 g of DL-methionine per 16 g of N usually makes up for the low concentration of methionine and cysteine in this ration.

With soya-bean meal and maize, two protein sources of remarkable constancy in protein content and amino acid pattern, an estimated mean deficit of 10–20% in the limiting amino acid can be safely assumed, and the appropriate addition made. The positive feedback on methionine production from the increasing acceptance of this practice has resulted in the price of feedgrade methionine falling to one-sixth of that prevailing in 1955.

For growing swine, the sulphur amino acid requirement is somewhat lower and is easily met by many common rations. Requiring less protein per unit of energy than chicks, that is a lower protein percentage in the feed, the ratio of grain protein to supplementary protein is reversed in swine feeding. In the case of soya-bean meal, broilers consume roughly two parts of soya-bean protein to one part of grain protein, whereas swine are given about two parts of grain protein to one part of soya-bean protein. Thus lysine becomes the limiting amino acid or—if maize is the grain used—possibly tryptophan.

This simple relationship should provide for a substantial demand for supplementary lysine and possibly, in maize growing areas, for tryptophan, if these amino acids could replace all or part of the protein supplements whose major functions seem to lie in supplying these two amino acids.

IV. ECONOMICS

Since neither the lysine nor the tryptophan requirement of swine has been agreed by potential users, the position is less satisfactory than that with the broilers given maize–soya-bean–methionine diets. Accordingly, another approach is chosen to illustrate some of the main economic factors which may indicate the potential usefulness of these amino acids as supplements for swine feeds.

"High-lysine maize", characterized by a somewhat increased protein content and 50% more lysine and tryptophan per 16 g N, has yielded growth rates and feed conversion figures similar to conventional maize–soya-bean rations in some experiments with pigs. Even with "high-lysine maize" there is still a requirement for some supplementary lysine. Moreover, normal hybrid maize, supplemented with lysine and tryptophan, gave results similar to those obtained from "high-lysine maize", as was shown first by Cromwell *et al.* (1967).

Assuming equivalence in nutritional performance from diets (a) 850 kg maize plus 150 kg soya-bean meal, and (b) 1000 kg maize plus 2·25 kg L-lysine plus 0·60 kg L-tryptophan, one can calculate under which set of cost conditions the amino acid version (b) is superior to the conventional maize–soya-bean mixture (a). Diet (a) would yield about 14% protein; (b) about 9% protein. (Necessary additions of minerals and vitamins are neglected, and differences in energy content ignored.) The additions of lysine and tryptophan lead to totals of 5 g and 1·4 g per 16 g N, respectively. These levels are on the higher side of the range of possible requirements.

In the accompanying illustrations, the advantage of using tryptophan is investigated by varying either the cost of maize (Figs 1–4) or of soya-bean meal (Figs 5 and 6), with prices for lysine set at different levels for each example. The cost advantage of using a tryptophan supplement (at zero cost for tryptophan) can be read from the ordinate for any chosen abscissa value. The lower line shows the maize plus lysine price as a function of increasing maize cost. The upper line indicates the price of the maize–soya-bean meal mixture (a) at the respective maize (soya-bean meal) prices. The difference between both lines is the cost allowable for 0·6 kg tryptophan.

In Fig. 1 soya-bean meal is fixed at \$100/ton. It can be seen that an increasing price of maize reduces scope for the use of tryptophan. At the low maize price of \$40/ton, tryptophan can cost up to \$11·50/kg, but its value becomes zero with maize costing \$80/ton (Fig. 1a).

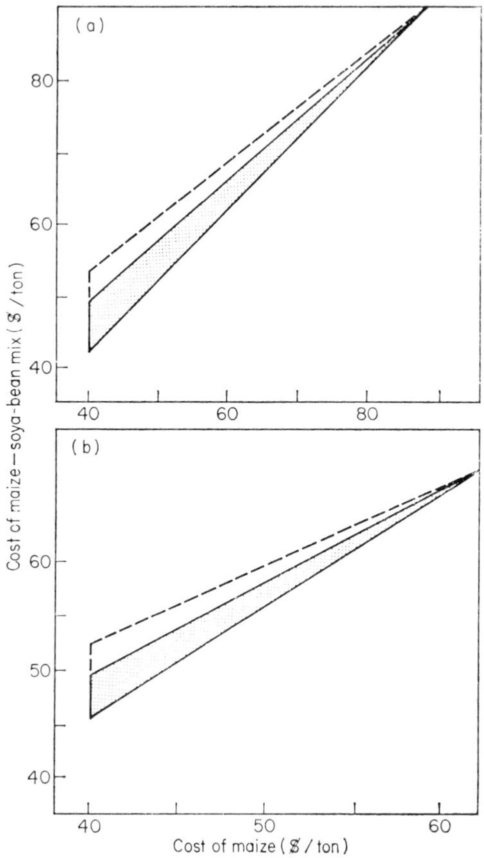

FIG. 1. Allowance for tryptophan, depending on the prices of maize and lysine. Soya-bean price fixed high (\$100/ton). a, lysine \$1.00/kg; b, lysine \$2.50/kg

With more expensive lysine (Fig. 1b), using tryptophan is less attractive. Even with maize costing only \$40/ton, its cost can only be \$7/kg and becomes zero with maize at \$62/ton. In this model, tryptophan can be afforded only if lysine is cheap.

Figure 2 presents the same two lysine prices, but with soya-bean meal reduced to \$80/ton. Even at the low lysine price, the allowance for tryptophan is only \$6/kg at the lowest maize price. Reducing soya-bean meal from \$100 to \$80/ton has about the same effect on tryptophan as lowering lysine from \$2.50 to \$1.00/kg. With soya-bean meal at \$80/ton and lysine at \$2.50/kg the use of tryptophan is uneconomic whatever the cost of maize (Fig. 2b).

In Fig. 3, soya-bean cost is the variable and maize is fixed at \$40/ton

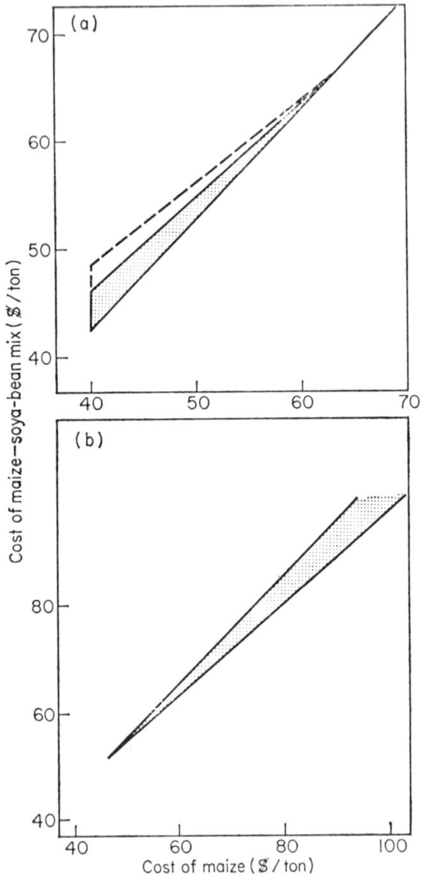

FIG. 2. Allowance for tryptophan depending on the price of maize and lysine. Soya-bean price fixed low (\$80/ton). a, lysine \$1.00/kg; b, lysine \$2.50/kg

and \$60/ton, respectively. With cheap lysine, tryptophan again can cost up to \$11.50/kg with soya-bean meal costing \$100/ton (cf. Fig. 1a). Here again, increasing lysine to \$2.50/kg restricts tryptophan use to high soya-bean meal prices. The higher maize price (Fig. 3b) further reduces scope for the use of tryptophan.

The assumed need for 0·6 kg of tryptophan may be an overestimate

(Baker *et al.*, 1971), and if 0·3 kg were sufficient to balance the diet, then using the same calculations, the cost of tryptophan could be twice as high.

These examples emphasize some basic features involved in quantifying the value of amino acid supplementation. The main factors are usually energy cost and the cost of competing protein sources which can supply

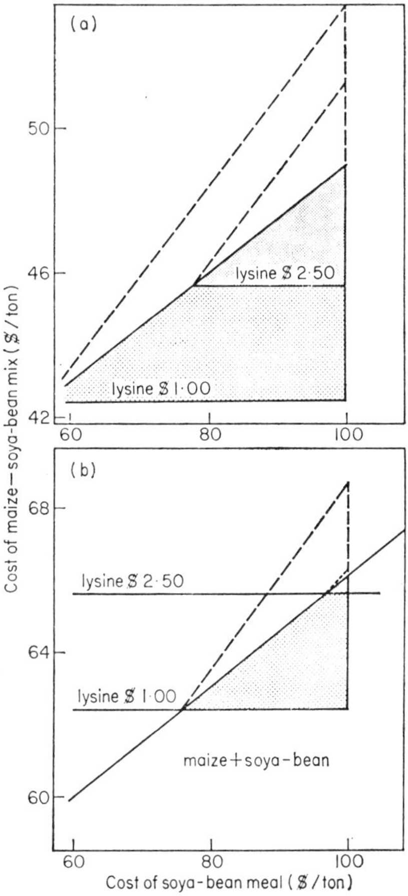

FIG. 3. Allowance for tryptophan depending on the price of soya-bean meal. Lysine $1.00/kg or $2.50/kg. a, maize $40/ton; b, maize $60/ton

the limiting amino acids. The cost of other limiting amino acids, contained in protein or added as free amino acids, can also affect the calculations, as was shown by varying the price of lysine.

In order to evaluate precisely the economic chances and limitations for supplementation in a more complicated situation, linear programming has to be employed. If correct estimates of ingredient composition and requirements are available, it provides an excellent tool for investigating a large number of possible formulations. Linear programming does not, of course, eliminate the need for feeding trials to test the performance of the various rations.

Since the effect of protein nutrition depends so much on the mutual supplementary action of proteins, amino acid supplementation usually implies good control of the whole diet. Such is the case in the manufacture of compounded feeds for pigs and poultry. In human nutrition, however, complete control of dietary intake is confined to exceptional situations, such as those in institutions.

V. PROTEIN EVALUATION MODELS AND LIMITING AMINO ACIDS

In conventional assays for protein quality, a response to amino acid supplementation can easily be demonstrated. Figure 4 shows the effects of combined lysine and methionine supplementation in a recent experiment in our laboratory. The mixed protein sources were typical in com-

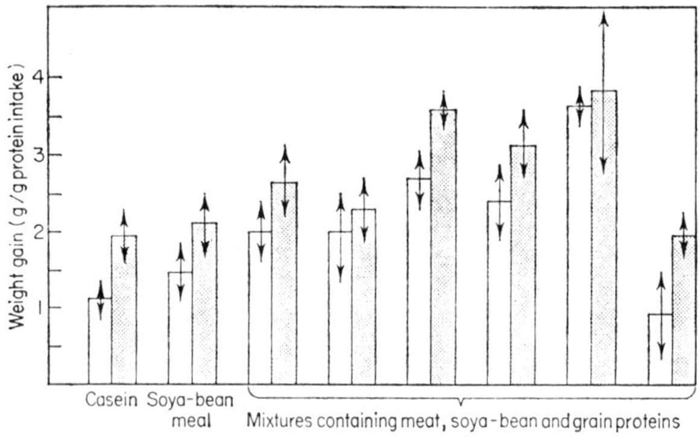

FIG. 4. Growth response of rats to addition of lysine and methionine to a semi-purified diet containing 7% protein.
□ without amino acids
::: with 0·135% lysine and 0·090% methionine added to the diet

position of many food and feed products and had been subjected to cooking. One could conclude that, at marginal protein intake, most of our foods would benefit from an addition of one or both of these frequently limiting amino acids. With increasing protein intake, such responses are usually gradually diminished. Therefore, the projection of such results to any practical situation is very questionable.

At near optimum performance, the growth responses to protein sources are often better than those expected from their calculated content of the limiting amino acid. Figure 5 is such an example from our earlier work. This is undoubtedly due to other "minor" limiting factors, or to inaccuracies in our assessment of requirements. Such findings imply that a very substantial advantage has to come from amino acid fortification of foods before it will be widely accepted as a practical alternative to the use of higher protein levels or combinations of proteins.

Investigation of specific, well-defined nutritional regimes of the species

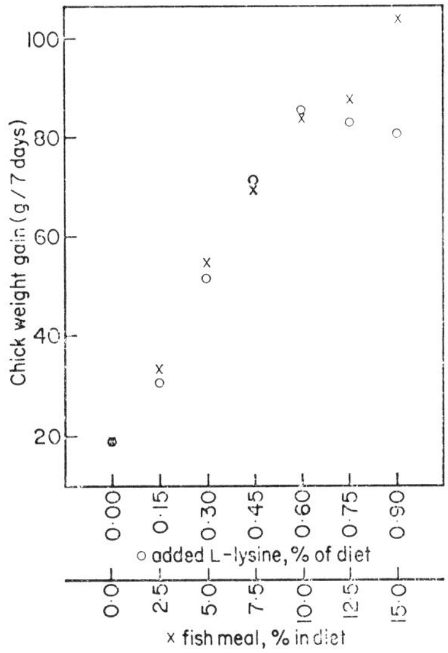

FIG. 5. Chick growth response to L-lysine or to the same amount given as fish meal added to a semi-purified diet containing 27% protein and 0·64% lysine (0·47% available lysine)

concerned seems much more rewarding than detailed studies of the protein quality of individual proteins. The series of comparisons of the biological values for human subjects and rats of a wide variety of combined N sources, conducted by Kofrânyi and his co-workers at the Max Planck Institute, Dortmund, is exemplified in Fig. 6. Such results should caution against too-liberal extrapolation of protein quality results.

One reason for considerable differences between species might be the different ratio of N turnover for maintenance to N requirement for tissue synthesis in growth, resulting from different growth rates. This is demonstrated by a comparison of man and pig in Fig. 7, two species of similar body weight but entirely different growth rate patterns. Synthesizing different kinds of proteins necessitates different amino acid requirements,

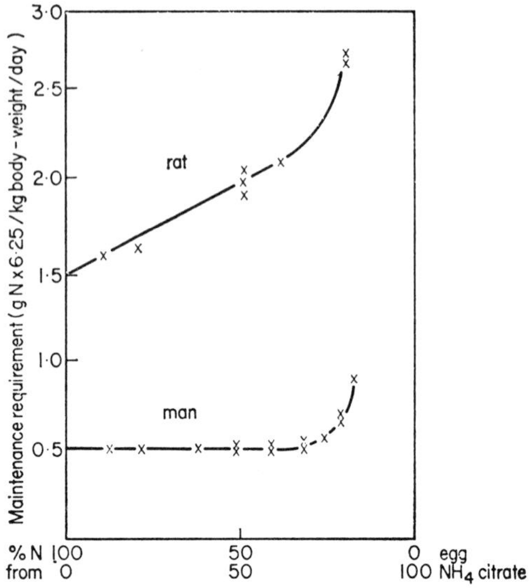

FIG. 6. Effect on protein quality for man and rat of diluting egg protein with ammonium citrate (Jekat and Pabst, 1969)

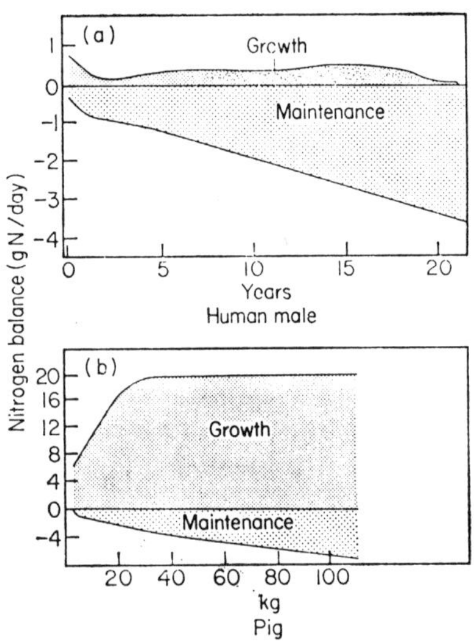

FIG. 7. Comparison of N requirement for growth and for maintenance in (a) a slow-growing species (man) and (b) a fast-growing species (pig)
a after Allison (1960)

as was shown by Rose in his comparisons of the amino acid requirements of growing and adult subjects.

There is little doubt that the supplementation of feeds and foods with synthetic amino acids will increase in importance. DL-methionine has already become an indispensable commodity. The production of L-lysine by a fermentation process is increasing. Ruminants, for which recent research shows benefit from high-quality proteins or essential amino acids if these materials by-pass rumen fermentation, may become major users of both methionine and lysine. Livestock as a whole, consuming 4–6 times as much protein as the human population, may trigger the demand for some other amino acids. Though initial commercial production and introduction is expensive, amino acids seem to find their way into nutrition via animal feeds rather than in the field of human food, where they could save protein of much higher cost. This paradoxical situation might continue if other amino acids besides lysine and methionine become available for use in diets.

With fast-changing production techniques, new plant crops and by-products, it is difficult to predict which amino acid may be found limiting on a scale large enough to induce commercial interest. Present knowledge of limiting amino acids would suggest tryptophan and threonine to be the most likely candidates. But the speed of such development will in any case be greatly influenced by the techniques used in the evaluation of efficiency, and by their precision.

REFERENCES

Allison, J. B. (1960). *Int. Congr. Nutr.* 5, Washington, D.C. **2**, 6–12.

Baker, D. H., Allen, N. K., Boomgaardt, J., Graber, G. and Norton, H. W. (1971). *J. Anim. Sci.* **33**, 42–46.

Carpenter, K. J. (1971). *Proc. Nutr. Soc.* **30**, 73–83.

Cromwell, G. L., Pickett, R. A. and Beeson, W. M. (1967). *J. Anim. Sci.* **26**, 1325–1331.

Jekat, F. and Pabst, W. (1969). *Z. ges. exp. Med.* **150**, 70–75.

Kwolek, W. F. and Cavins, J. F. (1971). *J. Ass. off. analyt. Chem.* **54**, 1283–1287.

CHAPTER 33

Toxic Factors in Protein Foods

IRVIN E. LIENER

University of Minnesota, USA

I. INTRODUCTION

One of the most dramatic and certainly controversial developments in the food industry has been the use of chemical additives for improving the functional properties, nutritional value, and shelf-life of food products. The introduction of these foreign chemicals into our food is under close surveillance by appropriate government agencies who are charged with the responsibility for protecting the health of the consumer. What is sometimes overlooked, however, is the fact that Nature herself has seen fit to contaminate our food with chemicals, which, although natural components of living tissue, may nevertheless be toxic to man. Unlike chemicals which are deliberately added to foods, these natural toxicants pose a special problem since their presence cannot be legislated out of existence. Unlike a chemical additive which should be assumed to be toxic until proved otherwise, the natural food is generally assumed to be safe if it has been consumed by man for centuries with relative impunity.

Although both plant and animal food products may contain these naturally occurring toxic factors, the emphasis here will be mainly on plant foodstuffs since our hope for feeding the exploding world population of the future will rest largely on the expanded use of plants as a source of protein. I have in mind here such important oil-bearing seeds as soya-bean, peanut and cottonseed, and a large variety of legumes which constitute an important component of the daily diet in many of the underdeveloped countries.

In addition to the naturally occurring toxic substances in plants, brief mention will be made of some examples of natural toxins in animal food products. In addition, brief consideration will be given to the problem of toxicity that may arise as a result of microbial activity or as a consequence of the manipulations which the food product may have received during processing or storage.

A note of explanation regarding the use of the term "toxic" would perhaps be in order at this point. In the context of our present discussion I wish to avoid the restrictive definition of a toxic substance such as might be used by a toxicologist—namely a substance which when administered to an animal (by some specified route) produces death at a certain level. Rather I would prefer to use the term "toxic" in its broadest sense, that is, to describe any adverse physiological response which detracts from the nutritive value of a particular foodstuff whether this be manifested simply as a retardation of growth or an interference with the utilization of protein or something more subtle and insidious such as cancer of the liver or kidneys.

As one who has been trained to think as a biochemist I am inclined to view the natural toxic substances in terms of their chemical structure. In so doing I find it convenient to classify the natural toxic factors into three main categories (Fig. 1):

Proteins or Amino acid derivatives	Trypsin inhibitors Haemagglutinins Lathyrogens
Glycosides	Goitrogens Cyanogens
Miscellaneous	Gossypol Metal-binding factors Anti-vitamin factors

FIG. 1. Classification of naturally occurring toxins

II. NATURALLY OCCURRING TOXICANTS IN PLANTS

A. Proteins and Amino Acid Derivatives

1. *Trypsin Inhibitors*

It was not long after soya-beans were introduced into the United States that Osborne and Mendel (1917) observed that soya-beans had to be heated in order to support the normal growth of rats. Kunitz (1946) subsequently isolated from raw soya-beans a protein which had the unique property of combining with trypsin to form an inactive complex. It was logical to assume that the trypsin inhibitor was the substance responsible for the poor nutritive value of unheated soya-beans. The hypothesis that its effect could be readily explained on the basis of its ability to inhibit intestinal proteolysis was an appealing one. The fact also that methionine

TABLE I. The effect of heat and methionine on the nutritive value of soya-bean for rats. (Data taken from Liener *et al.*, 1949.)

Diet	*Protein efficiency*
Raw soya-bean meal	1·33
Autoclaved soya-bean meal	2·62
Raw soya-bean meal + 0·6% methionine	2·42

exerted a marked improvement on the nutritive value of raw soya-beans (Table I) was taken to indicate that the trypsin inhibitor somehow interfered with the availability or utilization of methionine from the raw bean.

It now appears that the true explanation for the growth-inhibitory property of the trypsin inhibitor is not a simple one, and, although over 25 years have elapsed since Kunitz first isolated the trypsin inhibitor, there is still a lack of certainty regarding the mechanism whereby the trypsin inhibitor exerts its effect. There is little doubt that hypertrophy of the pancreas is one of the primary physiological effects produced by giving raw soya-beans (Booth *et al.*, 1960) or the isolated inhibitor (Nesheim *et al.*, 1962). Booth *et al.* (1960) are of the opinion that pancreatic hypertrophy leads to an excessive loss of endogenous protein secreted by the pancreas. Since this protein is quite rich in cystine, this represents a net loss of sulphur-containing amino acids from the body. This would explain why the need for methionine is so acute in diets containing raw soya-beans.

The situation is made even more complicated by the fact that there are known to be at least five different trypsin inhibitors in soya-beans (Liener and Kakade, 1969) whose physiological significance has yet to be established.

Trypsin inhibitors have also been found in a large number of other legumes including the peanut, navy bean and lima bean; in fact, all legumes which so far have been examined have been found to contain trypsin inhibitors in varying degrees. The exact nutritional significance of these inhibitors is not clear since there does not appear to be any clear-cut correlation between the trypsin inhibitor content of various legumes and the beneficial effect which heat has on their nutritional value (Borchers and Ackerson, 1950).

With the increased use of isolated soya-bean protein for the fabrication of textured meal analogues intended for human consumption, the question

TABLE II. Trypsin inhibitor activities of soya-bean flour, isolate, fibre, and finished textured products. (Data taken from Liener, 1971.)

	Antitrypsin activity	
Product	TIU/g *dry solids*[a] $\times 10^{-3}$	% *of soya-bean flour*
Soya-bean flour (unheated)	86·4	100
Soya-bean isolate	25·5	30
Soya-bean fibre	12·3	14
Chicken analogue	6·9	8
Ham analogue	10·2	12
Beef analogue	6·5	7

[a] Trypsin inhibitor activity determined by the method of Kakade *et al.* (1969). TIU = trypsin inhibitor units as defined in this reference.

has arisen as to whether such products contain appreciable levels of trypsin inhibitor, and, if so, whether they constitute a hazard to health. The first part of this question is very easy to answer (Table II). Soya-bean isolate and the fibre derived therefrom are surprisingly rich in trypsin inhibitor activity. Even the processed meat analogue has a fair amount of antitryptic activity. What this means in terms of human nutrition is very difficult to say. I am inclined to believe that the trypsin inhibitor has little significance as far as human nutrition is concerned. It is of interest to note that most of the activity values reported in the literature for the soya-bean inhibitors have been based on studies with *bovine* trypsin. *In vitro* studies (Feeney *et al.*, 1969; Travis and Roberts, 1969) with human trypsin, however, have demonstrated that this enzyme is only weakly inhibited by the soya-bean inhibitor. Furthermore, the trypsin inhibitor of egg white (ovomucoid) has virtually no effect on the nitrogen balance of human subjects (Scudamore *et al.*, 1949).

2. *Phytohaemagglutinins (PHA)*

Another kind of protein which appears to be universally distributed among the legumes is a protein which has the unique property of being able to agglutinate red blood cells, the so-called phytohaemagglutinins (PHA). A number of years ago we (Liener, 1953) showed that the purified PHA of soya-beans was in fact capable of producing a significant degree of growth inhibition in rats (Table III). We next turned our attention to

TABLE III. Growth inhibitory effect of the soya-bean haemagglutinin (SBH). (Data taken from Liener, 1953.)

Protein component of diet	*Weight gain g/2 weeks*	*% growth inhibition*
25% heated soya-bean meal	60	0
25% raw soya-bean meal	28	43
25% heated soya-bean meal + 0·8% SBH	45	26

PHA from other legumes. We were particularly interested in those legumes which enjoy popular consumption in some of the lesser-developed countries. For this purpose we obtained samples of a black bean from Guatemala, the Bengal and red gram from India, and the mung bean from the Philippines, and a domestic variety of the kidney bean. The effect of heat on the nutritive value of these beans is shown in Table IV; only the growth-promoting properties of the black and kidney beans were improved by heat. As shown in Table V, these same two beans were also the only ones which displayed a significant level of haemagglutinating activity. For these reasons PHA was purified from each of these beans and given at various levels to rats in a basal ration containing 10% casein. From the results presented in Table VI, it is evident that an inhibition of growth was obtained at levels as low as 0·5% of the diet, the kidney bean haemagglutinin at a level of 0·5% caused 100% mortality after about 2 weeks, whereas 1·2% of the black bean haemagglutinin was necessary to produce a similar mortality rate.

These results also show that the toxicity of both haemagglutinins may be destroyed by heat treatment. It would be well to point out here that in

TABLE IV. Effect of heat on nutritive value of some legumes. (Data taken from Honavar *et al.*, 1962.)

Source of protein	*Gain in weight* (g/day) *Raw*[a]	*Heated*
Phaseolus vulgaris		
Black bean	−1·94 (4–5)	+1·61
Kidney bean	−1·04 (11–13)	+1·48
Cicer arietinum		
Bengal gram	+1·25	+1·16
Cajanus cajan		
Red gram	+1·33	+1·74
Phaseolus aureus		
Mung bean	+1·05	+1·07

[a] 100% mortality observed during period (in days) shown in parentheses

our experience preliminary soaking prior to autoclaving or cooking of the bean is necessary for the complete destruction of PHA. Human cases of intoxication by partially cooked beans belonging to the genus *Phaseolus* have been reported from time to time (Jaffe, 1969). Recommendations for use of bean flours for baked goods, which involves the use of dry heat, should therefore be viewed with caution.

TABLE V. Haemagglutinating and antitryptic activities of crude extracts[a] of raw legumes. (Data taken from Honavar *et al.*, 1962.)

Legume	*Haemagglutinating activity* (HU/ml)	*Antitryptic activity* (TIU/ml)
Phaseolus vulgaris		
Black bean	2450	2050
Kidney bean	3560	1552
Cicer arietinum	0	220
Cajanus cajan	0	418
Phaseolus aureus	0	260

[a] A 10% suspension of the finely ground meal in 1% NaCl clarified by centrifugation

TABLE VI. Effect of purified haemagglutinin fractions from the black bean and kidney bean on the growth of rats. (Data taken from Honavar *et al.*, 1962.)

Source of haemagglutinin	*Purified haemagglutinin in diet* (%)	*Average gain in weight* (gm/day)	*Mortality*[a] (days)
Black bean	0	+2·51	
	0·5	+1·04	
	0·5[b]	+2·37	
	0·75	+0·20	
	1·2	−0·91	15–19
	2·3	−1·61	12–17
	4·6	−1·72	5–7
Kidney bean	0	+2·31	
	0·5	−0·60	13–16
	0·5[b]	+2·29	
	1·0	−0·87	11–13
	1·5	−1·22	4–7

[a] 100% mortality observed during period recorded here. Blank space indicates that no deaths were observed.

[b] Solution of haemagglutinin boiled for 30 min and dried coagulum fed at the level indicated. Haemagglutinating activity was completely destroyed by this treatment

3. *Lathyrogens*

Lathyrism is a disease associated with the consumption of certain species of peas belonging to the genus *Lathyrus*. It is particularly prevalent in India, especially during famine which results from periods of drought when the crop fields become blighted, and, as an alternate crop, a type of pea referred to as the chickling vetch or *L. sativus* is cultivated. Those who eat this plant frequently are afflicted with paralysis of the central nervous system and paralysis of the lower limbs.

Attempts to identify the causative agent of human lathyrism have been complicated by the fact that another species of *Lathyrus*, namely *L. odoratus* or sweet pea, produces in rats a type of lathyrism which is characterized by skeletal deformities. In contrast to this, rats thrive quite well on *L. sativus* and do not display the nervous disorder associated with the consumption of this species in man. Historically, the lathyrogen of the sweet pea was isolated first and identified as β-(N-γ-glutamyl)-aminopropionitrile

(McKay *et al.*, 1954) whose structure is shown in Fig. 2. It should be emphasized that this compound is not found in *L. sativus* and hence has little relevance to the pathogenesis of human lathyrism.

The isolation of a substance from *L. sativus* which produces neurotoxic effects when injected into chicks has been reported (Adiga *et al.*, 1964; Murti *et al.*, 1964) and identified as β-N-oxalyl-α,β-diaminopropionic acid (Fig. 3). Any conclusion that this compound is in fact the sole causative

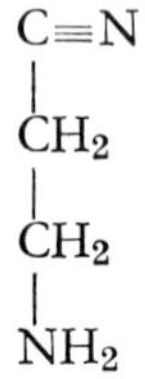

β-aminopropionitrile (BAPN)

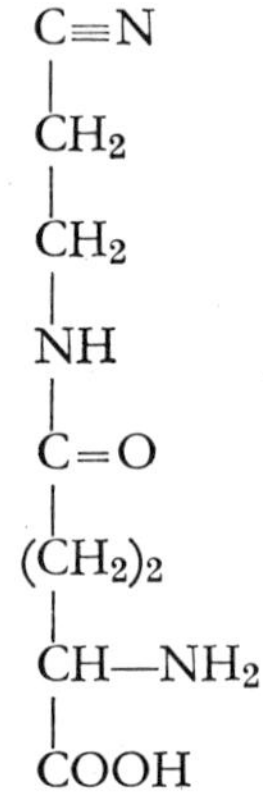

β-(N-γ-glutamyl)-aminopropionitrile

FIG. 2. Structure of osteolathyrogen in *L. odoratus* (sweet pea)

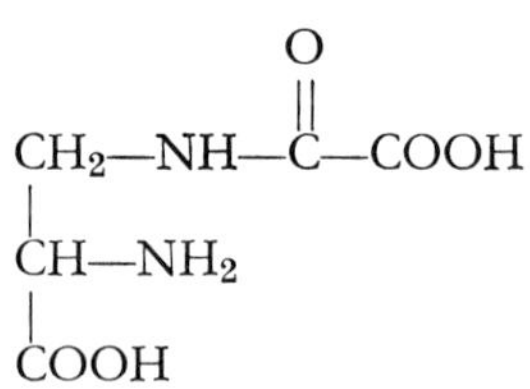

β-N-oxalyl-α,β-diaminopropionic acid

Found in: *L. sativus*

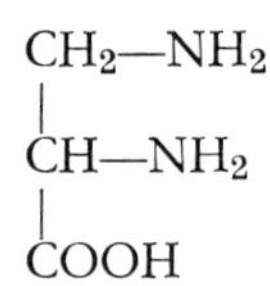

α,β-diaminopropionic acid

FIG. 3. Structure of neurolathyrogen in *L. sativus* (chickling vetch)

agent of human lathyrism must await the outcome of experiments involving the oral ingestion of this chemical by suitable experimental animals. Assuming that diaminopropionic acid is the culprit involved in human lathyrism, it may come as a surprise to learn that all of the misery in the past associated with the consumption of *L. sativus* could have been avoided by a relatively simple detoxification procedure involving soaking the dehusked seeds overnight followed by steaming for 30 min or roasting at

150° for 20 min (Sarma and Padmanaban, 1969). Actually this legume contains 24–28% protein which is rich in lysine (Sarma, 1968); so despite the tarnished name which the *Lathyrus* has had over the years, it may yet have potential as a protein supplement in a country which sorely needs it.

B. Glycosides

1. *Goitrogens*

Frequently the adverse physiological effects associated with the consumption of certain foods are not manifested in such obvious ways as retarded growth, paralysis, or, in the extreme case, death. A case in point is the observation that unheated soya-beans produce a marked enlargement of the thyroid gland of the rat and chick, an effect which can be counteracted, however, by the administration of iodide or partially eliminated by heat (Patton *et al.*, 1939). A typical experiment is shown in Fig. 4 where the thyroid enlargement produced by soya-bean milk has

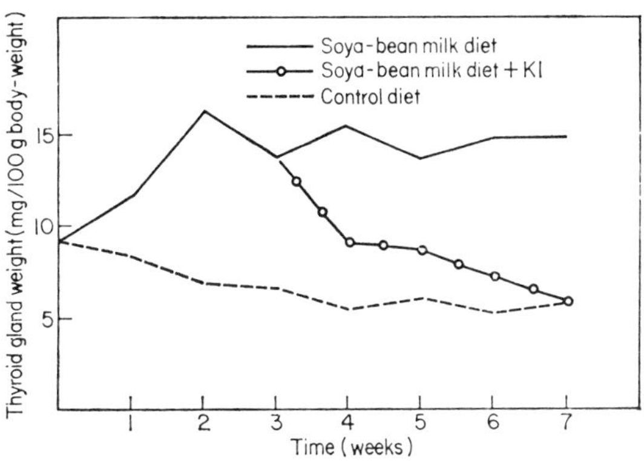

FIG. 4. Effect on the thyroid gland of the rat of a soya-bean milk diet with and without supplemental iodide (Taken from Anderson, 1961)

been largely counteracted by adding iodide to the diet at a level of 1·6 mg/kg of diet. The particular agent responsible for the goitrogenicity of improperly processed soya-bean protein has not yet been identified.

Goitrogenic agents are also widely distributed in the Brassicae or cabbage family, which includes such common edible plants as cabbage, turnip, cauliflower, kale, Brussels sprouts, broccoli, and rutabaga which are used in the human diet, and the rapeseed and mustardseed which, after extraction of the oil, are used largely for feeding animals. In most cases the chemical agents responsible for goitrogenicity have been isolated and characterized as sulphur-containing glycosides (VanEtten, 1969). An example of such a thioglycoside is *sinigrin*, which is widely distributed among plants of the cabbage family. This compound is hydrolysed by an enzyme contained in the plant tissue to produce allyl isothiocyanate which is the actual goitrogenic agent (Fig. 5). Goitrin or 5-vinyloxazolidine-2-thione is another potent antithyroid compound produced by hydrolysis of a thioglycoside also found in most members of the cabbage family. Since the release of these goitrogens is mediated by an enzyme already present in the plant, the destruction of these enzymes by cooking, autoclaving, or extraction with water serves to reduce the goitrogenicity of rapeseed and mustardseed meals. Steam distillation of

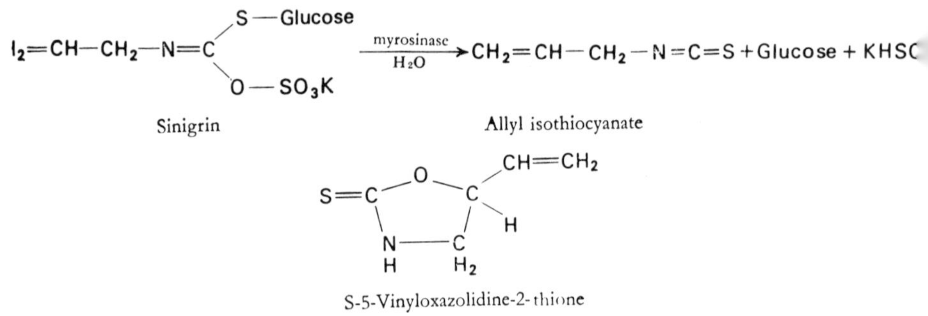

FIG. 5. Structure of the goitrogenic glycoside, sinigrin, and its hydrolysis products

cooked and solvent-extracted mustardseed serves to detoxify the meal so that the resulting product produces growth gains in animals essentially equivalent to properly heated soya-bean meal. In contrast to the goitrogenic effect of soya-beans, dietary supplementation with iodide is of little therapeutic value since these goitrogens are thyrotoxic because of their ability to inhibit the uptake of iodide by the thyroid gland. Lest we become too concerned about how much Brussels sprouts or broccoli we include in our diet, it has been estimated that it would take a daily intake of 10 kg of these plants to produce an effective goitrogenic concentration in the blood (Neuhaus, 1969).

2. *Cyanogens*

It has been known for a long time that a wide variety of plants is potentially toxic because they contain glycosides from which HCN is released by hydrolysis (Montgomery, 1969). Those most commonly eaten by man and animals are listed in Table VII in order of their potential cyanide content. In the early years of the present century, and again during World War I, lima beans imported into Europe from tropical countries (Java, Puerto Rico, and Burma) were responsible for serious outbreaks of cyanide poisoning, and cases of human intoxication from the consumption of certain varieties of lima beans are not uncommon today in some of the tropical countries. It is reassuring to note that most of the lima beans consumed in the US and UK at the present time are well below the toxic level implicated in fatal cases of poisoning. Sorghum has been responsible for the death of large numbers of livestock that consume the young green leaves of this plant which are rich in the cyanogen, *dhurrin*. The latter is absent in sorghum used for silage and in the dried seed which is sometimes consumed as food by man (Conn, 1969). The poisonous nature of improperly cooked cassava has been recognized for hundreds of years in the tropics where large quantities of these plants are consumed by the natives. The consumption of cassava is believed to be the cause of the

TABLE VII. Cyanide content of certain plants. (Data taken from Montgomery, 1969.)

Plant	*HCN yield* (mg/100 g)
Lima bean (*Phaseolus lunatus*)	
Samples incriminated in fatal human poisoning	210–312
Normal levels	14·4–16·7
Sorghum	250
Cassava	113
Linseed meal	53
Black-eyed pea (*Vigna sinensis*)	2·1
Garden pea (*Pisum sativum*)	2·3
Kidney bean (*Phaseolus vulgaris*)	2·0
Bengal gram (*Cicer arietinum*)	0·8
Red gram (*Cajanus cajan*)	0·5

high incidence of a degenerative disease, known as *ataxic neuropathy*, in Nigeria. The high levels of thiocyanate in blood associated with this disease are thought to be the result of the detoxification of the cyanide which is derived from cassava (Osuntokun, 1970).

Cyanide in the form of HCN is released from a glycoside through enzymic action as illustrated by the hydrolysis of *phaseolunatin* (also known as *linamarin*), the cyanide-containing glycoside of the lima bean (Fig. 6). Hydrolysis occurs when the plant is macerated in water, and the free HCN readily volatilizes on boiling. If, however, the cooking utensil is covered with a lid, condensation may occur, so that the cooking water may become heavily contaminated and should be discarded. If the cassava root becomes bruised, autohydrolysis of the glycoside may occur before it ever reaches the cooking pot. It is traditional, therefore, to wash

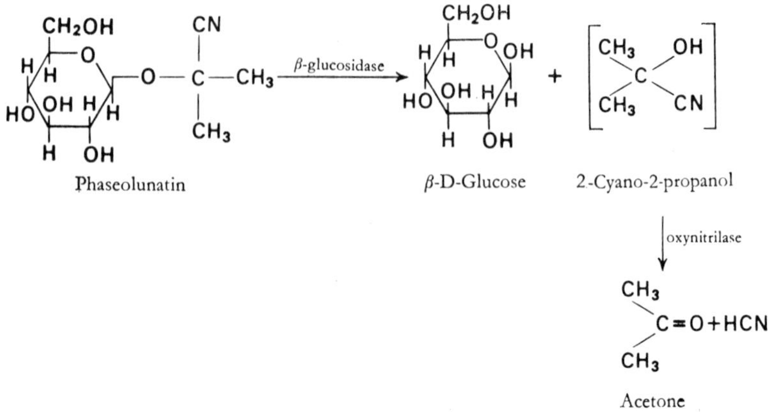

Fig. 6. Structure of the cyanogenetic glycoside, phaseolunatin, and its hydrolysis products

the plant in running water before cooking in order to eliminate any free cyanogen.

3. *Cycasin*

The seeds of the cycad plant (*Cycas circinalis*) provide a valuable source of starch for inhabitants of the Pacific islands, particularly Guam. It has been known for many years that these seeds, unless thoroughly soaked and extracted with water, can produce acute toxic effects in man and animals (Yang and Mickelsen, 1969). When rats are given diets containing several per cent of cycad seeds, a high proportion of the animals develops tumours in the kidney and liver. The carcinogenic principle of the cycad has been identified as a glycoside, *cycasin*, which has the structure shown in Fig. 7. Actually this glycoside is not toxic unless hydrolysed by the

$$CH_3\overset{\overset{O}{\uparrow}}{N}{=}NCH_2{-}O{-}\text{glucose}$$

Cycasin

$$CH_3{-}\overset{\overset{O}{\uparrow}}{N}{=}NCH_2{-}O{-}\text{primverose}$$

Macrozamin

$$CH_3\overset{\overset{O}{\uparrow}}{N}{=}NCH_2OH$$

Methyl azoxymethanol (MAM)

Fig. 7. Structure of cycasin and its hydrolysis product

microflora to form *methyl azoxymethanol* which is an extremely potent carcinogen. It is believed that methyl azomethanol is further metabolized by the liver to diazomethane which may initiate carcinogenesis by virtue of its ability to methylate nucleic acids.

C. Miscellaneous Toxic Factors

1. *Gossypol*

In contrast to the widespread distribution of most of the toxic substances mentioned so far, gossypol is found only in the pigment glands of the cottonseed. For many years, cottonseed meal was considered an undesirable protein supplement for monogastric animals, and certainly out of the question for human consumption. Modern technology has now given us the means for effectively reducing the gossypol content of cottonseed meal (Berardi and Goldblatt, 1969). Furthermore, glandless varieties of cottonseed which are virtually devoid of gossypol have been developed by plant breeders. All of these advances enhance the possibility that cottonseed flour can become an important source of protein in the human diet.

2. *Favism*

Favism is a disease characterized by haemolytic anaemia which affects certain individuals following ingestion of the broad bean (*Vicia faba*). This disease is confined largely to the inhabitants of countries surrounding the Mediterranean basin, although individuals of the same ethnic background residing in other countries frequently suffer from favism. Individual susceptibility to this disease is believed to be hereditary, and an attack is frequently precipitated simply by exposure to the pollen of the blossoms of this legume (Luisada, 1941).

Despite extensive studies on the clinical and biochemical manifestations of favism, the causative principle has not been identified with any degree of certainty. One of the difficulties lies in the fact that it has not been possible to reproduce this disease in experimental animals. Although heating improves the nutritive value of the broad bean for the rat (Borchers and Ackerson, 1950), no symptoms resembling human favism have been observed with the raw bean.

The causative principle of favism has been reported to be a glucose-

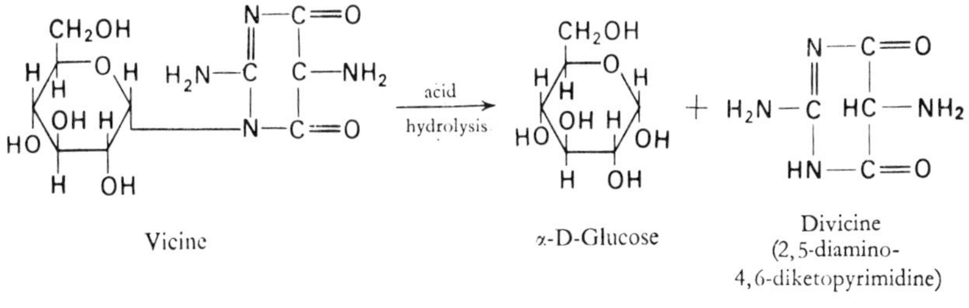

FIG. 8. Structure of vicine and its hydrolysis products

containing nucleoside called vicine (Lin and Ling, 1962) whose structure is shown in Fig. 8. This compound when eaten by rats at a level of 0·6% of the diet inhibited growth, and its administration by stomach tube to dogs at a level of 0·2 g/kg induced haemoglobinuria, indicative of haemolytic anaemia. The conclusion that vicine is indeed the cause of favism must be treated with scepticism in view of the fact that vicine is also found in such innocuous plants as the common vetch (*Vicia sativa*) and the garden pea (*Pisum sativum*) (Schulze, 1891). Why only certain individuals fall prey to favism likewise remains obscure.

3. *Metal-binding Factors*

The inclusion of isolated soya-bean protein in animal diets has been noted to lead to a decrease in the availability of certain trace minerals such as zinc, manganese, copper, and iron (Odell and Savage, 1960). In fact, an anaemia in monkeys due to a deficiency of iron may be induced by giving a soya-bean protein diet, an effect which may be eliminated by heat treatment or by chelating agents such as EDTA (Fitch *et al.*, 1964). Sesame meal and peas (*P. sativum*) have also been shown to interfere with the availability of zinc for chicks (Lease *et al.*, 1960; Kienholz *et al.*, 1962). The exact mechanism whereby certain plant proteins exert this effect is not known, although it may be related to the observation that a soya-bean protein–phytic acid complex has a special affinity for metal ions (Odell and Savage, 1960).

4. *Antivitamin factors*

The inclusion of unheated soya-bean meal, or the protein isolated therefrom, in diets for chicks may cause rickets unless higher than normal levels of vitamin D_3 are added to the diet (Carlson *et al.*, 1964). This rachitogenic effect could be eliminated by autoclaving the soya-bean meal, but supplementation with calcium or phosphorus was ineffective. Along the same lines, unheated kidney beans are believed to contain an antagonist to vitamin E as illustrated by their causing muscular dystrophy in chicks (Hintz and Hogue, 1964) and low levels of plasma tocopherol (Desai, 1966). The antivitamin E effect of kidney beans can be partially eliminated by heat treatment. Neither the identity of the antivitamin D factor of soya-beans nor that of the antivitamin E factor of kidney beans is known.

The identity of one antivitamin factor, however, has been determined, namely a compound in linseed meal which acts as an antagonist to pyridoxine (Klosterman *et al.*, 1967). This compound, whose structure is shown in Fig. 9, has been given the name of linatine and is actually a dipeptide comprised of L-amino-D-proline and glutamic acid. The toxicity of linatine resides in the aminoproline moiety which forms a complex

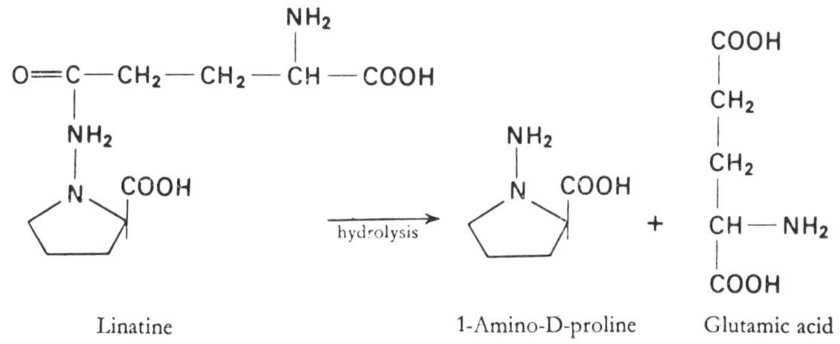

FIG. 9. Structure of linatine, the anti-pyridoxine factor in linseed meal

with pyridoxal phosphate *in vitro*, an observation that may explain its role as an antagonist of pyridoxine *in vivo*.

III. NATURALLY OCCURRING TOXICANTS IN ANIMALS

A. Fish Poisons

The number of naturally occurring toxic substances in animal protein is of course quite limited since its very presence would threaten the survival of the host. However, there are some examples of poisons in animal protein which do pose a hazard upon ingestion. Perhaps the most notable examples are certain marine organisms such as shell-fish which acquire their poisonous properties through the consumption of a poisonous alga or dinoflagellate, *Gonyaula catenella* (Schantz, 1967). The shell-fish are protected from self-intoxication by a special gland, referred to as the "dark gland" or hepatopancreas, which binds the toxic principle and prevents it from doing any harm to the organism. This bound poison, however, is readily released when consumed by man in whom it causes paralysis and possible death. It is possible for one small mussel weighing about 50 g to contain enough of the poison to be lethal to 10 people. The poisonous principle (saxitoxin) has been isolated but not fully characterized with respect to its structure. This poison is heat-stable, and there is thus far no known antidote. The pufferfish (*Tetraodontidae*) likewise possesses in its ovaries and testes an extremely poisonous principle (*tetrodotoxin*) which has accounted for nearly half of the fatal cases of food poisoning in Japan.

B. Biological Amines

Some foods which are normally considered to be non-toxic, and in fact quite nutritious, may prove to be harmful in special circumstances.

A case in point is the animal product cheese which contains large amounts of amines such as tyramine, histamine, and tryptamine which are derived from amino acids through the fermentative action of bacteria. Although these amines are known to elevate blood pressure, they are normally detoxified by monoamine oxidase. In patients who are receiving anti-depressant drugs which inhibit this enzyme, the consumption of cheese can lead to serious consequences because of the accumulation of tyramine. Even death from intracranial haemorrhage after the consumption of 1 oz of cheddar cheese has been reported (Sapeika, 1969).

The plantain fruit, which is a major article in the diet of many Africans, is known to contain large amounts of the pressor amine, serotonin. It has been estimated that the daily intake of serotonin from this source may reach levels as high as 100–200 mg. This has raised the question whether the consumption of plantain could be an aetiological factor in certain heart conditions among Africans (Foy and Parratt, 1962).

IV. ADVENTITIOUS TOXIC FACTORS

It would be manifestly impossible to deal in detail with the real or potential toxicity of substances which do not occur naturally in foods but are introduced inadvertently or, in some cases, deliberately. A list of such substances could include such things as pesticides, hormones, antibiotics, mercury, lead, polychlorobiphenyls, monosodium glutamate, cyclamates, saccharin, and many others. Experimental evidence may be marshalled to indicate that all of these substances can, under certain conditions and depending on the test animal, the dosage, the route of administration, and so on, exhibit carcinogenic, mutagenic, or teratogenic effects. All of which leads one to conclude that anything is toxic if you give a large enough dose, and anything is safe if you keep the dose low enough, or as one expert (Golberg, 1971) has put it, a food additive "remains under suspicion until such time as someone can discover an organism, devise a route of administration, or achieve a sufficiently heroic dose to produce some positive biological result, however bizarre".

Despite this note of cynicism, I should simply like to cite two examples of adventitious toxic substances that have given cause for genuine concern—(a) toxins that are introduced into food by microbial action, the so-called mycotoxins, and (b) the formation of nitrosamines, the result of man's efforts to improve the acceptability of a food product.

A. Mycotoxins

The contamination of foodstuffs by the microbial production of a toxic metabolite is best illustrated by the aflatoxin story, which is by now a very familiar one and needs no repeating here. The aflatoxins are a related group of compounds, two of which are shown in Fig. 10, that are produced by certain of the mould *Aspergillus flavus*; a large number of studies with various experimental animals have shown them to be potent carcinogens, the liver being the most likely target organ (Wogan, 1969). However, information on the occurrence of aflatoxins in human foods and raw materials is still fragmentary. Because of the initial discovery of these compounds as contaminants of peanut meals, there has been an

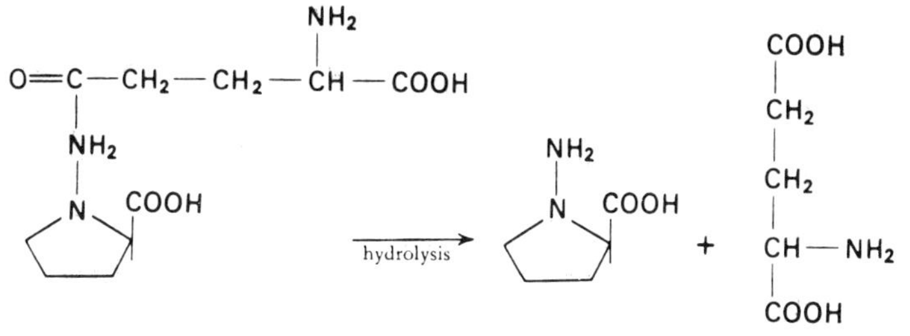

FIG. 10. Structure of aflatoxins B_1 and G_1.

unfortunate tendency to associate aflatoxin specifically with this commodity. However, subsequent studies have revealed the presence of aflatoxin in a wide variety of other food commodities from various parts of the world, particularly from Asia and Africa. One such survey recently conducted in Uganda showed a definite correlation of the distribution of aflatoxins in various cereals and legumes with the regional incidence of liver cancer (Alpert *et al.*, 1971). This list included many items which are dietary staples for some populations. These observations have given rise to considerable speculation as to the potential role of mycotoxins in the aetiology of liver cancer in man.

B. Nitrosamines

The use of nitrites and nitrates in the curing of meats for enhancement of colour and as a preservative has been a common practice in the meat industry for many years. This practice caused little concern until a liver disease in fur-bearing and other animals was traced to the formation of dimethylnitrosamine by the interaction of nitrite and various secondary and tertiary amines naturally occurring in the fish meal in the diet (Sakshaug *et al.*, 1965). Since dimethylnitrosamine is known to be a potent liver carcinogen, these findings have aroused a great deal of concern among food scientists and health officials about the possibility of the occurrence of nitrosamines in human foods. If enough dimethylnitrosamine could be formed in fish meal to show acute toxic effects, the presence of similar amounts of this compound in human foods known to contain amines and nitrite seems a real possibility. Meat products, for example, contain such naturally occurring quaternary ammonium compounds as choline, betaine, and carnitine which have been shown to react with nitrite to form small amounts of dimethylnitrosamine, and the conditions under which meat products such as sausage are cooked are known to enhance the formation of nitrosamines.

A number of surveys have been made to determine the dimethylnitrosamine content of various meat products such as bacon, ham, salami and sausage which are preserved with nitrate and nitrite. The available evidence indicates the presence of anything from 0·2–1·0 μg/kg (Sen, 1971). The question then arises as to what constitutes a "tolerable" level of nitrosamine in foods for human consumption. Work with animals has shown that the lowest level at which dimethylnitrosamine exerts its carcinogenic effect is about 0·2–0·5 mg/kg of the diet (Terracini *et al.*, 1967). Assuming that man is as sensitive as the rat to the carcinogenic effect of dimethylnitrosamine and allowing a safety margin of 100, one arrives at a value of about 2–5 μg/kg, which approximates the level of dimethylnitrosamine found in some samples of smoked meat products. While recognizing the inherent dangers in these extrapolations, it is nevertheless apparent that the possible public health hazard posed by the presence of dimethylnitrosamines in certain foodstuffs is one that will merit constant vigilance.

V. CONCLUSIONS

As long as our diet is varied, the chances are that we have a fairly large margin of safety with respect to the natural components of our diet. A diet consisting of a reasonable diversity of foods will provide many different potentially toxic constituents, each being present in such a small amount that little danger is involved. For most of us simple over-indulgence constitutes the principal hazard of the dinner table. Nevertheless there is the ever-present possibility that the prolonged consumption of any one kind of food could bring to the surface toxic effects that would otherwise not have become apparent in a more varied diet. As the shortage of protein becomes more acute, it is not unlikely that much of the population of the world will, in the future, be faced with a more limited selection of protein foods, most of which will undoubtedly be of plant origin and hence potential carriers of toxic constituents. The food scientist should at least be cognizant of such a possibility and be prepared to apply his technological skills to meeting this challenge should the occasion arise.

REFERENCES

Adiga, P. G., Padmanaban, G., Rao, S. L. N. and Sarma, P. S. (1964). *J. scient. ind. Res.* **21**, 284.

Alpert, M. E., Hutt, M. S. R., Wogan, G. N. and Davidson, C. S. (1971). *Cancer, N.Y.* **28**, 253–262.

Anderson, D. W. (1961). *Proc. Conf. Soybean Products for Proteins in Human Foods*, p. 173. Northern Regional Research Laboratory, Peoria, Ill.

Berardi, L. C. and Goldblatt, L. A. (1969). *In* "Toxic Constituents of Plant Foodstuffs" (I. E. Liener, ed.), p. 212. Academic Press, New York.

Booth, A. N., Robbins, D. J., Ribelin, W. E. and DeEds, F. (1960). *Proc. Soc. exp. Biol. Med.* **104**, 681–683.

Borchers, R. and Ackerson, C. W. (1950). *J. Nutr.* **41**, 339–345.

Carlson, C. W., Saxena, H. C., Jensen, L. S. and McGinnis, J. (1964). *J. Nutr.* **82**, 507–511.

Conn, E. R. (1969). *J. agric. Fd Chem.* **17**, 519–526.

Desai, I. D. (1966). *Nature, Lond.* **209**, 810.

Feeney, R. E., Means, G. E. and Bigler, J. C. (1969). *J. biol. Chem.* **244**, 1957–1960.

Fitch, C. D., Harville, W. F., Dinning, J. S. and Porter, F. S. (1964). *Proc. Soc. exp. Biol. Med.* **116**, 130–133.

Foy, J. M. and Parratt, J. R. (1962). *Lancet* **i**, 942–943.

Golberg, L. (1971). *Fd Cosmet. Toxic.* **9**, 65–80.

Hintz, H. F. and Hogue, D. E. (1964). *J. Nutr.* **84**, 283–287.

Honavar, P. M., Shih, C. V. and Liener, I. E. (1962). *J. Nutr.* **77**, 109–114.

Jaffe, W. G. (1969). *In* "Toxic Constituents of Plant Foodstuffs" (I. E. Liener, ed.), p. 93. Academic Press, New York.

Kakade, M. L., Simon, N. and Liener, I. E. (1969). *Cereal Chem.* **46**, 518–526.

Kienholz, E. W., Jensen, L. S. and McGinnis, J. (1962). *Poult. Sci.* **41**, 367–371.

Klosterman, H. J., Lamoreux, G. L. and Parsons, J. L. (1967). *Biochemistry, Easton* **6**, 170–177.

Kunitz, M. (1946). *J. gen. Physiol.* **29**, 149–154.

Lease, J. G., Barrett, B. D., Lease, E. J. and Turk, D. E. (1960). *J. Nutr.* **72**, 66–70.

Liener, I. E. (1953). *J. Nutr.* **49**, 527–539.

Liener, I. E. (1971). Unpublished results.

Liener, I. E. and Kakade, M. L. (1969). *In* "Toxic Constituents of Plant Foodstuffs" (I. E. Liener, ed.) p. 14. Academic Press, New York.

Liener, I. E., Deuel, H. J. and Fevold, H. L. (1949). *J. Nutr.* **39**, 325-339.

Lin, J.-Y. and Ling, L.-H. (1962). *J. Formosan med. Ass.* **61**, 484.

Luisada, A. (1941). *Medicine, Baltimore* **20**, 229–250.

McKay, G. F., Lalich, J. J., Schilling, E. D. and Strong, F. M. (1954). *Archs Biochem. Biophys.* **52**, 313–322.

Montgomery, R. D. (1969). *In* "Toxic Constituents of Plant Foodstuffs" (I. E. Liener, ed.), pp. 143–157. Academic Press, New York.

Murti, V. V. S., Seshadri, T. R. and Venkitasubramanian, T. A. (1964). *Phytochemistry* **3**, 73.

Nesheim, M. C., Garlich, J. D. and Hopkins, D. T. (1962). *J. Nutr.* **78**, 89–94.

Neuhaus, J. W. G. (1969). *J. Proc. R. Soc. N.S.W.* **102**, 163.

Odell, B. L. and Savage, J. E. (1960). *Proc. Soc. exp. Biol. Med.* **103**, 304–305.

Osborne, T. B. and Mendel, L. B. (1917). *J. biol. Chem.* **32**, 369–387.

Osuntokun, B. O. (1970). *Br. J. Nutr.* **24**, 797–800.

Patton, A. R., Wilgus, H. S., Jr. and Harshfield, G. S. (1939). *Science, N.Y.* **89**, 162.

Sakshaug, J., Sögnen, E., Hansen, M. A. and Koppang, N. (1965). *Nature, Lond.* **206**, 1261–1262.

Sapeika, N. (1969). "Food Pharmacology." Charles C. Thomas, Springfield, Ill.

Sarma, P. S. (1968). *J. Vitam.* **14**, 53–57.

Sarma, P. S. and Padmanaban, G. (1969). *In* "Toxic Constituents of Plant Foodstuffs" (I. E. Liener, ed.), p. 285. Academic Press, New York.

Schantz, E. J. (1967). *In* "Biochemistry of Some Foodborne Microbial Toxins" (R. I. Mateles and G. N. Wogan, eds.), p. 51. M.I.T. Press, Cambridge, Mass.

Schulze, E. (1891). *Hoppe-Seyler's Z. physiol. Chem.* **15**, 140.

Scudamore, H. H., Morey, G. R., Consolazio, C. F., Berryman, G. H., Gordon, L. E., Lightbody, H. D. and Fevold, H. L. (1949). *J. Nutr.* **39**, 555–565.

Sen, N. P. (1971). Personal communication.

Terracini, B., Magee, P. N. and Barnes, J. M. (1957). *Br. J. Cancer* **21**, 559.

Travis, J. and Roberts, R. C. (1969). *Biochemistry, Easton* **8**, 2884–2889.

VanEtten, C. H. (1969). *In* "Toxic Constituents of Plant Foodstuffs" (I. E. Liener, ed.), pp. 103–142. Academic Press, New York.

Wogan, G. N. (1969). *Prog. exp. Tumor Res.* **11**, 134–162.

Yang, M. G. and Mickelsen, O. (1969). *In* "Toxic Constituents of Plant Foodstuffs" (I. E. Liener, ed.), pp. 159–167. Academic Press, New York.

CHAPTER 34

Non-enzymic Browning

P. A. FINOT

Nestlé Products Technical Assistance Co. Ltd, La Tour de Peilz, Switzerland

Non-enzymic browning, also known as the Maillard reaction, is of great importance to the food industry since it is responsible for the formation of specific tastes and aromas. It also causes a decrease in the biological value of protein due to the blockage of lysine, which reacts with sugars during heat treatment.

I. CHEMISTRY OF THE MAILLARD REACTION

The chemistry of the Maillard reaction is not yet completely understood and several reaction mechanisms leading to melanoïdins have been proposed.

Hodge (1953) described the first steps of the reactions between amino-compounds and aldose leading to deoxy-ketosyl derivatives, through a Schiff base and an aldosylamine (Fig. 1).

He also described several possible reactions leading to melanoïdins from the deoxy-ketosyl derivative or its enol form through the Schiff base of hydroxymethylfurfural, reductones or the Strecker degradation.

Burton and McWeeny (1964) described two other routes leading to melanoïdins, the first one from a di-deoxy-ketosyl derivative previously identified by Anet (1959), the second one directly from the aldose-amino compound. One step in this second reaction should be a transamination of the Schiff base (Høltermand, 1966) giving a keto-acid and an amino-sugar. These reactions have been described between free amino acids and reducing sugars, but they can also take place between the ε-amino groups of lysine in protein and reducing sugars, leading to the blockage of lysine.

Another type of reaction capable of inactivating lysine has also been described between the ε-amino groups of lysine and non-reducing sugars. El-Nokrashy and Frampton (1967) demonstrated that raffinose, a non-reducing sugar, reacts with the ε-amino groups of lysine in cottonseed

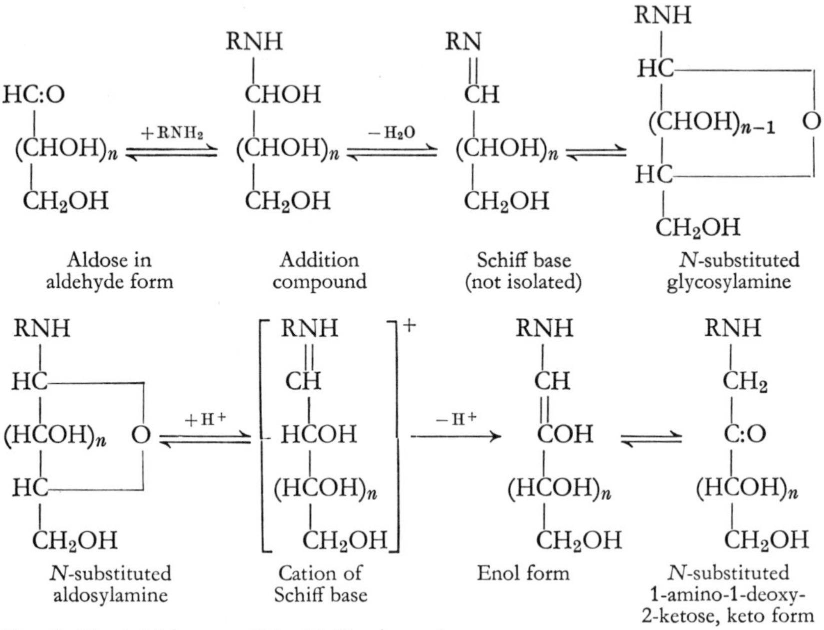

FIG. 1. The initial steps of the Maillard reaction

meals; this reaction is reported to be due to an aminolysis of the oligosaccharide. Karel and Labuza (1968) described also a Maillard-type reaction in freeze-dried systems containing sucrose, but in this case the reaction should be due to reducing sugars produced by acid-catalysed hydrolysis of sucrose.

In our laboratory, we have found that in extruded confections, containing only sucrose and starch as carbohydrates, 40% of the free lysine added to balance the protein became unavailable. From the study of the reducing properties of the lysine–sugar compound extracted from these products, it was not possible to determine whether the reaction involved was an aminolysis.

The chemical structure of blocked lysine in proteins is not very well known, but it is thought to be either in the form of a Schiff base, an aldosylamine, or a deoxyketosyl derivative; unless, of course, the reaction has reached the melanoïdin stage. We assume that this chemical structure must depend on several factors such as the nature of the sugar (aldose or ketose, pentose or hexose), the pH, the water content and the temperature, but the effect of each factor on the chemical structure is not yet known.

The nature of the chemical structure of unavailable lysine is of great importance from an analytical point of view, because the behaviour of the different forms of unavailable lysine can be different during acid hydrolysis and chemical analyses such as the determination of available lysine.

The chemical and the biological behaviour of one of these forms has been studied, namely the deoxy-ketosyl form, since it is the most stable and is therefore easily obtainable.

II. SYNTHESIS OF THE ε-*N*-DEOXY-KETOSYL-LYSINE DERIVATIVES

ε-*N*-deoxy-fructosyl-lysine has been synthesized according to the scheme of Fig. 2.

The reaction between α-*N*-formyl-lysine (α-F-Lys) and glucose was carried out in boiling methanol and the products deformylated in 2 M HCl (15 min at 100°). α-*N*-formyl-ε-*N*-deoxy-fructosyl-lysine (α-F-ε-DF-Lys) and ε-*N*-deoxy-fructosyl-lysine (ε-DF-Lys) have been purified by chromatography (Finot and Mauron, 1969). α-*N*-formyl-ε-*N*-deoxy-lactulosyl-lysine (α-F-ε-DL-Lys) has been prepared in a similar way, but its deformylated derivative has not been isolated because under the conditions for deformylation the lactulosyl residue is also hydrolysed, giving ε-DF-Lys + galactose.

III. BEHAVIOUR OF ε-*N*-DEOXY-KETOSYL-LYSINE DERIVATIVES DURING ACID HYDROLYSIS

A. Analysis of the Different Compounds Formed During Acid Hydrolysis

The measured total lysine content of overheated milks is lower than the theoretical value but higher than that of available lysine (Bujard *et al.*, 1967). This observation means that during analysis some of the unavailable lysine regenerates lysine. We can assume that the Schiff base and aldosylamine forms regenerate 100% of their lysine upon acid hydrolysis since the reactions leading to these compounds are reversible, but we do not know the percentage of lysine recovered from its deoxy-ketosyl derivative. When we hydrolyse the pure ε-*N*-deoxy-ketosyl-lysine derivatives synthesized from glucose and lactose, the three main

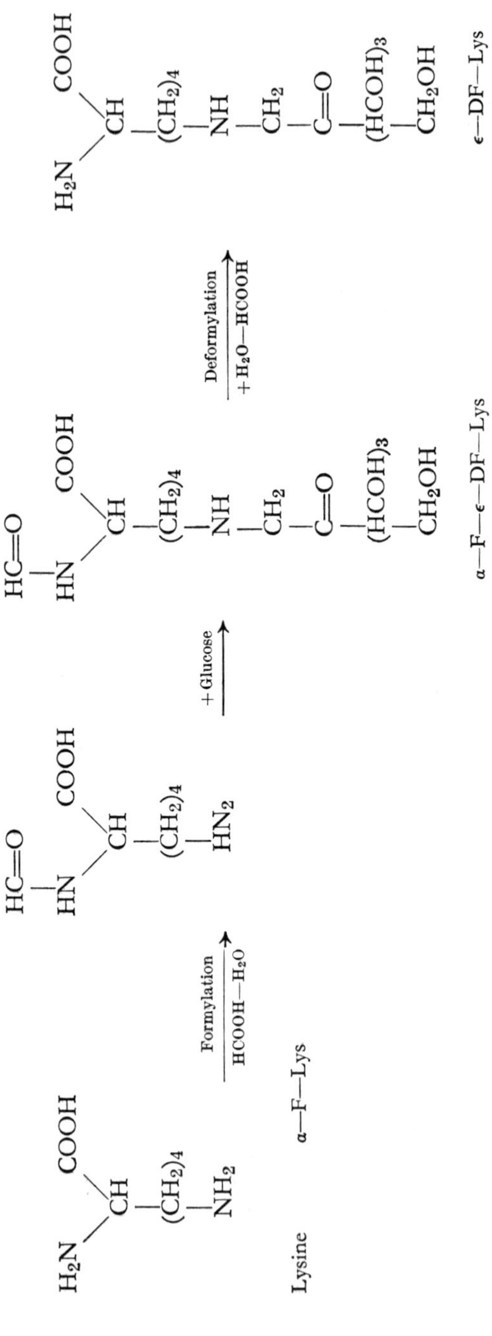

FIG. 2. The synthesis of ε-N-deoxy-fructosyl-lysine.

compounds obtained are lysine, furosine (ε-*N*-(2-furomylmethyl)-L-lysine) (Erbersdobler and Zucker, 1966; Heyns *et al.*, 1968; Finot *et al.*, 1968) and pyridosine (ε-[3-hydroxy-4-oxo-6-methyl-1-pyridinyl]-L-norleucine) (Finot *et al.*, 1969) (Fig. 3).

Furosine was first detected by Erbersdobler and Zucker (1966) on chromatograms of acid hydrolysates of overheated milk. Under normal conditions, pyridosine is not separated during the analysis of the basic

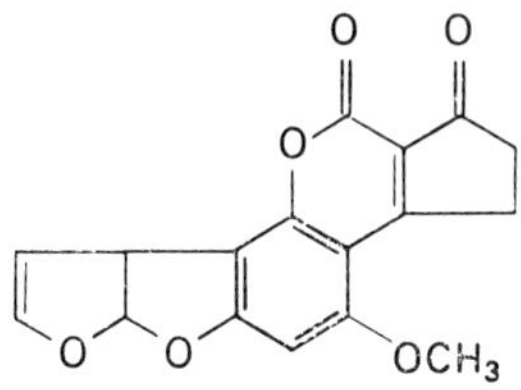

Aflatoxin B_1

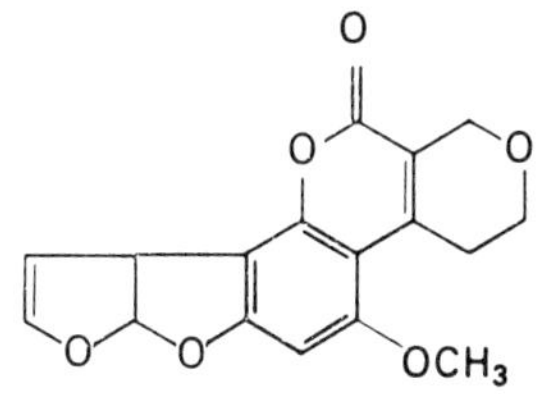

Aflatoxin G_1

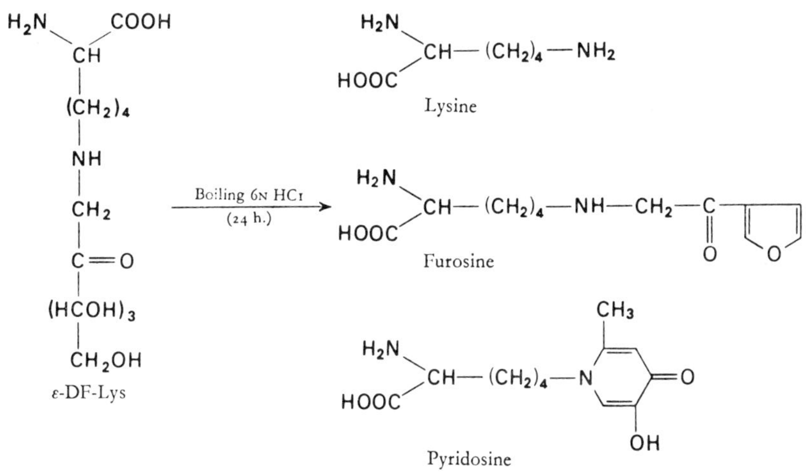

FIG. 3. Compounds obtained by acid hydrolysis of ε-*N*-deoxy-fructosyl-lysine (ε-DF-Lys)

amino acids but under special conditions (Finot *et al.*, 1969) pyridosine and furosine can be separated in the same run as lysine (Fig. 4). Lysine, furosine and pyridosine have been quantitatively determined in acid hydrolysates of ε-DF-Lys, α-F-ε-DF-Lys and α-F-ε-DL-Lys. It was found that on acid hydrolysis each of these deoxy-ketosyl derivatives yielded the same proportions of lysine, furosine and pyridosine. The yields of these three compounds were not affected by the method of hydrolysis (refluxing or in sealed tubes) or by the concentration of the substrate in the acid and the presence of reducing sugars in the medium, nor by the storage time of the compounds, which varied from 1 to 33 months.

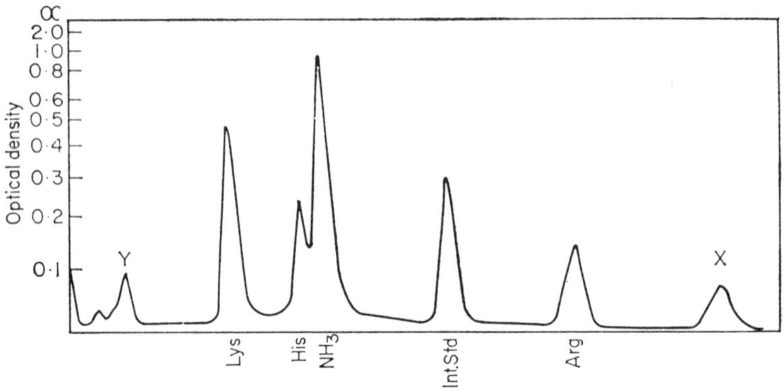

FIG. 4. Basic amino acid chromatogram of a scorched, roller-dried milk after 6 M HCl hydrolysis
X, furosine; Y, pyridoxine (Finot *et al.*, 1969)

However, the results were affected by the concentration of the acid used for hydrolysis (Finot and Mauron, 1972).

Two concentrations of hydrochloric acid have been tested: 6 M HCl, normally used in our laboratory to hydrolyse proteins, and 7·75 M HCl, used by Erbersdobler (1970) to measure furosine in milks. The results are summarized in Table I.

TABLE I. Regenerated lysine, furosine and pyridosine content found in the acid hydrolysates of the *N*-ε-deoxy-ketosyl-lysine derivatives of glucose and lactose

Acid hydrolysis in	6 M HCl	7·75 M HCl
Regenerated lysine (% of theoretical lysine)	49·5 ± 2·6	43·8 ± 0·20
$\frac{\text{Furosine}}{\text{lysine}}$ (ratio of the areas of the chromatographic peaks)	0·41 ± 0·01	0·67 ± 0·03
$\frac{\text{Pyridosine}}{\text{lysine}}$ (ratio of the areas of the chromatographic peaks)	0·21 ± 0·01	0·26 ± 0·03
Furosine (% of theoretical lysine)	20·3	29·3
Pyridosine (% of theoretical lysine)	10·4	11·4

Since it was not possible to get samples of furosine and pyridosine of sufficient purity to obtain exact colorimetric factor values, and since furosine and pyridosine are not readily available, we have expressed the results in terms of lysine. The ratios of the areas of the chromatographic peaks furosine/lysine and pyridosine/lysine and the value obtained for lysine regenerated from its deoxy-ketosyl derivative enable one to calculate the percentage of furosine and pyridosine formed during acid hydrolysis of the deoxy-ketosyl-lysine derivatives.

With these values, it is possible to calculate directly from any hydrolysate the quantity of lysine blocked in the deoxy-ketosyl form and the amount of lysine regenerated from this deoxy-ketosyl form. Thus, a new method for the evaluation of available lysine in milk can be based on the determination of lysine and furosine.

B. Chemical Structure of Unavailable Lysine in Milk

1. Calculations using Measured Lysine Content

We can assume that in overheated milk some of the unavailable lysine is in the aldosylamine or Schiff base form and that the rest is in the deoxy–ketosyl form. During acid hydrolysis, all of the lysine blocked in the aldosylamine or Schiff base form regenerates into lysine but only 49·5% of lysine in the deoxy–ketosyl form is recovered (Fig. 5).

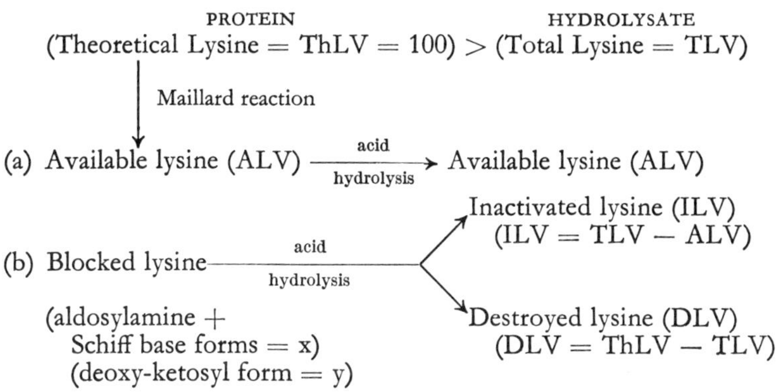

FIG. 5. Behaviour of available and unavailable lysine during acid hydrolysis

If we analyse the figures published by Mauron *et al.* (1955), Mauron and Mottu (1958) and Bujard *et al.* (1967) we find a very good correlation equation between inactivated lysine (ILV) and destroyed lysine (DLV):

$$\text{ILV} = 1{\cdot}93\ \text{DLV} - 6{\cdot}2$$

We assume that ILV $= x + 0{\cdot}495y$
we know that DLV $= 0{\cdot}505y$ (Table I)
If we solve these equations we find

$$y = \text{deoxy-ketosyl form} = 71{\cdot}5\%$$
$$x = \text{aldosylamine} + \text{Schiff base forms} = 28{\cdot}5\%$$

This result shows that in milk the main part of blocked lysine (71·5%) is in the chemical form of a deoxy-ketosyl derivative.

2. *Calculations using Measured Furosine Content*

(a) *Relation between contents of furosine* (*FUR*) *and total lysine* (*TLV*). Using a model system in which casein and glucose are heated under different conditions, and then hydrolysed in 6 M HCl, the following regression equation was obtained:

$$FUR_{Cas} = -0{\cdot}408\ TLV + 42{\cdot}9 \qquad r = 0{\cdot}80 \tag{1}$$

This equation is very similar to the theoretical equation calculated from the pure deoxy-ketosyl-lysine derivatives hydrolysed under the same conditions:

$$FUR_{6M} = -0{\cdot}402\ TLV + 40{\cdot}2 \tag{2}$$

From the results of Erbersdobler (1970) obtained from milks hydrolysed in 7·75 M HCl, the following regression equation has been calculated:

$$FUR_{Erb} = -0{\cdot}586\ TLV + 59{\cdot}6 \qquad r = 0{\cdot}90 \tag{3}$$

whereas the theoretical equation calculated from the pure deoxy-ketosyl-lysine derivatives hydrolysed under the same conditions would be:

$$FUR_{7{\cdot}75M} = -0{\cdot}522\ TLV + 52{\cdot}2 \tag{4}$$

These results show that during acid hydrolysis, free deoxy-ketosyl-lysine behaves in a similar way to deoxy-ketosyl-lysine combined in protein.

(b) *Relation between contents of furosine and available lysine* (*ALV*). It is important to know whether it is possible to determine available lysine by using the measured furosine content (FUR) in acid hydrolysates of proteins. Furosine has been found only in acid hydrolysates of protein which has been heated with glucose and lactose, and is derived from deoxy-ketosyl lysine. This observation limits the use of this method to milk and milk products.

(i) Calculations using available lysine values measured by the enzymic method (ALV_{enz}). We have done no experiments in which furosine content and available lysine have been determined. However, Bujard *et al.* (1967) found a good correlation between available lysine measured by an enzymic method (ALU_{enz}) and total lysine (TLV) measured after acid hydrolysis.

$$ALV_{enz} = 2{\cdot}70\ TLV - 167 \qquad r = 0{\cdot}99 \tag{5}$$

In this equation, it is possible to replace TLV by its equivalent of furosine, calculated from eqn (2). Eqn (5) becomes:

$$ALV_{enz} = 2{\cdot}70\left(\frac{40{\cdot}2 - FUR}{0{\cdot}402}\right) - 167$$

$$ALV_{enz} = 103 - 6{\cdot}72\ FUR \tag{6}$$

The theoretical relationship between ALV and furosine content would be

$$\text{ALV} = 100 - \text{unavailable lysine}$$

If we suppose that 100% of the unavailable lysine is in the deoxy-ketosyl form, we must have

$$\text{ALV} = 100 - 4{\cdot}92\ \text{FUR} \tag{7}$$

since

$$\text{deoxy-ketosyl-lysine} = \frac{\text{FUR}}{0{\cdot}203} \qquad \text{(Table I)}$$

The content of available lysine measured by the enzymic method (ALV_{enz}) is lower than that calculated theoretically. This means that in milk a certain amount of unavailable lysine is in a form other than deoxy-ketosyl-lysine. The difference observed in the coefficients of these two equations corresponds to this other chemical form of unavailable lysine which does not give furosine; this difference is equal to 26·8%, corresponding to the percentage of aldosylamine or Schiff base forms determined earlier (see p. 507). The percentages of lysine blocked in the form of an aldosylamine or a Schiff base determined in milk by using the total lysine values or the furosine values were found to be 28·5% and 26·8%, respectively. We decided to take the mean of these two figures, 27·6, as the correct percentage.

(ii) Calculations using content of available lysine measured by Carpenter's method. Correlations can be calculated between available lysine contents measured according to Carpenter (1960), and total lysine or furosine values. Unfortunately, the regression equations calculated from the results published by Bujard *et al.* (1967) and Erbersdobler (1970) are so different that it is not possible to draw any conclusions.

C. Suggestion for a New Method for the Determination of Available Lysine

Eqns (5) and (6) can already be used to calculate available lysine in milk, but the results given by these equations are related to an enzymic method only used in one laboratory. We should like to propose a more general method for calculating available lysine from the total lysine and furosine contents measured after acid hydrolysis of the protein. An example is given below for milk: in an acid hydrolysate of overheated milk, total lysine (TLV) is equal to:

$$\text{TLV} = \text{ALV} + 100\%\ \text{(aldosylamine)} + 49{\cdot}5\%\ \text{(deoxy-ketosyl-lysine} + \text{Schiff base forms)}$$

$$\text{TLV} = \text{ALV} + x + 0{\cdot}495y \tag{8}$$

On the other hand we have determined the following ratios

$$\frac{x}{y} = \frac{27{\cdot}6}{72{\cdot}4} = 0{\cdot}381 \qquad (9)$$

$$\frac{\text{FUR}}{y} = 0{\cdot}203 \quad \text{(Table I)}$$

$$\text{ALV} = \text{TLV} - (0{\cdot}381y + 0{\cdot}495y) = \text{TLV} - 0{\cdot}876y$$

$$\text{ALV} = \text{TLV} - 0{\cdot}876\,\frac{\text{FUR}}{0{\cdot}203}$$

$$\text{ALV} = \text{TLV} - 4{\cdot}31\ \text{FUR}$$

The coefficient of this equation can vary according to the respective percentage of lysine in the forms of an aldosylamine or a Schiff base and of a deoxy-ketosyl derivative. The minimum value of the coefficient would be 2·44 if all the unavailable lysine were in the form of a deoxy-ketosyl derivative.

The determination of this coefficient according to the heat treatment or the type of product would be very helpful in calculating available lysine in proteins more easily.

IV. BEHAVIOUR OF THE *N*-ε-DEOXY-KETOSYL DERIVATIVES OF LYSINE DURING CHEMICAL DETERMINATIONS OF AVAILABLE LYSINE

The following chemical methods were used for the assay of available lysine in α-F-ε-DF-Lys and α-F-ε-DL-Lys: with FDNB (Carpenter, 1960), with TNBS (Kakade and Liener, 1969) and with *O*-methyl-isourea (Mauron and Bujard, 1963).

It was surprising to find how easily FDNB reacted with the *N*-ε-deoxy-ketosyl-lysine derivatives to give three dinitrophenylated compounds (Finot and Mauron, 1972). It was also surprising to find, in acid hydrolysates of these compounds, *N*-ε-dinitrophenyl-lysine (ε-DNP-Lys) and free lysine. The reaction with FDNB can be explained as follows: the hydrogen atom linked to the ε-nitrogen is still reactive and can be substituted by a DNP group and the hydrogen atom linked to the oxygen of the enol form of the deoxy-ketosyl moiety can also be substituted (Fig. 6). The three compounds obtained would be two mono-substituted derivatives (*O*- and *N*-derivative) and a di-substituted derivative. During acid hydrolysis, ε-DNP-Lys and free lysine are released.

When Carpenter's method was applied to the pure *N*-α-formyl-*N*-ε-deoxy-fructosyl derivative of lysine we found that 14–28% of this unavailable form was determined as available lysine. The same estimation of

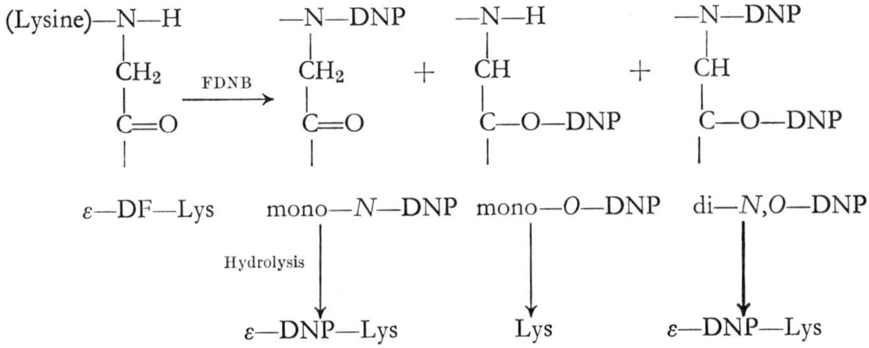

FIG. 6. Hypothetical reactions between FDNB and the deoxy-ketosyl derivatives of lysine, and transformations during acid hydrolysis

available lysine was repeated using other methods with reagents that are claimed to be more specific for the ε-amino group (Table II). The guanidination method using *O*-methyl-isourea would be the most specific, whereas the TNBS method is completely non-specific.

The Silcock method (Roach *et al.*, 1967) in which available lysine is calculated as follows: total lysine (TLV) − inaccessible lysine (lysine value obtained after hydrolysis of the dinitrophenylated protein), is not suitable for measuring deoxy-ketosyl derivatives of lysine since 50% is determined as total lysine (Table I) and 6–10% as inaccessible lysine (Table II).

TABLE II. Available lysine values obtained with pure deoxy-ketosyl derivatives of lysine (*N*-α-formyl form) by different chemical methods

Reagent	*Worker*	*Deoxy-ketosyl-lysine derivatives obtained from*	*Available lysine* % *theoretical lysine*	*Available lysine Chemical form*
FDNB	Carpenter	glucose	25–28	ε-DNP-Lys
			14–19	
			(regenerated lysine: 6–10%)	
		lactose	10·2–6·2	ε-DNP-Lys
	Roach	glucose	40–44	lysine
TNBS	Kakade	glucose	82–89	ε-TNP-Lys
O-methyl-isourea	Bujard	glucose	0	homoarginine

V. BIOLOGICAL ACTION OF THE *N*-ε-DEOXY-KETOSYL DERIVATIVES OF LYSINE

A. Biological Action of Free *N*-ε-Deoxy-Fructosyl-Lysine (fructoselysine)

Free fructoselysine, given to rats receiving a lysine-deficient diet, appeared not to be used as a source of lysine (Mottu *et al.*, 1972), and a considerable quantity was excreted unchanged in the urine. The faeces contained a variable amount of fructoselysine, probably because it was partly destroyed by the intestinal flora (Erbersdobler *et al.*, 1970).

TABLE III. Balance sheet of free *N*-ε-deoxy-fructosyl-lysine in rats

	Percentage of ingested fructoselysine[a]		
Rat no.	*Urine*	*Faeces*	*Recovery*
214	60·7	8·4	69·1
215	72·2	2·5	74·7
216	60·0	26·4	86·4

[a] Determination by measurement of furosine in the hydrolysed samples

B. Biological Action of ε-*N*-Deoxy-Lactulosyl-Lysine (Lactuloselysine) Bound to Protein

Rats were given a cereal-based diet cooked with milk and then roller-dried; about 50% of the lysine was unavailable in the resulting product.

Deoxy-ketosyl derivatives of lysine were determined by measuring the furosine content, after acid hydrolysis, of the faeces and urine of these

TABLE IV. Balance sheet of deoxy-ketosyl-lysine bound to protein

	Percentage of the ingested lactuloselysine[a]		
Rat no.	*Urine*	*Faeces*	*Recovery*
15	6·7	24·6	31·3
21	5·9	6·3	12·2
22	8·8	10·0	18·8

[a] Determined by measurement of furosine in the hydrolysed samples

animals. Only a small amount of the total blocked lysine was recovered (12–30%) (Table IV).

The chemical structure was determined of the sugar-lysine derivatives in the faeces and urine.

Urine was found to contain only free deoxy-fructosyl-lysine whereas faeces contained free deoxy-fructosyl-lysine (fructoselysine), free deoxy-lactulosyl-lysine (lactuloselysine) and peptides containing deoxy-lactulosyl-lysine.

The digestion of proteins containing lactuloselysine probably proceeds by the stages outlined in Fig. 7.

This study shows that free blocked lysine does not behave in the same way as blocked lysine bound to proteins; if free lysine is added to foodstuffs before heat treatment, the part which is blocked will largely be excreted in the urine, whereas blocked lysine bound to protein will be only partly excreted in the urine.

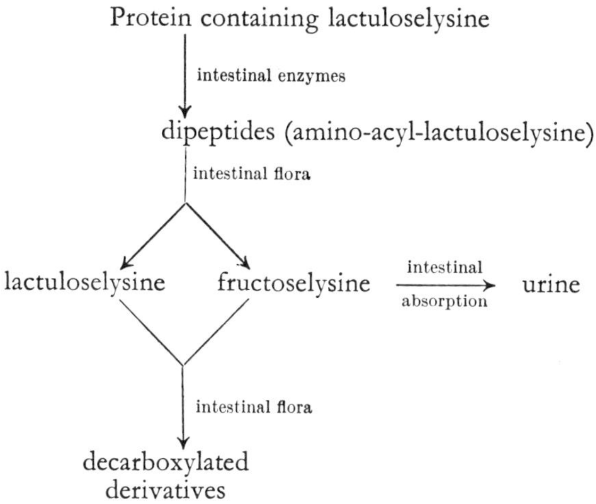

FIG. 7. Digestion of lactuloselysine bound to protein.

REFERENCES

ANET, E. F. L. J. (1959). *Aust. J. Chem.* **12**, 280–287.

BUJARD, E., HANDWERCK, V. and MAURON, J. (1967). *J. Sci. Fd Agric.* **18**, 52–57.

BURTON, H. S. and MCWEENY, D. J. (1964). *Chemy Ind.* pp. 462–463.

CARPENTER, K. J. (1960). *Biochem. J.* **77**, 604–610.

EL-NOCKRASHY, A. S. and FRAMPTON, V. L. (1967). *Biochem. biophys. Res. Commun.* **28**, 675–681.

ERBERSDOBLER, H. (1970). *Milchwissenschaft* **25**, 280–284.

ERBERSDOBLER, H. and ZUCKER, H. (1966). *Milchwissenschaft* **21**, 564–568.

Erbersdobler, H., Gunsser, I. and Weber, G. (1970). *Zentbl. Vet Med. A* **17**, 573–575.

Finot, P. A., Bricout, J., Viani, R. and Mauron, J. (1968). *Experientia* **24**, 1097–1099.

Finot, P. A. and Mauron, J. (1969). *Helv. chim. Acta* **52**, 1488–1495.

Finot, P. A. and Mauron, J. (1972). *Helv. chim. Acta* (In press).

Finot, P. A., Viani, R., Bricout, J. and Mauron, J. (1969). *Experientia* **25**, 134–135.

Heyns, K., Heukeshoven, J. and Brose, K.-H. (1968). *Angew. Chem.* **80**, 627.

Hodge, J. E. (1953). *J. agric. Fd Chem.* **1**, 928–943.

Høltermand, A. (1966). *Stärke* **10**, 319–328.

Kakade, M. L. and Liener, I. E. (1969). *Analyt. Biochem.* **27**, 273–280.

Karel, M. and Labuza, T. P. (1968). *J. agric. Fd Chem.* **16**, 717–719.

Mauron, J. and Bujard, E. (1963). *Int. Congr. Nutr. 6*, Edinburgh. pp. 489–490.

Mauron, J. and Mottu, F. (1958). *Archs Biochem. Biophys.* **77**, 312–327.

Mauron, J., Mottu, F., Bujard, E. and Egli, R. H. (1955). *Archs Biochem. Biophys.* **59**, 433–451.

Mottu, F., Finot, P. A. and Mauron, J. (1972). *Helv. chim. Acta* (In press).

Roach, A. G., Sanderson, P. and Williams, D. R. (1967). *J. Sci. Fd Agric.* **18**, 274–278.

CHAPTER 35

Some Effects of Processing on Nutritive Value

J. E. FORD

National Institute for Research in Dairying, Shinfield, Reading, England

I. INTRODUCTION

The amino acid composition of food protein is of fundamental importance in determining its nutritional quality; but other characteristics may also be important, especially in proteins that have been heated during manufacture. Thus, in meat meals and fish meals, for example, we can take the amino acid analysis as representing the *potential* nutritive quality, but we also have to take into account the digestibility of the meals and the biological availability of some of their constituent amino acids.

II. POSSIBLE MECHANISMS OF HEAT DAMAGE

Susceptibility to heat damage varies among different protein sources. It is increased in the presence of various carbohydrates and other food constituents. But even in isolated pure proteins, and in protein foods that are essentially free from carbohydrate, heat treatment can impair the nutritional quality, and yet have little or no apparent effect on the amino acid composition. There is very little precise information on the nature of the chemical changes that take place; there are many possibilities of interaction between functional groups, and perhaps the most important nutritionally are those that result in the formation of a tangle of new linkages within and between the peptide chains. We can suppose that these new linkages are resistant to hydrolysis by the proteases of the gut, and also that they will impair the digestibility of adjacent peptide bonds.

Mecham and Olcott (1947) made a detailed study of the effects of dry heat on a variety of proteins. They observed marked losses of amino nitrogen, and decreased solubility and digestibility which they attributed to the loss of polar groups through internal formation of amides or esters. Figure 1 illustrates just three of several possibilities. It shows (1) an ester link between the carboxyl of aspartic or glutamic acid and the hydroxyl group of a hydroxy-amino acid; (2) a thioester link between aspartic or glutamic acid and the thiol group of cysteine; (3) an imide link between asparagine or glutamine and aspartic or glutamic acid. Fuller discussion

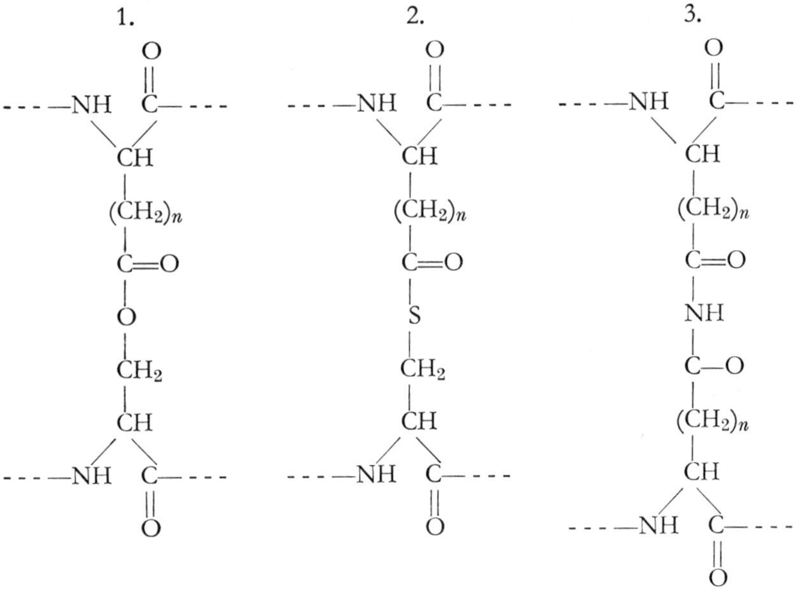

FIG. 1. Some examples of possible intramolecular linkages

of these and other intramolecular reactions is given by Bjarnason and Carpenter (1970) and Mauron (1970).

The damaging effect of heat processing on the availability of lysine is of special nutritional importance and has been much investigated. It has been suggested that the inactivation of lysine is caused by reaction between the ε-amino group of lysine and carboyxl groups, but Bjarnason and Carpenter (1970) concluded that this reaction is not very likely on thermodynamic grounds, and provided strong evidence that the main reaction is with the amide groups of asparagine or glutamine (Fig. 2). It is of interest that ε(γ-glutamyl)lysine occurs naturally in wool keratin (Asquith *et al.*, 1970), and that its content increases on heating the wool.

III. ANALYSIS OF PROTEIN DIGESTS

This paper presents some results of experiments on the effects of severe heat treatment on the course of digestion of protein. Freeze-dried cod muscle was taken as the test protein. It was heated in an air oven for 18 h at 130°C, and then digested for successive 24 h periods with pepsin, trypsin and erepsin (Ford and Salter, 1966). For comparison, a similar digest of the unheated material was also prepared.

For analysing protein digests, Sephadex gel filtration has proved a useful technique. It gives us a simple means of separating different solutes

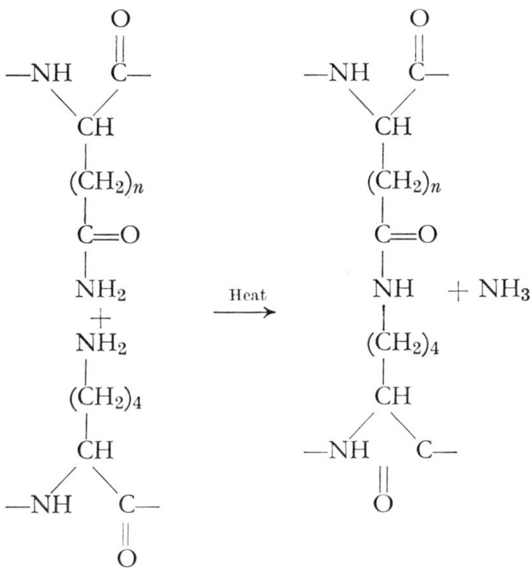

FIG. 2. Formation of internal amide by interaction of the ε-amino group of lysine and the amide group of asparagine (n = 1) or glutamine (n = 2)

from mixed solution, and grading them in approximate order of molecular size. Figure 3 shows the calibration of a column of Sephadex gel grade G-25, by the use of marker compounds of known molecular weight. With G-25 the elution volume is roughly proportional to log (mol. wt) over the molecular weight range 100–5000. If now we pass an enzymic digest of a protein through the column, undigested protein and large peptides are eluted first, and they are followed in turn by progressively smaller peptides and free amino acids. Figure 4 shows the elution profile of the digest of heat-damaged cod muscle, compared with that for the unheated material. The fractions were hydrolysed and their amino acid content was estimated

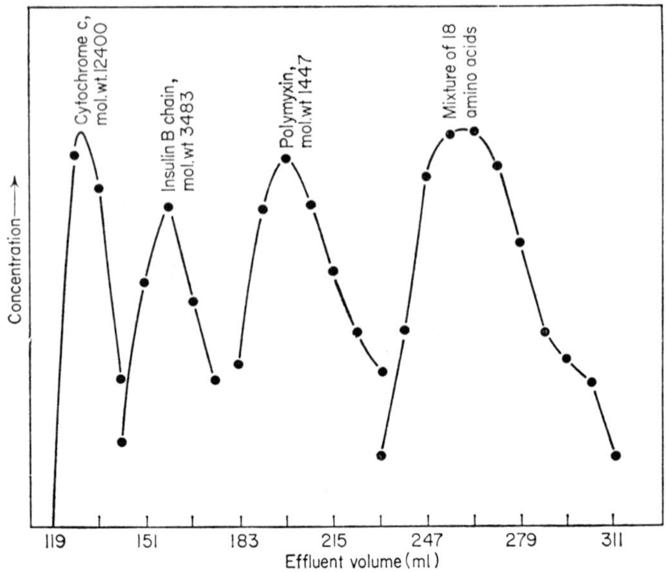

FIG. 3. Calibration of Sephadex G-25 column

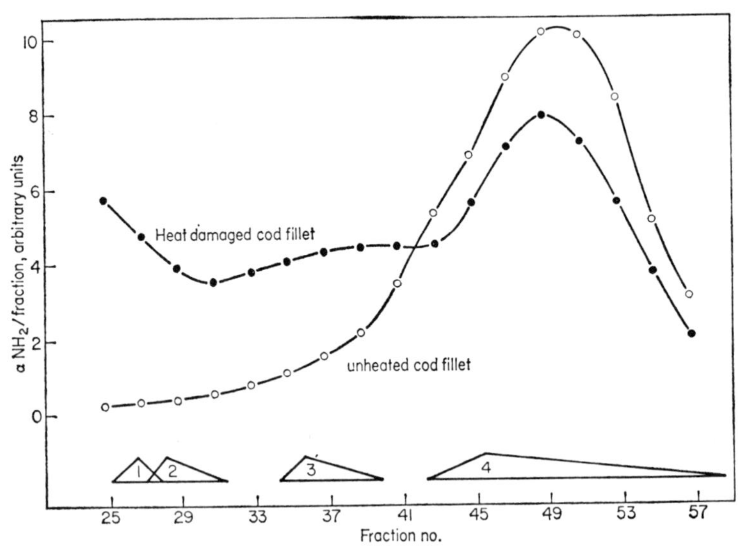

1, Cytochrome C, mol. wt. 12,400; 2, Insulin B chain, mol.wt. 3483; 3, Bacitracin A, mol.wt. 1470
4, A mixture of 18 amino acids

FIG. 4. Fractionation of enzymic digests of cod muscle in a column of Sephadex G-25

by reaction with ninhydrin and expressed as "leucine equivalent". On digestion, the unheated cod muscle yielded predominantly free amino acids with some small peptides, the heated material gave less free amino acids and more of the larger peptide species.

The difference between these two patterns was not simply an indication of the lower overall digestibility of the heated meal, as is evident in Fig. 5, which shows that there were marked differences between the composition of the "free amino acids" component of the digest of a good quality fish meal and that of a heat-damaged meal. The total amino acid analysis showed very little effect of the heat-damage, but lysine and the sulphur

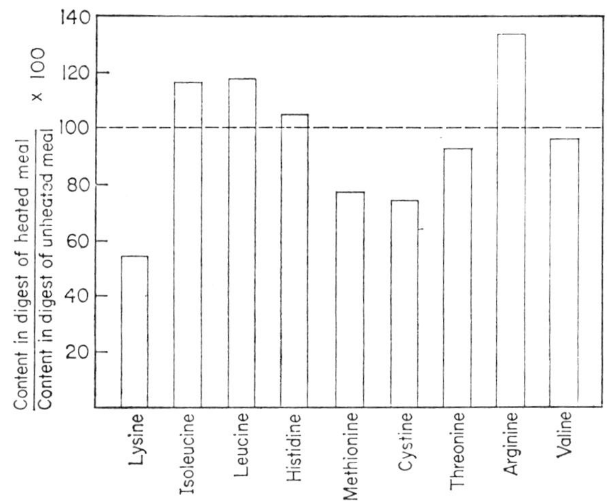

FIG. 5. Concentrations of free amino acids (g/16 g N) in an enzymic digest of heat-damaged cod muscle, shown as percentages of the corresponding values for the unheated material

amino acids were relatively deficient in the free amino acids component from the heated meal. Thus the biologically effective amino acid composition may be considerably altered by the heat treatment, as is evident again in Fig. 6, which shows a fractionation of a pepsin–pancreatin–erepsin digest of the heat-damaged cod muscle. There were clear differences in the extent of the release of different amino acids. The free amino acids component was comparatively poor in lysine and rich in arginine and leucine. Conversely, the undigested peptide was depleted of arginine and leucine, and relatively rich in lysine. Aspartic acid, and also glutamic acid, were present largely as small peptides, in a broad peak about mol. wt 1000.

The finding that different amino acids in the heat-damaged protein were

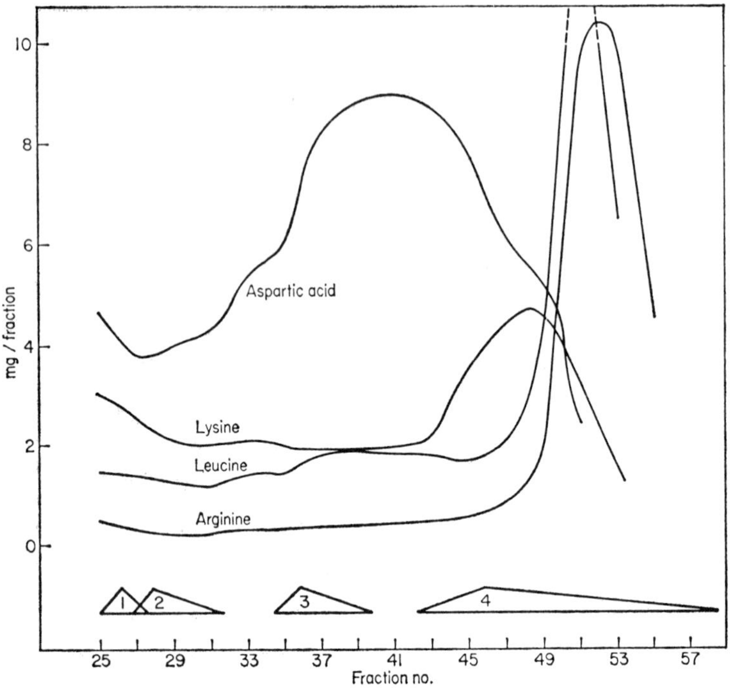

FIG. 6. Fractionation of an enzymic digest of heat-damaged cod muscle in a column of Sephadex G-25, showing the relative concentration of leucine, lysine, aspartic acid and arginine in the effluent fractions. 1, cytochrome *c*, mol. wt 12 400; 2, insulin B chain, mol. wt 3483; 3, bacitracin, mol. wt 1470; 4, a mixture of eighteen amino acids

released at widely different rates was not peculiar to the pepsin–pancreatin–erepsin system. Much the same results were obtained with pepsin–papain, and with pronase—a proteolytic enzyme of *Streptomyces griseus* that has an unusually broad substrate specificity.

Growth tests with rats also indicated that the biological availability of the lysine was very much lower than that of the methionine and isoleucine (Table I) and analysis of the contents of the small intestine showed an

TABLE I. Available lysine, methionine and isoleucine in fish meals (g/16 g N), measured in growth tests with rats

Cod fillet	N *digestibility*	*Lys*	*Met*	*Ileu*
Unheated	0·999	10·9	3·64	5·57
Heated	0·561	1·3	1·22	2·06

accumulation of undigested protein and peptide which, like the *in vitro* digests, was enriched in lysine and in aspartic and glutamic acids (Buraczewski *et al.*, 1967; Buraczewski, 1966). Similarly, in studies on the digestion of heat-damaged casein in rats, Erbersdobler *et al.* (1969) found differences in the availability of different amino acids, and lysine, asparagine and glutamine were the most reduced in availability.

Study of the amino acid composition of the undigested peptide residues provides some clues to the chemical changes that have occurred in the protein during heating. Figure 7 shows the "profile" that was obtained on

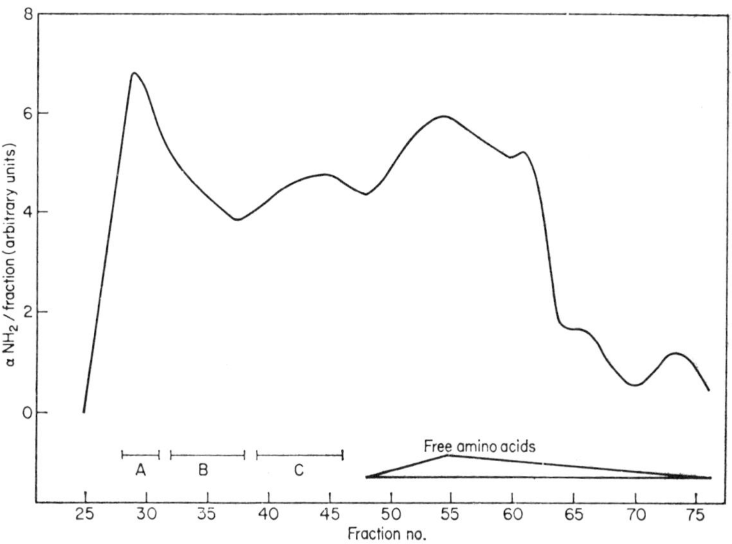

FIG. 7. Fractionation of an enzymic digest of heat-damaged cod muscle in a column of Sephadex G-25. Peptides: A, "large"; B, "medium"; C, "small"

gel filtration of a pepsin–pancreatin–erepsin digest of heat-damaged cod muscle. The fractions were combined arbitrarily into groups containing large, medium and small peptides, with molecular weights around 3500, 2000 and 1000 as judged by their behaviour on gel filtration.

Table II shows the amino acid composition of acid hydrolysates of the heated cod muscle, and of these different peptide classes (large, medium, small) separated from the enzymic digest. If we compare the composition of the different peptide classes with that of the heated cod muscle from which they were prepared, it seems that all the peptides were enriched in glutamic and aspartic acids and in proline, and the "large" and "medium" classes also in lysine, methionine and glycine. In contrast, they were severely depleted of leucine, tyrosine, phenylalanine, arginine and histidine.

The analyses tell us nothing about the reasons for the low biological availability of the peptides: the classes were each composed of highly complex mixtures of peptides, which must next be resolved into their components.

A point of interest about these peptide fractions is that they were all strongly yellow-brown in colour, especially the large peptides. It seems very likely that they contained products of the interaction of protein and

TABLE II. Amino acid composition of peptides separated from an enzyme digest of heat-damaged cod muscle protein

	Amino acids (moles %)			
	Heated cod muscle	*Peptide classes*		
	(before digestion)	*Large*	*Medium*	*Small*
Glu	15·7	18·2	19·2	21·2
Asp	10·9	15·0	15·8	16·5
Lys	7·0	7·8	7·9	5·3
Thr	4·9	4·1	4·0	4·8
Ser	4·8	3·9	3·8	3·8
Pro	1·7	4·2	5·2	6·4
Gly	8·8	10·0	11·8	8·7
Ala	11·0	9·7	10·6	10·7
Val	6·1	6·0	5·9	5·8
Met	2·1	2·7	2·6	2·1
Ileu	5·0	5·4	4·7	4·9
Leu	8·5	7·1	5·4	4·8
Tyr	2·5	1·6	0·9	0·58
Phe	3·2	2·1	1·0	0·99
His	2·2	nr[a]	nr	1·45
Arg	4·5	2·0	1·1	1·14

[a] nr = not resolved

reducing sugars. Table III shows that the freeze-dried muscle contained 335 mg ribose/100 g, as compared with 142 mg after heat treatment. This residual ribose was present with the peptide-containing fractions, and it may be that some of their resistance to enzymic digestion resulted from the presence of sugar-containing substituents—possibly products of nucleic acid breakdown.

As mentioned above, we now had to resolve the complex mixtures of peptides in the different size classes. With the small peptide class we have obtained a further separation into five "families" of peptides, by column

TABLE III. Carbohydrate analysis of fish meals

	Ribose	*Mannose*	*Arabinose*	*Galactose* (mg/100 g)	*Xylose*	*Glucose*	*Total*
Freeze-dried cod muscle:							
unheated	335	18		45		56	454
heated 18 h at 140°	142	21		14		53	230
Commercial white fish meal	79	61	29	130	22	255	546

chromatography on cation-exchange Sephadex (SP-Sephadex, grade C-25), using gradient elution over the pH range 2·4–4·0 with volatile buffers containing formic and acetic acids and pyridine. Figure 8 shows the elution pattern. Two well defined and strongly acidic peaks (K and L) were eluted with the starting buffer at pH 2·4. They were followed by a larger peak (M), and then by a long and irregular peak that we subdivided into two families (N and O). The next stage will be to rechromatograph

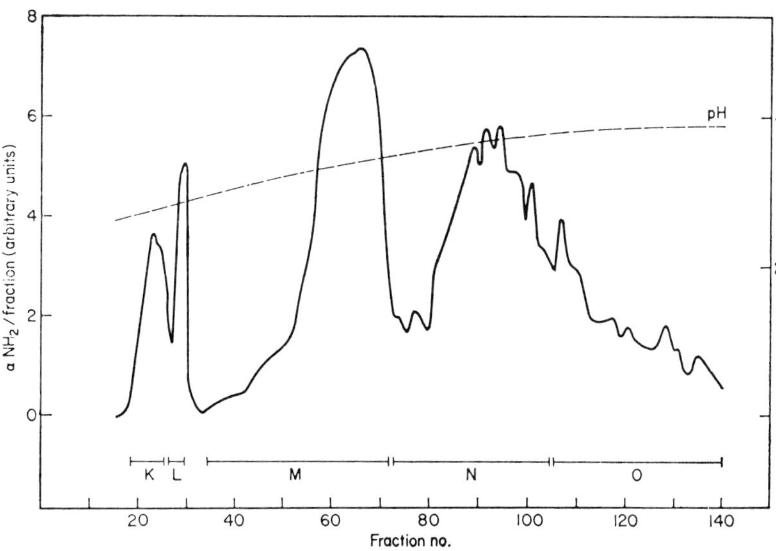

FIG. 8. Further separation of small peptides of group C by chromatography on cation exchange Sephadex

these families under modified conditions. The amino acid composition of these peptides is of some interest and is shown in Table IV. Comparing again with the original fish meal, peak K was greatly enriched in glutamic and aspartic acids, and in proline. It also contained a high concentration of cysteic acid (4%) and no cystine. This raises the interesting question whether cysteic acid was present as such in the peptide, or whether it was

TABLE IV. Amino acid composition of peptide families separated from the "small peptide" fraction by cation exchange chromatography

	Amino acids (moles %)				
	K	*L*	*M*	*N*	*O*
Glu	25·0	14·6	20·1	15·0	19·3
Asp	16·3	22·1	14·3	12·9	13·6
Lys	2·4	3·8	3·5	12·3	12·3
Thr	4·4	5·1	4·9	3·5	4·4
Ser	3·8	4·5	4·2	2·8	3·4
Pro	5·7	4·7	7·5	6·6	6·0
Gly	9·2	12·9	12·2	9·1	9·5
Ala	10·5	8·9	11·2	9·1	9·0
Val	5·5	6·5	6·3	4·9	3·8
Met	1·6	1·4	1·5	1·8	1·7
Ileu	4·0	3·8	5·2	4·5	5·1
Leu	4·6	4·1	5·5	4·4	5·1
Tyr	0·53	0·02	0·08	0·07	0·12
Phe	0·79	0·99	0·94	0·86	1·4
His	nr[a]	0·91	nr	5·5	nr
Arg	0·23	0·42	0·49	4·1	4·0
Cys	0	0	0·82	0·24	0·55
Cysteic acid	4·0	4·0	1·0	1·7	nr
Met sulphoxide	trace	0·15	0·14	trace	trace

[a] nr = not resolved

formed during the acid hydrolysis. It is difficult to be certain on this point. We hydrolysed the peptide under nitrogen in sealed ampoules, and it seems likely that the cysteic acid was indeed present in the peptides. If so, it indicates a possible specific mechanism whereby the cystine in some proteins might be damaged during heat processing, and in consequence hinder the enzymic release of the adjacent amino acids.

Ellinger and Palmer (1969) suggested that methionine might become unavailable in the same way, through conversion to sulphoxide. They found that methionine sulphoxide in peroxide-treated casein was of much lower biological availability than was the free sulphoxide, and concluded that the presence of the sulphoxide residues impaired the digestibility. We found very little sulphoxide in the acid hydrolysates of our peptides—there was generally less than 10%. But it is probable that this methionine, like the cystine, was present in the oxidized form in the peptide but was largely reduced during the acid hydrolysis (cf. Njaa, 1962a,b).

The very high content of glutamic and aspartic acid in peak K was not matched by a correspondingly high level of lysine. The lysine content in fact was very low, like that of leucine, tyrosine, phenylalanine and arginine.

Peak L was even richer in aspartic acid but poorer in glutamic. Its composition, like that of the next peak, M, was broadly similar to that of peak K.

In peaks N and O a significant feature was the high content of lysine, accompanying an increase in the content of the other basic amino acids. This is of particular interest in relation to the concept (Bjarnason and Carpenter, 1970) that most of the unavailable lysine in heat-damaged proteins of this type is amide linked to aspartic and glutamic acid residues. What is also evident, however, from the composition of the peptides in peaks K, L and M is that much, and perhaps most, of the glutamine and aspartic acids in the small peptide class was not associated with lysine.

On chromatography of the medium peptide class under similar conditions, two sharply defined and strongly acidic peaks were eluted in the starting buffer at pH 2·4. Each represented about 20% of the total amino acid residues. They were followed by a broad peak at around pH 3·8 which contained most of the remainder. The amino acid composition of these peaks is shown in Table V. The two strongly acid peaks (X and Y) were similar in composition to the corresponding peaks from the small peptide class. They were rich in glutamic and aspartic acids and rather poor in lysine. Peak Y was noticeably dark brown in colour. Peak Z was much richer in lysine, and somewhat poorer in glutamic and aspartic acids. In all three peaks the methionine content was higher than in the original fish meal, and also higher than in the small peptides. Again, as in the small peptides, it is possible that this methionine was an artefact, and that the peptide contained the sulphoxide.

All these findings indicate that severe heating had a marked differential effect in retarding the enzymic release of different amino acids. The free amino acids component in the enzymic digests was deficient in several amino acids relative to their content in the original protein, and notably in lysine and the sulphur-containing amino acids. For most of the amino

TABLE V. Amino acid composition of peptide families separated from the "medium peptide" fraction by cation exchange chromatography

	Amino acids (moles %)		
	X	*Y*	*Z*
Glu	25·1	24·7	19·0
Asp	19·6	18·6	15·4
Lys	3·9	5·0	10·6
Thr	3·5	2·8	1·3
Ser	2·1	2·3	0·87
Pro	4·7	2·9	6·3
Gly	10·5	10·9	10·2
Ala	10·2	10·0	7·9
Val	5·8	5·8	5·8
Met	2·3	2·7	2·8
Ileu	4·2	5·3	6·1
Leu	4·6	6·1	5·8
Tyr	0·39	0·15	0·75
Phe	0·99	0·99	1·2
His	0·99	0·38	2·7
Arg	0·52	0·99	1·8

acids the harmful effects of the heat processing were probably indirect, and resulted from the formation during heating of new intramolecular linkages that were not amenable to enzymic hydrolysis and involved mainly glutamine and asparagine and perhaps also the corresponding acids, and lysine.

IV. THE NUTRITIONAL IMPLICATIONS OF HEAT DAMAGE

Turning now briefly to the nutritional effects of heat damage: we have seen that these are not explained simply by the lowered digestibility. It is an interesting question whether the lowered biological value of heat-damaged protein is entirely due simply to the poorer pattern of amino acids that it yields on digestion. A further possibility is that some of the amino acids that are absorbed from the gut are still locked up in indigestible peptides. Ford and Shorrock (1971) examined the effects of feeding heat-damaged cod muscle to rats on the content of peptides and free amino acids in the urine. They found a marked increase in the excretion of peptide-bound amino acids, but it represented only a very small proportion—about 0·2%—of the nitrogen absorbed from the gut, and it was evident that urinary losses of undigested peptide residues could be of only marginal nutritional importance. The composition of this urinary peptide was perhaps significant: it was rich in lysine and in glutamic and aspartic acids, which together comprised about 70% of the amino acid residues. Ford and Shorrock (1971) suggested that the peptide might represent the biologically unavailable residues based on amide-linked asparagine or glutamine and lysine (Bjarnason and Carpenter, 1970) but this now seems less likely, since Mauron (1970) and Waibel and Carpenter (1972) have shown that the lysine in ε-(γ-L-glutamyl)-L-lysine is fully available to the rat, although the compound is probably not hydrolysed in the lumen of the gut (Pisano *et al.*, 1969; Asquith *et al.*, 1970). Waibel and Carpenter (1972) also showed that glutamyl-lysine is not completely hydrolysed during its passage through the gut wall, as are normal dipeptides, and appears in the blood plasma. They suggest that its hydrolysis may occur in the kidney, which contains enzymes that will hydrolyse a variety of ε-acyl derivatives of lysine.

The hypothesis that much of the deterioration in nutritive quality that occurs during severe heating is attributable to the formation of cross-linkages between glutamine and lysine (Bjarnason and Carpenter, 1970) is not impaired by the finding that ε-(γ-glutamyl)-lysine itself is absorbed and efficiently utilized as a source of lysine. An essential feature of the hypothesis is that each new glutamyl-lysine linkage hinders the access of peptidases to the several adjacent peptide bonds, so that little or no free glutamyl-lysine would in fact be liberated into the gut. The demonstration that glutamyl-lysine is biologically available is therefore probably not directly relevant. It may be, of course, that there is some absorption and subsequent utilization of these larger peptides containing the glutamyl-lysine moiety, but evidence on this point is lacking.

If we accept that there is no evidence for any considerable uptake of unavailable peptide from the gut, the question remains whether the nutritive quality of the heat-damaged protein is determined simply by the extent and relative rates of release of its constituent amino acids. For several amino acids—for example lysine and cystine—we can identify chemical processes that are specifically damaging but, for the most part, the amino acids in a heat-damaged protein are "unavailable" only in the sense that they are slow to digest, presumably because of steric hindrance to the access of proteolytic enzymes. The distinctions we make between "available" and "unavailable" are arbitrary and they relate to the particular conditions of the tests. Thus, assay results from biological tests may vary with the species of animal used, and with several other factors not directly related to the intrinsic availability of the amino acids in the test protein.

When we compared rat growth assays for lysine, methionine and isoleucine in severely heated cod muscle with results obtained from microbiological assay after prolonged *in vitro* digestion with various proteolytic enzymes, we were surprised to find that much more of these amino acids was susceptible to enzymic release and utilized by the test microorganisms than was biologically available to the rat (Ford and Salter, 1966). About 71% of the methionine, 81% of the isoleucine and 28% of the lysine were recovered in the *in vitro* digests, as against only 42, 39 and 18% measured in the rat growth tests (Table VI). It appears that for

TABLE VI. Availability of methionine, isoleucine and lysine (g/16 g N) in heat-damaged cod muscle, measured in growth tests with rats and by microbiological assay of *in vitro* enzymic digests

	Predigestion	*Met*	*Ileu*	*Lys*
Rat assay		1·22	2·06	1·30
Microbiological	pepsin–pancreatin–erepsin	2·06	4·56	2·18
assay, after	pepsin–papain	1·94	3·95	2·64
predigestion	pronase	2·16	4·37	1·92
with:	HCl	2·90	5·30	7·30

lysine, as well as for isoleucine and methionine, the rate of digestion is critically important in determining the biological availability.

It is interesting that digestion *in vivo* was comparatively so inefficient. Because of this slower digestion, the guts of rats given heat-damaged fish meal contained a high concentration of undigested peptides. One consequence of this might have been to increase the losses of endogenous protein, of which there is a considerable secretion into the gut, mostly as digestive enzymes, mucus and desquamated epithelial cells; in man it has been estimated that the total amount is probably not much less than the dietary intake (Munro, 1964). It is normally digested and reabsorbed along with the food protein, but Buraczewski (1966) suggested that the presence of unavailable food protein residues might retard this process. In evidence for this, he reported that in rats given heat-damaged fish meal the proteolytic activity of the middle and distal lengths of the small intestine was nearly double that in rats given the unheated meal. A more surprising finding was that the content of free amino acids and small peptides was also very high—much higher than in rats given unheated fish meal—and yet despite this the levels of free amino acids in the portal blood were much lower (Buraczewski *et al.*, 1967). One possible explanation for this finding is that the presence of unavailable peptides in high concentration saturates absorption sites involved in the transport of amino acids across the mucosal barrier. Some support for this hypothesis comes from experiments on the influence of unavailable peptides on the uptake of ^{14}C leucine by everted sacs of rat small intestine. Shorrock (1972) found that unavailable peptides, isolated from an enzymic digest of heat-damaged fish meal, strongly depressed the uptake of leucine. Another possibility is that the unavailable peptides interfere with peptide uptake. It is now recognized that uptake of intact peptides by intestinal mucosal cells is an important process in protein digestion, and may indeed be the predominant mode of protein absorption (cf. Crampton *et al.*, 1971). The intestine probably has a much higher capacity for the absorption of peptides than of amino acids, and we can picture an "unavailable" peptide as competing for absorption sites where, because of its failure to digest, it hinders the flux of digestible peptides. However, further speculation on this aspect of the metabolism of unavailable peptides must await further study and confirmation of these findings of Buraczewski *et al.* (1967).

REFERENCES

Asquith, R. S., Otterburn, M. S., Buchanan, J. H., Cole, M., Fletcher, J. C. and Gardner, K. L. (1970). *Biochim. biophys. Acta* **221**, 342–348.

Bjarnason, J. and Carpenter, K. J. (1970). *Br. J. Nutr.* **24**, 313–329.

Buraczewski, S. (1966). Ph.D. Thesis: University of Reading, England.

Buraczewski, S., Buraczewska, L. and Ford, J. E. (1967). *Acta biochim. pol.* **14**, 121–133.

Crampton, R. F., Gangolli, S. D., Simson, P. and Matthews, D. M. (1971). *Clin. Sci.* **41**, 409–417.

Ellinger, G. M. and Palmer, R. (1969). *Proc. Nutr. Soc.* **28**, 42A.

Erbersdobler, H., Dümmer, H. and Zucker, H. (1968). *Z. Tierphysiol. Tierernähr. Futtermittelk.* **24**, 136–152.

Ford, J. E. and Salter, D. N. (1966). *Br. J. Nutr.* **20**, 843–860.

Ford, J. E. and Shorrock, C. (1971). *Br. J. Nutr.* **26**, 311–322.

Mauron, J. (1970). *Int. Z. VitamForsch.* **40**, 209–227.

Mecham, D. K. and Olcott, H. S. (1947). *Ind. Engng Chem.* **39**, 1023–1027.

Munro, H. N. (1964). *In* "Mammalian Protein Metabolism" (H. N. Munro and J. B. Allison, eds), Vol. II, p. 21. Academic Press, New York.

Njaa, L. R. (1962a). *Acta chem. scand.* **16**, 1359–1362.

Njaa, L. R. (1962b). *Br. J. Nutr.* **16**, 571–577.

Pisano, J. J., Finlayson, J. S. and Peyton, M. P. (1968). *Science, N.Y.* **160**, 892–893.

Shorrock, C. (1972). Ph.D. Thesis: University of Reading, England.

Waibel, P. E. and Carpenter, K. J. (1972). *Br. J. Nutr.* **27**, 509–515.

CHAPTER 36 (DISCUSSION)

What are the Important Factors Affecting Protein Utilization?

K. J. CARPENTER
Department of Applied Biology, University of Cambridge, England

I. REVIEW

A. The Need for a Balanced Assessment

The present discussion is concerned with the detailed changes that take place in protein foods that have been heat-damaged, work that has occupied professional people in leading laboratories for several years. And yet it has been claimed (Chapter 6) that studies of protein quality are of little practical importance. How can we reconcile these two points of view or put them into perspective?

Like everything else, the war on world malnutrition demands specialization. First there are the "front line" men who are waging it directly in the developing countries through education, increased food production and medical services. They, in turn, need help from all kinds of people: economists, land tenure specialists, psychologists and so on. Among all these they look to the back-room, academic nutritionists for help with ideas and background information as to the relative value of one food compared with another, or one method of processing compared with another, or the possible explanation of "odd" observations. The back-room nutritionist has to be ready to give such advice from his experience of controlled experiments.

What is out of place is for an academic nutritionist working on one specialized aspect of nutrition to believe that this qualifies him to be an "instant expert" in a foreign culture that he does not understand, and to diagnose overall solutions to complex practical problems. But our immediate task is to consider specifically the chemistry, biology and physics of protein evaluation.

It is unfortunate that "protein" was adopted, oversimplified and popularized as the one world nutrition problem; and there is now an understandable reaction in the other direction, since energy is equally limiting in children's diets where there is malnutrition. Of course, if the bulkiness of the "problem" diets is to be reduced, and the extra energy has to come from fat, this, in turn, will have to be balanced by adding high-protein constituents to the diet, and there will then be a renewed interest as to what these can be. In the meantime, we have a continuing application for protein quality work in the formulation of animal diets; this is in itself a means of providing valuable human food, and also an area in which ideas are being tested and developed which may prove eventually to be of direct use in human nutrition.

B. Some Problems of Protein Utilization

It is now accepted that processed materials can be damaged without this being shown up by ordinary amino acid analysis. A practical consequence of this is a need for analytical procedures that will act as indicators of the extent of this damage so that manufacturing procedures may be controlled. Even to develop these in a rational way, however, we need to understand what the essential changes are that have occurred in the processed proteins. The study of the Maillard reactions has led to improved control of milk products, as we have already seen. But, from work on the feeding to calves of UHT milks, it seems that there may also be more subtle changes in milk proteins that affect their value for the young suckling; changes that have still to be understood.

There can be no doubt of the importance of studying the naturally occurring toxicants associated with food proteins. We are fortunate that there is even *one* person who tries to keep this field of knowledge under constant review. A few years ago it seemed that the presence of trypsin inhibitors in uncooked soya-beans was a sufficient (and therefore full) explanation of their growth-depressing effect. We know now that there are several growth-depressing factors present in soya- and other beans—haemagglutenins, saponins and goitrogens—and that the growth depression may still not be explained by any of them. Yet we have the responsibility of trying to help plant breeders to select lines of beans that are of improved nutritional quality and with less need for specific heat treatments to overcome inhibitors.

We are not creating the complexity of nature, only trying to understand it. The complexity is such that the individual human brain can only cope with trying to understand one small segment of the whole, and progress is therefore dependent on specialization. Although we must not exaggerate the importance of any particular portion of knowledge, we must also believe it to be likely that there are useful things still to be discovered in the critical evaluation of foods and the interpretation of biological responses to foods in terms of their chemistry.

II. GENERAL DISCUSSION

Dr E. Dworschak (Institute of Nutrition, Budapest, Hungary) outlined some of his results which offered an opportunity of decreasing the protein damage caused by the Maillard reaction which Dr Finot had discussed (Chapter 34). Some chemical agents, such as sulphur dioxide, could not be used because of their danger to human health. However, there were certain additives widely used in the bakery industry which were completely harmless but with a remarkable and little-known effect on the nutritive value of proteins. Additives promoting the fermentation (e.g. enzyme preparations of high amylase activity, small amounts of sugar) of flours themselves of high amylase activity, reduced the degradation of lysine and tryptophan during the baking process. The extent of this sparing effect was about 10–20% in bread, which was significant in terms of human nutrition.

There could be two explanations of this phenomenon. Firstly, the increased fermentation lowered the pH of the dough as compared with the older methods. The increased fermentation enhanced the brown pigments in the crust and promoted sugar caramelization and hydroxymethylfuraldehyde production, while the lower pH reduced amino acid decomposition. It was his opinion, therefore, that non-enzymic browning and the degradation of proteins could have different pathways in different circumstances. The other explanation could be that increased fermentation enhanced carbon dioxide production which reduced the effect of the Strecker degradation of amino acids.

In support of Dr K. J. Carpenter's observations on the fermentation of amino acids in the hind-gut of chicks, Dr V. C. Mason (Landskonomisk Forsøglaboratorium, Copenhagen, Denmark) drew attention to his own work conducted at the Rowett Research Institute with Dr F. White and Mr R. Palmer. In these studies, it was demonstrated in both sheep and rats that over 50% of the faecal nitrogen was incorporated in bacterial residues, and that bacterial mucopeptide synthesized in the rumen or given in a diet is not digested in the small intestine but is extensively degraded in the hind-gut in these species. He further pointed out that any undigested starches reaching the hind-gut stimulated fermentation and resulted in an increase in faecal nitrogen and a decrease in urinary nitrogen excretion. Although such effects may not influence n.p.u. estimation, they do influence the apparent digestibility of dietary nitrogen and estimates of b.v. Potato starch is particularly effective in this regard. Rats given rumen bacteria demonstrated increased digestibility of certain peptides and this occurred mainly in the hind-gut.

Dr H. Erbersdobler wondered whether it was essential to separate faeces and urine in digestibility tests, a procedure which would be difficult with germ-free chicks. He presumed it would depend upon the level of amino acid (and unavailable peptide) excreted in the urine. Dr K. J. Carpenter replied that he had seen one paper which suggested that no separation was necessary with chicks, but these workers had dealt only with high-quality proteins, and heat-damaged proteins might behave very differently.

Dr L. R. Njaa (Government Vitamin Laboratory, Bergen, Norway) referred to some of Dr Eggum's results which showed that methionine was liberated more slowly from fish meals than from other foods during digestion. He wondered if this were general, since he had obtained similar results with fish meals supplemented with methionine. Dr B. O. Eggum replied that these results were obtained with only one particular fish meal. Slow digestion curves for some amino acids had been observed for certain proteins, and it was possible that supplementation with free amino acids might be different with proteins of different digestibility.

Dr B. O. Eggum wondered whether the influence of the microflora of the lower gut was affected by the age of the animal. Dr H. Erbersdobler said that there were no precise results, but he felt that in his comparisons of germ-free and conventional chicks the animals used may have been too young. The variability between individuals was very high. Dr M. Turner (University of Southampton, England) asked whether the increased absorption of amino acids in animals adapted to high-protein diets was a result of the number of carrier sites or was due to changes in the properties of the carrier system and whether this would result in any effect on the protein value of food consumed in view of the reserve capacity?

Dr H. Erbersdobler said that the number of available sites increased, not their affinity for amino acids. He did not think that these results had any significance for human beings as high-protein diets of this type were not eaten by man, but the regulatory mechanism might be of interest in, say, the regulation of appetite.

Dr J. Schou (Institute of Protein Chemistry, Copenhagen, Denmark) asked whether the effect of the position of the N atom on the reactions between lysine and sugar had been studied. He also wondered whether the residue of the lysine could be accounted for, since the fate of only 80% had been explained, and whether the lag in reaction of FDNB with fructoselysine was due to steric hindrance.

Dr P. Finot said that he had carried out no work on stereospecificity.

He could not account for the unrecovered lysine. He assumed that FDNB reacted in the same way as the sugar, but he did not know the mechanism. In reply to questions from Dr J. Peret (CNRS, Bellevue-Meudon, France) on the duration of feeding and fasting periods, Dr Erbersdobler said that the time of adaptation varied, even at the same protein level of 75%. He found that the transport system adapted rapidly, within hours, although de-adaptation took 4–5 days. The enzymes took a rather longer time. He fasted his rats for 24 h.

Dr J. Peret said that in his own work in which rats were fed 75% protein diets, they took 8–12 days to adapt, and only the pancreas had adapted within 24 h. He had found that very high dietary levels of protein caused falls in liver glycogen and altered the circadian rhythm. He found it difficult to relate amino acids with appetite, perhaps this was more related to glycogen and enzyme levels in the liver.

Dr Erbersdobler added that he had generally used adaptation periods of 14 days. He had found that adaptation in the gut wall was much more rapid than in other enzyme systems.

CHAPTER 37

The Way Ahead?

N. W. PIRIE

Rothamsted Experimental Station, Harpenden, Herts, England

I. INTRODUCTION

Problems connected with the world's protein needs can be arranged under the headings: Why? Who? How Much? What? and How? This is not the place to discuss the first of these issues. The second seems to me simple. We are not concerned with the welfare of rats in spite of our preoccupation with them. Nor are most of us concerned with people wealthy enough to be part of a market economy and legitimate targets for the blandishments of advertisers of processed and packaged foods. Most of us are concerned with the welfare of those people, especially the young, who have advanced far enough from primitive conditions to be able to use a simple tractor but not much further than that. By the end of the century that group will probably still number 1 000 000 000. Foods made by industrialized processes, e.g. solvent-extracted fish without smell or taste, or yeast grown on petroleum products, are not likely to contribute directly to the welfare of that group. Products of this type will make a useful contribution by satisfying some of the food and fodder demands of the wealthy countries, thus enabling the poorer ones to retain more of their own protein. Furthermore, if the prestige of microbial products is increased, traditional fermentative methods of food processing will be used more widely.

II. HOW MUCH?

It is easy to decide how much protein a domestic animal needs in its diet: it needs the amount that gives the financially optimal growth rate, or rate of production of milk or eggs. It is not so easy to decide how much protein children should get because we do not know whether quick growth is advantageous. A protein-rich diet probably protects from infection and certainly promotes recovery after infection, but it may shorten life. Some people see this as an ethical dilemma; it seems to me that the advantages of health and quick recovery in youth outweigh any probable ultimate curtailment of life. It may even cost less to prevent disease by better nutrition rather than to cope with it medically later, but I deplore any attempt to look on the two approaches as alternatives—both are needed.

There is even less evidence about the protein needs of adults. A naive approach is to measure N balance and assume that as soon as someone is not being depleted, protein intake is optimal. The mechanistically-minded advocates of evidence from N balance seem aware that their conclusions are apt to be absurd, so they add on various factors to get a more reasonable result. It would be wiser to look at what the more productive, enthusiastic, and mentally and physiologically responsive people eat when given a free choice, and consider the possibility that their diet is about optimal and that the presence of amino acids in the blood is, perhaps pharmacologically, beneficial. It can, therefore, be argued that we need twice as much protein as is being produced now; it can on the other hand be argued that the world would get on better if some people and nations were less productive and enthusiastic. Disagreement on this issue cannot be resolved by physiological studies.

III. WHAT?

If it is agreed that most attention should be given to the needs of fairly primitive communities, it would seem to follow logically that the most important protein sources are those that can be made locally with little continuing aid from outside. There is space to mention only a few of the sources that could be more fully exploited. The advent of protein-rich strains of cereals makes it less reasonable to keep more pigs and chickens than can be maintained on household wastes. Ruminants should be confined to non-arable land, and the merits of goats, if adequately contained, should be more widely recognized. Much of the effort put into work on fish seems to be misdirected: it would be better to ensure that fresh or lightly preserved fish could move a few miles further inland rather than try to make fish products with an indefinite shelf-life. Because of the importance of legume seeds as protein sources, it was very encouraging to learn from Liener (Chapter 33) that, although trypsin inhibitors are widely distributed among them, the inhibitor in soya-bean at any rate does not act on human trypsin. This gives an added incentive to research on improved methods for making traditional bean curds. Leaf protein is one of the potential sources on which much more work is needed because it can be made in regions with such regular rainfall that it is difficult to ripen a seed crop; the yield attainable is unequalled by any other method for making a protein concentrate, and the extraction procedure is simple and cheap. Figure 1 gives our yields at Rothamsted during the past 15 years. With irrigation, we expect to be able to get 3 tons of dry extracted protein per hectare per year. That yield has already been reached in

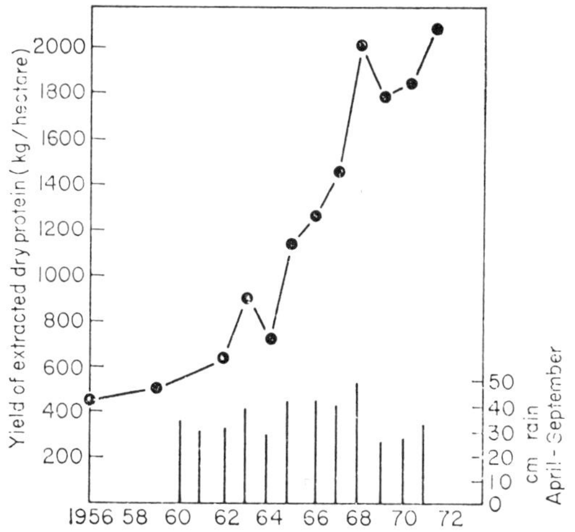

Fig. 1. Improvements in the annual yields of extracted leaf protein. The cropping year in these experiments ran from October to October and a succession of crops was grown on the same plot. The sequence varied, but always started with winter wheat (*Triticum aestivum*). This was followed by mustard (*Sinapis alba*), fodder radish (*Raphanus sativus*) or vetch (*Vicia sativa*). The plot was not irrigated; breaks in the improvement curve were probably caused by dry summers

India; 5 tons should be attainable there. These issues, and the use of the by-products, are discussed by Pirie (1971).

The categories "First Class" and "Second Class" were established soon after the recognition, a century ago, of differences in the nutritional value of proteins. The simple dichotomy has been given up. Unfortunately, several people have invented an equally fallacious one: animal protein and plant protein. Admittedly many seed proteins are poor; so are some animal proteins, but the protein in leaves and some tubers is as good as most animal proteins. The words *good* and *poor* in sentences such as the last distress many scientists. Surely we can manage something that at least looks more quantitative? Many attempts have been made. Thirty years ago it became apparent to some of us that it would no more be possible to assign numerical merit to proteins than to alloy steels. Food proteins, like steels, are used for many different purposes and operate in many different environments. Different contexts call for different compositions. This nihilist attitude has obviously not yet been accepted by most authorities in this field.

IV. HOW?

Whatever the theoretical merits of a protein, and however valuable it may be because it is rich in an amino acid that is scanty in most other food proteins, it will not contribute to nutrition until it becomes part of the normal diet. Marketing surveys are a waste of time; they supply no more than snap judgements on the extent to which a novelty resembles an existing food. If our ancestors had relied on market surveys, the potato, tomato and grapefruit would not have entered Britain. Food preferences are so bizarre and varied that a taste for anything that is wholesome and is not a tasteless impalpable powder could probably be built up. The slow progress made by some valuable novel foods is not surprising, because less money has been spent on publicizing all of them than a commercial concern would devote to promoting a new type of chocolate. Furthermore, if the novelty is intended for infants, it would be a pity if it were made so attractive to adults that they consumed more than their share.

People in the communities most in need of improved nutrition are being exposed to many forms of cultural change and exhortation. The idea is spreading that the traditional foods are barbarous relics that ought to be replaced by the types of food eaten in affluent countries. This is unfortunate, though understandable, because some of the more easily produced protein concentrates would fit easily into traditional dishes whereas it will not be possible quickly, if ever, to organize throughout the world adequate supplies of the present foods of the affluent. We are in danger of destroying old ideas about food before we can satisfy new ones. This destruction is profitable and causes what Jelliffe calls "commerciogenic malnutrition". Health was for centuries the domain of charity and private enterprise, in many countries it is now managed as a national service; the consequences are widely accepted as beneficial. Is there any valid reason why the basic foodstuffs should not similarly be regarded as a fundamental human right?

REFERENCE

Pirie, N. W. (ed.) (1971). "Leaf Protein: Its Agronomy, Preparation, Quality and Use", IBP Handbook no 20. Blackwell Scientific Publications, Oxford.

Author Index

(numbers in italics indicate those pages where references are given in full)

Subject Index